# Community Preparedness and Response to Terrorism

# Community Preparedness and Response to Terrorism

## III  Communication and the Media

*Edited by*

*H. Dan O'Hair, Robert L. Heath, and Gerald R. Ledlow*

*General Editors*

*James A. Johnson, Gerald R. Ledlow, and Mark A. Cwiek*

PRAEGER PERSPECTIVES

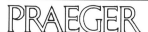

Westport, Connecticut
London

**Library of Congress Cataloging-in-Publication Data**

Community preparedness and response to terrorism / James A. Johnson, Gerald R.
  Ledlow, and Mark A. Cwiek, general editors.
    p. cm.
  Includes bibliographical references and index.
  Contents: v. 1. The terrorist threat and community response / edited by Gerald R.
Ledlow, James A. Johnson, and Walter J. Jones—v. 2. The role of community
organizations and business / edited by James A. Johnson, Michael H. Kennedy, and
Nejdet Delener—v. 3. Communication and the media / edited by H. Dan O'Hair,
Robert L. Heath, and Gerald R. Ledlow.
  ISBN 0–275–98366–8 (set : alk. paper)—ISBN 0–275–98365–X (v. 1 : alk. paper)—
ISBN 0–275–98369–2 (v. 2 : alk. paper)—ISBN 0–275–98373–0 (v. 3 : alk. paper)
  1. Terrorism—United States—Prevention. 2. Emergency management—United
States. 3. Civil defense—United States. 4. Community organization—United States.
5. Terrorism and mass media—United States. 6. Preparedness—United States.
I. Johnson, James A., 1954– II. Ledlow, Gerald R. III. Cwiek, Mark A.
HV6432.C654 2004
363.34'97–dc22          2004042290

British Library Cataloguing in Publication Data is available.

Library of Congress Catalog Card Number: 2004042290
ISBN: 0–275–98366–8 (set)
        0–275–98365–X (Volume I)
        0–275–98369–2 (Volume II)
        0–275–98373–0 (Volume III)

First published in 2005

Praeger Publishers, 88 Post Road West, Westport, CT 06881
An imprint of Greenwood Publishing Group, Inc.
www.praeger.com

Printed in the United States of America

The paper used in this book complies with the
Permanent Paper Standard issued by the National
Information Standards Organization (Z39.48–1984).

10 9 8 7 6 5 4 3 2 1

# Contents

# Acknowledgments

The editors wish to thank the contributors for their wisdom, creativity, and extraordinary work ethic for bringing this volume to a successful conclusion. The tight deadlines and requested revisions were met with professionalism and promptness that exceeded expectations. We are deeply grateful to our families for giving up private time, especially over weekends and holidays, so that we could devote attention to this project. We thank Hilary Claggett and Sarah Coe from Praeger Publishing for their masterful expertise in helping us bring this volume to publication. Finally, thanks go to Aamna Qamar, Bolanle Oyefesobi, and Olawaale Adjenor for developing the index, to Ritva Carlson of Capital City Press for her outstanding editorial guidance, and to Cheryl Reen for her invaluable administrative support throughout the project.

# Introduction

## *H. Dan O'Hair*

For the third volume in this series on community preparedness, deterrence, and response to terrorism, the editors and contributors took on the task of examining the complex interplay among messages, symbolism, communicators, media, communities, and agencies in the context of terrorism. As ideas poured in for chapters and exchanges among editors and contributors became elevated, it was obvious that capturing and creating a composite of notions about communication and terrorism would be out of reach, especially in one volume.

What is represented here is a compendium of chapters that best reflects the approaches to communication that are most familiar to the editors and contributors, while keeping an eye on new twists and turns unlikely to be found in other works on communication and terrorism. The highly select group of contributors, who offer their insights, opinions, and suggestions concerning the inextricable link between communication and terrorism go beyond the normal offerings from the lay press and governmental officials. At times, the ideas represented are unusual, counterintuitive, and risky. At other times, they apply new paths and creative thinking to what is considered standard operating procedure. At all times, the approach is simple: Terrorism is a communication act, and it is only through competent communication that terrorism can be managed.

# 1 Conceptualizing Communication and Terrorism

## *H. Dan O'Hair and Robert L. Heath*

Terrorism is a complex, controversial, and contested concept, as evidenced by the diverse entries in this volume. The contributors, and at times the editors, do not completely agree on definitions, concepts, approaches, plans, and implications of terrorism and communication. Moreover, discussants of concepts such as terrorism always risk stepping into traps of oversimplification and reductionism. While we would like to avoid such traps, we know that readers' perspectives vary, and viewpoints can be difficult to manage. Our goal is to present information and analysis limited to specific aspects of communication and terrorism, and let readers infer their own implications from the ideas offered here.

## DEFINING TERRORISM

A key process in conceptualizing the link between communication and terrorism involves developing a clearer understanding of how terrorism is viewed or defined. We are not uninfluenced by the contributions of others who have conceptualized terrorism. We also understand that definitions can be relative, contingent on who is focusing on terrorism at the time. For example, Hacker identifies three types of terrorist: criminals, crazies, and crusaders.[1] All acts of terrorism are likely to be criminal assaults on a person or property. They violate criminal codes in many ways. Some acts are purely criminal; one of the most iconic is the murders using Tylenol capsules as weapons. The distinction between crazy and crusader is likely to be a matter similar to the fact that beauty is in the eye of the beholder. In order to establish some common ground for the purposes of delineating the relationship between terrorism and communication, we can turn to some widely held notions of terrorism. According to Stevens,[2] the definition of terrorism most frequently relied upon is the one advanced by the U.S. State Department, which defines acts of *international* terrorism as "involving citizens or the territory of more than one country." Thus, excluded here would be major *domestic* terrorist acts that might have major national or international impact. "Terrorism" is defined as "premeditated, politically motivated violence perpetrated against noncombatant targets by subnational groups or clandestine agents, usually intended to influence an audience."[3]

Other examples, representing both official and unofficial views of terrorism, are offered in table 1.1. Notice that a number of common elements link these descriptions.

**Table 1.1**
**Definitions of Terrorism**

| Definition | Source |
| --- | --- |
| The unlawful use of force or violence against persons or property to intimidate or coerce a government, the civilian population, or any segment thereof, in furtherance of political or social objectives. | Federal Bureau of Investigation |
| The use or threat, for the purpose of advancing a political, religious or ideological cause, of action that involves serious violence against any person or property. | United Kingdom Government |
| A strategy of violence designed to promote desired outcomes by instilling fear in the public at large. | Walter Reich |
| The deliberate, systematic murder, maiming, and menacing of the innocent to inspire fear in order to gain political ends. . . . Terrorism . . . is intrinsically evil, necessarily evil, and wholly evil. | Paul Johnson |
| [International terrorism is] the threat or use of violence for political purposes when (1) such action is intended to influence the attitude and behavior of a target group wider than its immediate victim, and (2) its ramifications transcend national boundaries. | Peter Sederberg |
| Terrorism is ineluctably political in aims and motives; violent—or, equally important, threatens violence; designed to have far-reaching psychological repercussions beyond the immediate victim or target; conducted by an organization with an identifiable chain of command or conspiratorial cell structure (whose members wear no uniform or identifying insignia); and perpetrated by a subnational group or nonstate entity. | David J. Whittaker |

*Source*: Whittaker DJ, editor. The terrorism reader. 2nd ed. New York: Routledge; 2003. p. 3.

Common to these definitions are criteria that distinguish terrorist acts from those that are simply violent, illegal transgressions. First, fear is the ultimate goal. Second, the violence only has to be threatened. Third, the victims are not always the ultimate targets. Fourth, primary audience members are those who observe the terrorist act. Fifth, political or social change is the primary objective of terrorists.[4] Terrorism, then, means deliberately inflicting pain, suffering, and death on civilians for the purpose of accomplishing specific goals, without regard for human rights, and creating a climate of fear through violent means.[5]

## THE MOTIVES OF TERRORISTS

Terrorists are motivated by a variety of psychosocial and communicative dispositions and goals. Psychological experts seem to agree that potential terrorists feel trapped by their circumstances. Vengeance and retribution are spawned by feelings of intense anger—an anger emanating from hurt, pain, and suffering. Traditional avenues for expressing their concerns seem closed. Terrorists believe that their voices go unheard. These feelings of frustration turn to perceptions of powerlessness. Paradoxically, terrorists perceive themselves as victims. They sense it is they who are threatened and violated. In many cases, terrorists feel that they have nothing left to lose. Acts of terrorism become their final recourse when circumstances are irreparably stacked against them.[5]

Although terrorists are motivated, in large part, by psychological and political aims, successful terrorists are also motivated by practical ends. These motives include the following pragmatic goals:[6]

- Causing disruption—instilling fear and creating confusion in the target.
- Draining resources—causing resources to be redirected to outcomes of terrorism.
- Grabbing attention—creating attention, publicity, and/or some public communication spectacle.
- Generating profit—engaging in activities that serve the well-being of the terrorist group.

Other, more traditional motives of terrorists have been reported as being politically and spiritually based. This view was emphasized by Stevens, who summarizes several scholars who adopt an evolutionary view of terrorism, in which globalism and spiritual fanaticism serve to ignite or invigorate religious and political causes that previously had lain dormant. Factors that expand opportunities for terrorists to act include greater access to the Internet and weapons of mass destruction, a larger gap between rich and poor nations, and increased links to organized crime.[2]

Whether we acquiesce to Stevens' claim that other regions of the world are particularly disposed toward violence against the West, it is clear that recent events illustrate distaste for Western values and for globalized goals involving military occupation, exploitation of natural resources, and terrorists' political aversion. By emphasizing their victimhood, terrorists and their sympathizers can blame terrorism on the targets of violence. It is worth noting that many ordinary people in countries other than the United States view terrorist attacks on this country as a response to its presence and activity in other nations. This is especially true of Arab and Muslim countries (76 percent felt the United States was responsible for creating terrorism against its own country); but even in Western Europe, more than a third felt this way. Obviously, only a fraction of Americans were reported to feel this way.[7]

## BINDING THE TIE BETWEEN TERRORISM AND COMMUNICATION

At no time in this volume do the contributors condone terrorists. On the contrary, they recognize that terrorism is a reprehensible act. It is violence motivated by the myopic needs of individuals or groups who seek specific responses including any combination of the following: publicity, terror, fear, reciprocation, identification, sympathy, and hatred. Terrorists' primary motive is the elicitation of feedback, and this is where the current volume situates itself among other books on terrorism. *Terrorism is an inherently communicative process.* Terrorism is germinated through intrapersonal communication, it is incubated in interpersonal communication processes, it is nurtured through group communication, it is promoted during public communication, organized and enriched by organizational communication, and publicized and perpetuated through mass communication. Frequently, intercultural communication is a primary goal of terrorists. Make no mistake; the response and reaction to terrorism follow the same path. Communication serves as the lens through which responses to terrorism are identified and strategized, and communication becomes a primary tool for counterterrorist activities. In essence, terrorists and counterterrorists become communication interactants, locked in a fray of moves and countermoves that ends only when the communication cycle becomes interrupted.

The media, as communication agents, propel this process along in the name of free speech, open access, and the right to know. Public officials, feeling the pressure of public exposure, stand ready to play their roles (usually as counterterrorists), with further investment in the terrorism and communication cycle. Terrorists feel empowered in their cause, based on the resultant media exposure they sought. The media are often flagged with a reputation of promoting terrorism because their mission of serving media consumers—the public—intersects with the desires of terrorists who seek public exposure.

This volume takes no side save for the perspective that communication is at the heart of terrorism. Terrorism is symbolic, message based, and fully predicts a communication response. Its goals are both simple and convoluted. Simply, terrorism seeks to direct attention to the perpetrators and their causes. A terrorist act must be a simple act. Thus, regardless of the magnitude and complexity of planning—to say nothing of the luck in execution—the attack on the World Trade Center buildings in New York City in 2001 was simple. It made a simple statement. We are here. We can strike. We can hit at your mind, soul, and operations. You cannot prevent us from acting in this manner. We may not always win, but we will win often enough so that you cannot say you are invincible.

At a more complex level, terrorism sets in motion a cascade of communicative events, starting with awareness; then moving to more emotional communication processes such as condemnation, anger management, resentment; and eventually progressing to postevent processes such as accounting, curiosity, and retaliation. Is it appropriate to elevate communication to a primary means of how we conceptualize terrorism? Our answer is an unequivocal yes. Terrorism is an act, a process, a plot intended to garner a response. It is inherently communicative. Communication serves as the conduit for expressing terrorism motives. Until we acknowledge, and then seek to understand, the primacy of communication within terrorism, we will continue to slave at the mercy of its communicative influence on our lives.

Understand that we fully acknowledge those that precede us in our thinking; we are not the first to expose terrorists as communicators. We offer a fresh perspective by agreeing to see terrorism for what it is. Contributions to this volume are balanced among those that are controversial and those that are practical. We embrace this balance, or tension, as an opportunity to expose the righteous indignation of terrorists and the fallacies of those who communicatively react to them. At the same time, contributors offer some of the best thinking about how to prepare for, and react to these violent communication acts. Some of these challenges are framed as ethical concerns: How should the media balance the value of news coverage against the risk that attention will give terrorists undue visibility and legitimacy? How should the appeals and arguments of terrorists be framed? Is violence justified by the value position advocated? Is society, through media and other response and reaction options, unnecessarily provoking terrorists by not acknowledging their grievances and seeking remedies to problems that can otherwise only be forced into public attention through violence?

Conventional wisdom views terrorists as persons who attack corporate, governmental, or NGO facilities and personnel; or create havoc by causing collateral damage to civilian populations. The fundamental assumption of this view is that terrorists use terror to publicize their cause and intimidate some aspect of established authority in society. Thus, recognition of terrorists and managing the risks they can create provides rationale for the study of terrorist and the development of protocols for awareness and preemption.[8]

Terrorists may not refer to themselves as such, even though their acts and statements fit a profile that leads them to be so called. Identifying terrorists and their potential for harm is a vital part of risk management. It is typical that some group, however large or small, sets out to commit criminal acts and make statements that are intended to attract media attention. The act needs to be so symbolic that it attracts this attention, or the statements won't be heard. Thus, a substantial issue addressed in this volume is how the goals of terrorists and the services of the media fabricate a cyclical trap.

Terrorism resides at the end of the communication continuum occupied by reprehensibility, malevolence, and virulence. We must launch collective efforts to reduce exhortation and other similar types of communication. What this volume represents is a diversity of options for accomplishing just that. While this volume reaches into an ominous box with no fixed boundaries or firm edges to guide our understanding, its ideas are compelling enough for us to pull from that container insights and questions that can ultimately facilitate successful management of terrorism.

## PLAN OF THE BOOK

The chapters that follow coalesce into four areas of communication and terrorism: (1) Identity and Sense Making: Having to Deal with Terrorism; (2) Media, Public-Information Strategy, and Terrorism; (3) Crisis Preparation and Response to Terrorist Attacks; and (4) Peering into the Future. In the first of these sections, three chapters focus on identity and sense making as means of dealing with terrorism. Sparks' chapter, "Social Identity and Perceptions of Terrorist Groups: How Others See Them and How They See Themselves," examines the role of social group membership in terrorist events. One of her goals was to describe the ways in which group identifications and stereotypes can facilitate understanding of mass communicated representations of terrorist groups. Using social identity theory, Sparks' chapter describes the means through which we come to understand primary identities, secondary identities, and tertiary identities that help explain terrorism-related social processes. Because the media play a critical role in forming identities, they serve to alter the phenomenon of terrorism itself. This is directly in line with our thoughts earlier.

The chapter entitled "Terrorism and Political Socialization: Young Adults' Perspectives on the Anniversary of 9/11," by Horowitz and Wanstrom, reports a study that demonstrates a number of political socialization challenges that exist in America. Their study found only 15 percent of undergraduate students knew the nationality of the 9/11 terrorists, and the undergraduate students' general knowledge about U.S. involvement in the Middle East was very limited. This lack of knowledge stems from a variety of factors. The authors argue that not only has the educational system neglected issues of terrorism and Middle Eastern politics, but also parents were ill equipped to provide this kind of information. As a result, political socialization regarding international terrorism is left to the media—which constitute an institution whose goal is presenting spectacular, horrific stories. Media were generally effective in describing the sensational aspects of terrorism stories, but failed to give the public opportunities to understand the international context of terrorism.

Becker and Thompson, in their chapter, "The Intersection of Terrorism, Interpersonal Communication, and Health," argue that terrorism influences the way people talk to their families and friends and how they develop relationships with others who were also victimized. By relating to significant others, individuals find a means of obtaining basic and interpersonal needs. Supportive communication enhances feelings of security and safety, because it promotes connecting to others. It can also help people make sense of the meaning and significance of a terrorist event and can enhance feelings of security and comfort. Targets of terrorism can communicate to "reconnect" to their social world and restore some sense of normalcy. This chapter is a special offering of some of the more basic feelings following terrorist acts.

Three chapters comprise the subsequent section, which delves into how media and public-information strategy are related to terrorist acts, both conceptually and practically. Bowen's chapter, "Communication Ethics in the Wake of Terrorism" focuses on the ethics of media communication about terrorist acts, and the legitimacy the media confer on terrorists. This situation becomes complex in that the media not only have the power to convey legitimacy, but also to influence public opinion through their choice of newsworthy events. Since terrorists use violence to gain publicity and legitimacy through media coverage, "communication plays a large role in the aftermath of terrorism, and media coverage is highly sought after, both by members of the affected public and by terrorists themselves." Bowen goes on to suggest that media framing creates a perspective for thinking about topics covered in the news. Through framing, the media can legitimize certain events or highlight specific aspects of the event that lead to predetermined conclusions. How a terrorist act is communicated, then, can convey inalterable ethical interpretations of the act.

The chapter by Ryan and Switzer, "Using Binary Language to Sell the War in Afghanistan," contends that terrorists use violence rhetorically and understand that they cannot achieve their goals if the media do not cooperate. They go on to argue that terrorists have much less success in societies where the media are not allowed to report terrorist acts. Like others in the volume, the authors argue that media framing is a critical factor in the world of terrorism, since how the media frame an incident determines how it is reported. Ryan and Switzer report that frames may be divided into four categories based on their function: defining problems and issues, determining causes, presenting value judgments, and suggesting solutions. In a study reported in the chapter, government officials used words that were judgmental, inflammatory, and sensational in describing the terrorist perpetrators of 127 incidents of political violence from 1980 to 1985. The study went on to examine the extent of media framing in the war against terrorism between September 11 and October 8, 2001, when the United States began bombing Afghanistan. A troubling finding of this chapter concerns media coverage of terrorism as a means to boost ratings. Ryan and Switzer also suggest that "some journalists allowed themselves to be used by those who wanted to stifle dissent about the military strikes."

In "Community Right-to-Know vs. Terrorists' Exploitation of Public Information," Heath, McKinney, and Palenchar argue that "while an open stream of communication is the essence of community right-to-know, information could, in fact, harm the community if it were made available in such ways that it easily could be obtained by terrorists." This chapter takes up the thorny issue of the risk that terrorists can use information that citizens have a right to know. Potentially, this information can be turned against citizens by terrorists who want to make a statement through violence that endangers the livelihoods, health, and even lives of those individuals.

The fourth section offers seven distinct but overlapping perspectives for crisis preparations and responses to terrorist attacks. In the chapter by Sellnow, Seeger, and Ulmer, "Constructing the 'New Normal' through Post-Crisis Discourse," the authors recount events of the CDC anthrax crisis as a means of exploring the ways in which organizational learning is inspired by a crisis event, and how such learning leads to changes in the structure and planning of an organization. They describe the process by which learning can generate the emergence of a "new normal," following a crisis situation. In the case of the anthrax crisis, new normal involves the stockpiling of antibiotics and gas masks, as well as acts of civility and selflessness that emerged following the attacks. The CDC learned that uncertainty is an ever-present component of crisis situations and that organizations need to understand that they cannot rely on their past experiences. The new normal at the CDC involves identifying, accepting, and acknowledging uncertainty, and placing communication at the center of its strategy.

Kreps, Alibek, Bailey, Neuhauser, Rowan, and Sparks, in a chapter entitled "The Critical Role of Communication to Prepare for Biological Threats: Prevention, Mobilization, and Response," describe a multistage communication process for biodefense. Based on arguments that effective biodefense efforts depend on coordinating communications to promote awareness, surveillance, mobilization, and response; their model includes the essential steps of preventing, preparing for, and responding to biological threats. Discussion includes issues related to media management and message and channel characteristics.

Coombs engages in a discussion of the crisis-management process in the chapter, "The Terrorist Threat: Shifts in Crisis-Management Thinking and Planning Post-9/11." A number of risk-assessment issues are discussed, with emphasis placed on business continuity. He recommends that those involved in crisis-prevention plans must coordinate their crisis-management plans (CMP) with the Community Emergency Operation Plan (EOP). This will entail shifts and accommodations in various planning and preparation strategies.

Rhoads, in his chapter, "Thinking the Unthinkable: How Industry Is Reinventing and Communicating Disaster Recovery in a Post-9/11 World," presents a model for crisis preparation and response, termed $P^2R^2$. He distinguishes between this model and the Federal Emergency Management

4. Why are others or we a symbolic target—primary or secondary?
5. What is the ideological rationale for terrorism?
6. What ideological rationale is likely to guide the way terrorism is framed by the media, opinion leaders, and other influential groups in society?
7. How can we best conduct surveillance—alone and in coordination with others—to reduce the likelihood of becoming a successful target?
8. Do our surveillance and security measures increase or decrease our vulnerability?
9. Do our surveillance and security measures serve as useful preconditions for crisis-response messages that may be required in the event that we are a primary or secondary target?
10. How well prepared are we with our total crisis planning and communication program to deal with the possibility of being a primary or secondary target?

We ask that you consider these questions and add your own, as you reflect on the issues raised in the following chapters. Ultimately, this volume is asking for greater awareness of perspectives that will lead to the management of terrorism.

## NOTES

1. Hacker FJ. Crusaders, criminals, and crazies: terror and terrorism in our time. New York: Norton; 1976.
2. Stevens MJ. The unanticipated consequences of globalization: contextualizing terrorism. In: Stout CE, editor. Theoretical understandings and perspectives. Westport, CT: Praeger Publishers; 2002. p. 31–56. (The psychology of terrorism; vol 3).
3. 22 United States Code, s.2656f(d).
4. Buck G, Buck L, Mogil B. Preparing for terrorism: the public safety communicator's guide. Clifton Park, NY: Delmar Learning; 2003. p. 2.
5. Abdullah S. The soul of a terrorist: reflections on our war with the "other." In: Stout CE, editor. Theoretical understandings and perspectives. Westport, CT: Praeger Publishers; 2002. p. 129–42. (The psychology of terrorism; vol 3).
6. Reid WH. Controlling political terrorism: practicality, not psychology. In: Stout CE, editor. Theoretical understandings and perspectives. Westport, CT: Praeger Publishers; 2002. p. 1–8. (The psychology of terrorism; vol 3).
7. McCauley C. Psychological issues in understanding terrorism and the response to terrorism. In: Stout CE, editor. Theoretical understandings and perspectives. Westport, CT: Praeger Publishers; 2002. p. 3–30. (The psychology of terrorism; vol 3).
8. Heng Y. Unraveling the "war" on terrorism: a risk-management exercise in war clothing? Secur Dialogue 2002;33(2):227–42.

# 2 Social Identity and Perceptions of Terrorist Groups: How Others See Them and How They See Themselves

## Lisa Sparks

When the two aircrafts attacked the twin towers of the World Trade Center in New York on September 11, 2001, all the elements of a catastrophic event were present. The tragic day could be considered a turning point for American society, in terms of marking a transition in how we conduct our daily lives, what we think about, and how we live. The 9/11 terrorist attacks have also dramatically changed how organizations deal with crisis management.[1] Crisis management consists of the four-step communicative process of prevention, preparation, response, and learning, which are typically used to combat crises and lessen the damage such crises can impose.[2] Crisis-management communicators are most often responsible for identifying, confirming, and investigating crises; developing strategies for managing crises; and developing strategies for recovering from crisis incidents—with "crisis communications" defined as communicating with the public before, during, and after a negative event, such as 9/11.[3] Two special conditions of a crisis are victims and a high level of visibility. Communication is the key to understanding such crises. Until the 9/11 attacks, terrorism was not a leading concern in risk- and crisis-communication planning in the United States, but since the attacks, has become a significant topic in crisis management.[1]

As crisis communication, the events of September 11, and the experience of a city and nation, were brought to the international public eye via the media. Once such an attack occurs, community members are inundated with a barrage of mass-media representations of the attack (i.e., television, Internet); opinions, reading and information gathering; and discussions among friends. These representations may result in distorted by a terrorist act. Understanding these three identity types can help explain certain terrorism-related social processes.

## SOCIAL IDENTITY AND CRISIS COMMUNICATION IN THE TERRORISM CONTEXT

This chapter examines the role of social-group memberships in crisis communication surrounding the American terrorism experience. Much work has focused on how individuals are influenced by their group memberships. People orient to one another not only in terms of individual characteristics, but also group identifications. This orientation occurs in terms of individuals' perceptions of their own groups (social identities), and of others' (stereotypes). Identities and stereotypes influence how we communicate with others—typically referred to as an intergroup approach, grounded in the pioneering work of Tajfel.[13,14] In this chapter, it is argued that intergroup processes are germane to crisis communication, certainly following terrorist acts. While previous work has touched on these processes, it has not provided an integrative intergroup theoretical framework. This chapter suggests that the three levels of identity discussed above must be considered in establishing a meaningful agenda for intergroup work during terrorist events. Primary identities, which traditionally have been at the center of intergroup research, need to receive attention. The chapter also attends to secondary identities. The two most obvious of these identities are direct victims of terrorism, and terrorists themselves, but there are others, including some with more positive connotations (e.g., identification as a survivor of an attack). Finally, the chapter addresses tertiary identities, or those unique to individuals who have indirectly experienced a terrorist attack. Tertiary identities help explain certain terrorism-related social processes. Identification as one indirectly affected by a terrorist, identification as an indirect victim of terrorism (e.g., having a friend, co-worker, or family member who has been attacked), and identification as a terrorism survivor (e.g., Americans collectively, who are psychologically connected via the new media) are all relevant here. The chapter provides some context for understanding communication issues as they relate to terrorism. Following this, the chapter describes how examining processes at each level of identity will aid in understanding the impact of terrorism and/or terrorism outcomes. Propositions surrounding each level will be advanced. At the outset it is important to briefly define "group identification." Individuals who identify with a group are those who see their group membership as central to who they are. They are proud of their group memberships and act according to group norms. Identification is also indicated by specific behaviors (e.g., members of the AARP generally have higher levels of aging identification than similar nonmembers).

## PRIMARY IDENTITIES

Most work in intergroup communication and social psychology has examined identities stemming from large social groups such as ethnic identity,[15,16] age identity,[17] and health identity.[18] This line of research has provided suggestive evidence for the propositions related to secondary and tertiary identities below. Links exist between the primary identities as members of large-scale social groups, and the identities with specific behaviors as outlined in the next section.

## SECONDARY IDENTITIES

An intergroup perspective leads to an examination of the extent to which identification with those behaviors, or with groups that are associated with those behaviors, might influence terrorism risks and outcomes. The following two propositions are put forth.

*a) Identification as a terrorist victim (directly) will have positive consequences in terms of encouraging information seeking, social support seeking, and attention to terrorist related coping behaviors (e.g., information-seeking). It will have negative consequences to the extent that it encourages a sense of being victimized as an intrinsic part of the self as an American or one who lives in America.*

Acts of terrorism have caused psychological disorders such as post-traumatic stress disorder and psychosomatic illness, and have been linked to increased exhibition of chronic physical health problems in those directly and indirectly affected.[19,20] Furthermore, the impact of terrorist acts on American soil appears to create a shift in many American's social identity. For instance, in the case of the terrorist attacks on the Twin Towers on September 11, 2001, issues of safety have entered the American psyche on some level. While the level by which Americans are impacted is not clearly understood, it is most certainly present now in a way that did not exist before 9/11.

On first attack, most individuals will make efforts to understand more about terrorism and risk, particularly those who have been directly impacted through the death of a loved one or friend. For some, this will develop into seeking information from other terrorist victims and survivors and new media consumption (i.e., Internet) and joining together with them (either in person, phones or cell phones, or in virtual environments such as online chat rooms). Such joining together may well be driven in part by a growing sense of identity with the group, and in a cyclical fashion will also lead to greater identification. Online forums might be particularly associated with increased identification, given the relative anonymity and reduced opportunities for perception of individuating information.[21] As individuals identify with others with similar problems, they are likely to conform to group practices in terms of health care, knowledge, and the like.[22] Such social pressures would be likely to have positive consequences in the current context.

*b) Individuals who feel a sense of identification with others who engage in terrorist victim/survivor related behaviors (or terrorist acts) will find it harder to change those behaviors, and be more likely to suffer negative consequences than those who engage in the behaviors without such a sense of identification.*

The most prominent behavior associated with terrorism is violence. Terrorist victims and survivors identify with being a "terrorist victim or survivor" to various degrees—that is, for many this is a meaningful social category to which they belong and with which they identify. Websites saving the history of such events should be examined to further understand the voices behind such events (see e.g., 911digitalarchive.org or The September 11 Digital Archive: Saving the Histories of September 11, 2001, at the Center for History and New Media, George Mason University), which might provide insight into intergroup behavior in this context.

Terrorists themselves have an increased sense of being oppressed,[23] which might build group solidarity. Based on research grounded in intergroup theory, this chapter argues that individuals who are highly identified as terrorists are less likely to want to stop and will find it harder to stop even if they want to. They may have a higher awareness of the risks associated with terrorism (see earlier), but will also have more elaborate rationales for continuing to participate.[20]

*c) Individuals who feel a sense of identification with others who engage in terrorist victim/survivor related behaviors (or terrorist acts) will find it easier to maintain those behaviors, and be less likely to suffer negative consequences than those who engage in the behaviors without such a sense of identification.*

Conversely, this argument is proposed for those who engage in terrorist victim/survivor related behaviors—those who can easily maintain such behaviors over time and as a result will be less likely to experience negative effects. For instance, identifying as a heroic victim or survivor, civil servant to the community, an upstanding member of society, or as an activist against terrorism and seeing this identification as an important element of self-concept are likely to lead to maintenance of those behaviors. The concept of Alcoholics Anonymous is similar in that group participants are more likely to maintain a positive self-image and sobriety by getting support from and relating to others in their groups with similar circumstances.[24]

## TERTIARY IDENTITIES

Tertiary identities are unique to those who have experienced a terrorist attack indirectly. This chapter argues that *indirectly affected* terrorist victim/survivorship behaviors or the indirect impact of terrorist acts can help explain certain terrorism-related social processes. Identification as one indirectly impacted by a terrorist, identification as an indirect victim of terrorism (e.g., friend, coworker, or family member who has been attacked), and identification as a terrorism survivor (e.g., collective Americans indirectly impacted but psychologically connected via the new media) are all relevant here. As noted at the outset, it is very important to attend to the ways in which individuals identify with their position as terrorist *victims* as well as their identification as *survivors*. A related area here is the extent to which they identify as members of a *specific* group of survivors (e.g., in the form of a support group). Thus, the following propositions are proposed.

*d) Identification as a terrorist victim (indirectly) will have positive consequences in terms of encouraging information seeking, social support seeking, attention to terrorist related coping behaviors (e.g., information-seeking). It will have negative consequences to the extent that it encourages a sense of being victimized as an intrinsic part of the self as an American or one who lives in America.*

As noted previously in the section on direct impacts of terrorist attacks, many people impacted indirectly via massive amounts of media exposure and interpersonal channels will follow similar behaviors in terms of information seeking and social support. Those impacted indirectly are likely to have similar emotions, but may be less intense at least initially. Community-based social support as well as online forums might also be associated with increased identification, given the relative anonymity and reduced opportunities for perception of individuating information.[18] As van Knippenberg[19] points out, individuals are likely to begin conforming to the group as they identify with the collective experiencing similar problems (e.g., terrorist attack on the nation). Such social pressures would be likely to have positive consequences in the current context. As noted earlier, daily interactions and stress can indirectly influence individuals in mysterious ways including coping behaviors related to terrorist attacks, and potentially subsequent interactions with those fitting the terrorist profile following such attacks.[17] The extent to which individuals are *indirectly affected* by a terrorist attack may bring about differences in levels of group identification. As Contrada and Ashmore[25] state, group identification may provide social support resources similar to close personal relationships. Attributions for discrimination are also relevant and worth considering. Whether directly or indirectly impacted, the notion of what it means to be an American or to live in America post-9/11 is likely to be fraught with safety concerns, unknown social identity shifts, and fear of interacting with individuals fitting media-enhanced stereotypes and the like—an added aspect of identification with the terrorism experience that most Americans had not experienced prior to such a life-changing event. To what extent does one conceal or embrace one's American identity when conversing with those from other parts of the world? Tajfel's work, while not explicitly addressing terrorism or crisis issues, does point to other negative consequences of concealing group identity ("passing," or in social identity theory terms, "social mobility").[10]

In contrast to the argument in the previous paragraphs, it is suggested that there may be unhealthy consequences related to identification as a terrorist victim or survivor. In particular, the degree to which victims identify with a "victim role" may lead to reduced feelings of control, a tendency to defer to authorities and the like.[26,27] In addition, identification with being terrorized may override or overwhelm other important social identifications that may serve positive functions for one's health.[24] In part, the extent to which identification as a terrorist victim or survivor has positive or negative consequences may well depend on the cognitive representations that are most salient with regard to the identity. Self-stereotyping research suggests that identification with a group leads to a view of the self that is in accord with a prototypical representation of the group.[28,29] If the prototypical cognitive representation is of an empowered, active person successfully surviving the terrorist attack (e.g., 9/11 survivors), the consequences of identification are likely to be positive. However, if the prototypical cognitive representation is of a terrorist victim or nonsurvivor, then the consequences of identification will probably be negative.

*e) Terrorist-related discrimination/stigma will be associated with terrorism-related outcomes.*

Very little work exists looking at social representations (stereotypes) of terrorist victims/survivors. It is clear that there is a certain differentiation associated with victims of terrorism.[6] Hence, once an individual has been attacked in some way by a terrorist or terrorist groups, they may well experience or perceive themselves as victims of discrimination, and for some individuals it may be their first experience of such treatment. Research needs to examine more about the stereotypes of terrorist victims and survivors post-9/11 (and other relevant crisis communication contexts). It seems likely, following from other research on stereotypes[30,31] that multiple stereotypes of terrorist victims/survivors exist (e.g., a "battling to the death" heroic stereotype; the frail young female).

It would be useful to examine the extent to which such stereotypes and differing worldviews are shared in the population and portrayed in all aspects of the new media. McLuhan and Powers,[32] for instance, noted that violence arises when there is no room made (in our society) for different points of view and that the key to peace is to understand both ways of thinking *simultaneously*. McLuhan and Powers[30] initially uncovered their tetradic structure while investigating the formal aspects of (linguistic) communication and found that all media forms simultaneously undergo change through four fundamental components. Thus, all media forms: (a) *intensify* something in a culture, while, at the same time, (b) *obsolescing* something else. They also (c) *retrieve* a phase or factor long ago pushed aside and (d) undergo a modification (or *reversal*) when extended beyond the limits of their potential. To put it simply, as a stereotype or worldview *intensifies*, parts of the stereotype or worldview become *obsolete*. However, at the same time individuals and members of societies (or countries) are discovering new information about the other (*retrieval* on some level). As this information seeking and discovery increases, the stereotypes and worldviews are going through a constant *modification* (or even reversal). Depending upon the nature of the stereotype or worldview at a given time, certain aspects appear to be highlighted more at different points in time. Thus, all four elements of the tetrad exist in motion simultaneously, however, one or more of the four may be more dominant than another at a given time depending upon the nature and state of the transformation process. The tetradic structure was originally formulated to explain transformations in world life and media in the 21st century. In other words, this structure was developed to bring about a visual understanding of McLuhan's[33] characterization of today's world as a "global village" because of the accelerated expansion of technology, communication networks, and worldwide transportation. McLuhan and Powers[30] explain the tetrad through the view that the world has been going through "a vast and material psychic shift between the values of linear thinking, of visual, proportional space, and that of the values of the multisensory life, the experience of acoustic space" (p. ix). Visual space is viewed as a more linear Western way of communicating and making sense of the world, whereas acoustic space is defined as a more holistic Eastern way of approaching the world. Thus, once we understand the different ways individuals think and operate, we can achieve greater satisfaction and happiness in our relationships, our organizations, our places of worship, our society, and ultimately survive.

Once these are better understood, additional work should examine the ways in which communication with terrorist victims/survivors is driven by such stereotypes. It is important to know whether crisis communication interactants are exercising such stereotypes when interacting with victims of terrorism. Likewise, it will be important to discover the extent to which terrorist victims and survivors themselves may be self-stereotyping into such categories, and whether that self-stereotyping might be influencing their communication with others, and so forth. In some cases this might be positive. Self-stereotyping as a "battler" might have positive consequences in terms of not giving up, trying multiple support groups, taking a proactive approach to terrorism, by becoming an activist, joining the military, and the like.

*f) Simultaneous identity is constructed with the media (i.e., television) and new media (i.e., Internet) via shared experiences.*

Television and the Internet allow the American public to experience events as the news is unfolding. News coverage has undergone a dramatic shift since the arrival of 24 hours news coverage (e.g., Fox, CNN). As a result, it is argued that the American identity is not only shaped by the media, but is simultaneously constructed along with the new media with supplemental information-seeking strategies ranging from Internet surfing to interpersonal channels, and so forth. The way in which information seeking can be driven by stereotypes has been documented.[34] Further, the American public learns about such catastrophic events much more quickly and via multiple channels. We define and redefine such events through these multiple channels and thus, cocreate shifts in identity (e.g., what it now means to be an American, fight for American rights and freedom!). Perceptions formed by the public based on representations or misrepresentations of people or groups portrayed in the mass media carry over into personal interactions and can have effects, either positive or negative, on future communication or interactions based on these perceptions.[8]

g) *Stereotypes and representation of heroes are redefined via media and new media (e.g., firefighters and victims).*

Mediated representations have been found to reveal stereotypes.[8,9] The media and new media simultaneously help us to redefine our notion of "hero" via images that are shown over and over again both on television and the Internet. One dimension of "hero" is the person/persons who commit the terrorist act. Viewers and reporters alike may report some perpetrators as heroes, while others may see them as villains. Hero and other identities of the terrorist(s) as well as the individuals who either side with or oppose that person is certainly an identity issue. Furthermore, persons who respond in "noble" ways to terrorism become heroes and tend to produce enormous amounts of identification (e.g., the police and fire department personnel in New York City on 9/11).

Victims of such terrorist acts are often depicted as "heroes" via the media in ways rarely seen before. Of course, the role of the reporter as interpreter is often more important in regard to television and less so in regard to the Internet. However, both the media and new media continually reinforce stereotypes by showing a few images again and again. As a result, the American public may start to think of "heroes" and "victims" of terrorism through a narrower lens that is defined and redefined, negotiated, and renegotiated through the visual choices depicted. A current cautionary example of this phenomenon is the media coverage of Pfc. Jessica Lynch in April 2003. She was depicted as a hero of the Iraq War by the media for "fighting to the death" rather than being captured by the enemy even after sustaining multiple gunshot and stab wounds. The Jessica Lynch story was the perfect opportunity for the media (and military) to build morale for the war; however, three months later, the media found that reports of her story were severely exaggerated, and she suffered no gunshot wounds and did not gun down any Iraqi soldiers during her capture.[35] Experts have even accused Pentagon officials of deliberately feeding reporters a completely false account of Lynch's capture experience to build support for the war.[33]

h) *Increased contact with terrorist victims/survivors may reduce or modify damaging stereotypes.*

Research on the "contact hypothesis" has yielded a wealth of findings over the past 50 years.[36,37] The evidence suggests that contact with members of a stigmatized outgroup can ameliorate negative attitudes, particularly under certain conditions (e.g., contact is equal status, cooperative, pleasant.[38,39] Most recently, work has suggested that group memberships need to be salient in such contact.[40,41] Hence, to improve attitudes toward terrorist victims in general, we should encourage contact in which the status of victims/survivors is salient and they are seen as *typical* of terrorist victims/survivors as a group. Such contact might lead to generalization from pleasant contact with one individual to more positive attitudes towards all victims and survivors of terrorism.

*i) Identification as a survivor will have a positive influence on continued survival.*

In general, positive consequences stem from identification with other terrorist survivors, as well as a tendency to view the self in terms of survivorship. Identification as a survivor should link to internal locus of control and more general feelings of self-esteem,[42] which are themselves associated with increased survival.[43] Identification with other survivors may also enhance preventive measures, such as obtaining a supply of antibiotics.[44] Thus, it seems likely that continued involvement with support groups might serve positive functions.

## CONCLUSIONS AND THEORETICAL DIRECTIONS

The above discussion is intended to illustrate the range of important issues surrounding terrorism that can be addressed using an intergroup framework. More theoretical and empirical work will be necessary to tease apart such complex issues.[45,46] There are certainly others. For instance (chemical and biological) terrorism can result in physical changes, and some terrorist attacks result in profound socio-relational impacts (e.g., 9/11, Oklahoma City Bombing). The current chapter is more concerned with the identity *consequences* of terrorism and related issues surrounding the experience of terrorism.

This chapter has provided an understanding of how social identities are created by means of the American terrorism experience. It is now important that we move forward in terms of better understanding how an intergroup approach utilizing social identity theory will impact the way in which we communicate during times of terrorism crisis. The goal of the current chapter has been to begin the discussion, to provide a framework, and to present some propositions emerging from prior research and theory in this area. Much work has already addressed some of these issues (e.g., discrimination and health related stress). In other cases, an intergroup framework suggests areas of research that appear to be relatively untapped (e.g., terrorist victims' levels of identification with one another; the content and pervasiveness of stereotypes of terrorist victims/survivors). Future work in this area should investigate the extent to which heavy viewers of crisis related new media coverage differ from light viewers of such coverage and the degree to which such viewers differentially support related public policy decisions connected to the crisis or terrorist acts. Further, to what extent does cultural and national identity affect support for fighting terrorism (e.g., war, etc.).

Some of the identities discussed here deal with what are traditionally thought of as collective identities. Other identities are somewhat beyond the confines of social identity theory, but are also relevant. Family identity, for instance, may be crucial among those who have a family member who has experienced a terrorist attack. However, the extent to which such individuals identify with the family may be crucial. People who are less involved and identified with their family may dissociate from the experience and perhaps perceive themselves as less vulnerable.

Similar to Harwood and Sparks[15] suggestions on health identity and cancer, identification with support groups is worth examining from this perspective, despite the fact that a specific support group is a somewhat smaller "group" than is traditionally the focus of intergroup research. An intergroup perspective would predict that such stress would be particularly powerful for those who identify most strongly with the support group. At the same time, identification with the group may serve positive functions in terms of valuing the support received, following guidance, attending support group meetings regularly, and maintaining group life. This double-edged sword of support group identification is worth further examination.

The current chapter is put forth as a beginning step toward theoretical development in the crisis communication area. First, it would be possible to generate an identity-based theory of communication and crisis-related behavior. Such a theory might incorporate the propositions described above, developing and integrating them in ways that emphasize the processes common to them all. This intergroup perspective, initially derived from Harwood and Sparks[15] work on health identity, would embrace such research and offer new resources. For example, intergroup theory makes it clear that abandoning a particular identity is possible for the weakly identified. For the more strongly identified, a strategy like that described by Harwood and Sparks may result in enhanced identification and social activism (e.g., for "terrorist victims/survivors' rights!"; "God Bless America!") to battle the perceived identity threat. Thus, it is vitally important that we better understand the construction and interpretation of interpersonal and mediated crisis communication messages and how such messages influence our lives. Terrorism always has been and will remain a risk for which we all should prepare and to which we should pay closer attention. We must pay critical attention to the powerful and relevant role the media play in the shaping and shifting our identities as well as the impact and modification of the phenomenon of terrorism itself. Communicating with the public about crises can be a problematic and complex endeavor, but training and support from research can help scholars, practitioners, and the public to communicate with each other in more systematic ways that translate theory and research into practical application when such crises arise.

## NOTES

1. Coombs WT. The terrorist threat: shifts in crisis-management thinking and planning post 9/11. In O'Hair HD, Heath R, Ledlow G, editors. Communication, communities, and terrorism. Westport, CT: Praeger Publishers; forthcoming.

2. Coombs WT. Ongoing crisis communication: planning, managing, and responding. Thousand Oaks, CA: Sage Publications; 1999.

3. Fearn-Banks K. Crisis communications: a casebook approach. Mahwah, NJ: Erlbaum; 1996.

4. Nacos B. Terrorism as breaking news: attack on America. Pol Sci Q 2003;118(1):23–53.

5. Nacos B. Accomplice or witness? The media's role in terrorism. Curr Hist 2000;99:174–78.

6. National Center for Post-Traumatic Stress Disorder. Surviviors of human-caused and natural disasters. Available at: www.ncptsd.org/facts/disasters/fs_survivors_disaster.html. Accessed November 12, 2003.

7. Roots R. Terrorized into absurdity: the creation of the transportation security administration. Independent Rev 2003;7(4):503–18.

8. Florida Museum of Natural History of the University of Florida; 2002.

9. Shark bites man. Sci Am 286(6):28–9.

10. Altheide DL. The impact of television news formats on social policy. J Broadcasting Electron Media 1991;35(1):3–21.

11. Harwood J, Anderson K. The presence and portrayal of social groups on prime-time television. Commun Rep 2002;15(2):81–97.

12. Lule J. Myth and terror on the editorial page: The New York Times responds to September 11th. J Mass Commun Q 2002;79(2):275–94.

13. Tajfel H, Turner JC. The social identity theory of intergroup behavior. In: Worschel S, Austin WG, editors. The social psychology of intergroup relations. 2nd ed. Chicago: Nelson-Hall; 1986. p. 7–24.

14. Robinson WP, editor. Social groups and identities: developing the legacy of Henri Tajfel. Boston, MA: Butterworth Heinemann; 1996.

15. Branscombe NR, Schmitt MT, Harvey RD. Perceiving pervasive discrimination among African Americans: implications for group identification and well-being. J Pers Soc Psychol 1999;77:135–49.

16. Hecht ML. 2002—a research odyssey: toward the development of a communication theory of identity. Commun Monogr 1993;60:76–82.

17. Harwood J, Giles H, Ryan EB. Aging, communication, and intergroup theory: social identity and intergenerational communication. In: Nussbaum JF, Coupland J, editors. Handbook of communication and aging research. Hillsdale, NJ: Lawrence Erlbaum; 1995. p. 133–59.

18. Harwood J, Sparks L. Social identity and health: an intergroupcommunication approach to cancer. Health Commun 2003;15(2):145–70.

19. Lacy TJ, Benedek DM. Terrorism and weapons of mass destruction: managing the behavioral reaction in primary care. South Med J 2003;96(4):394–9.

20. Yehuda R. Changes in the concept of PTSD and trauma. Psychiatr Times 2003 April 1;35.

21. Postmes T, Spears R, Lea M. Breaching or building social boundaries? SIDE-effects of computer-mediated communication. Commun Res 1998;25: 689–715.

22. Van Knippenberg D. Social identity and persuasion: reconsidering the role of group membership. In: Abrams D, Hogg MA, editors. Social identity and social cognition. Malden, MA: Basil Blackwell; 1999. p. 315–31.

23. Federal Research Division, Library of Congress. Social psychology of terrorism: who becomes a terrorist? 1999. Available from: www.loc.gov/rr/frd/pdf-files/Soc_Psych_of_Terrorism.pdf. Accessed November 11, 2003.

24. Dunlop J. Peer groups support seniors fighting alcohol and drugs. Aging 1990;361:28–32.

25. Contrada RJ, Ashmore RD. Introduction: self and social identity: key to understanding social and behavioral aspects of physical health and disease? In: Contrada RJ, Ashmore RD, editors. Self, social identity, and physical health: interdisciplinary explorations. New York: Oxford University Press; 1999. p. 3–21.

26. Parsons T. The social system. Glencoe, IL: The Free Press; 1951.

27. Charmaz K. From the "sick role" to stories of self: understanding the self in illness. In: Contrada RJ, Ashmore RD, editors. Self, social identity, and physical health. New York: Oxford University Press; 1999. p. 209–39.

28. Levy B. Improving memory in old age through implicit self-stereotyping. J Pers Soc Psychol 1996;71:1092–1107.

29. Reicher SD. Crowd behavior as social action. In: Turner JC, Hogg MA, Oakes PJ, Reicher SD, Wetherell MS, editors. Rediscovering the social group: a self-categorization theory. Oxford: Blackwell; 1987. p. 171–202.

30. Hummert ML, Garstka TA, Shaner JL, Strahm S. Stereotypes of the elderly held by the young, middle aged, and elderly adults. J Gerontol Psychol Sci 1994;49:240–49.

31. Eckes T. Explorations in gender cognition: content and structure of female and male subtypes. Soc Cogn 1994;12:37–60.

32. McLuhan M, Powers BR. The global village: transformations in world life and media in the 21st century. Oxford: Oxford University Press; 1989.

33. McLuhan M. The Gutenberg Galaxy. New York: New American Library; 1962.

34. Ng SH, Giles H, Moody J. Information-seeking triggered by age. Int J Aging and Hum Dev 1991;33:269–77.

35. Ritea S. Jessica Lynch's story: a little too perfect? Am J Rev 2003;25(6): 10–11.

36. Allport GW. The nature of prejudice. Reading, MA: Addison-Wesley; 1954.

37. Pettigrew T. Intergroup contact theory. Annu Rev Psychol 1998;49:65–85.

38. Amir Y. The role of intergroup contact in change of prejudice and race relations. In: Katz PA, editor. Toward the elimination of prejudice. New York: Pergamon; 1976. p. 245–80.

39. Brewer MB, Miller N. Contact and cooperation: when do they work? In: Katz PA, Taylor DA, editors. Eliminating racism. New York: Plenum Press; 1988. p. 315–26.

40. Hewstone M, Brown RJ. Contact is not enough: an intergroup perspective on the contact hypothesis: In: Hewstone M, Brown RJ, editors. Contact and conflict in intergroup encounters. Oxford: Basil Blackwell; 1986. p. 1–44.

41. Harwood J, Hewstone M, Paolini S, Hurd R. Grandparent-grandchild contact and attitudes towards older adults: moderator and mediator effects. [unpublished manuscript]. University of Arizona; 2002.

42. Deimling G, Kahana B, Schumacher J. Life threatening illness: the transition from victim to survivor. J Aging Identity 1997;2(3):165–86.

43. Contrada RJ. Type A behavior, personality hardiness, and cardiovascular responses to stress. J Pers Soc Psychol 1989;57:895–903

44. Mears JB. The cultural construction of breast cancer. [dissertation] Dissertation Abstr Int A 1997;58(6A):2273.

45. Herd D, Grube J. Black identity and drinking in the U.S.: a national study. Addict 1996;91:845–57.

46. Morman MT. The influence of fear appeals, message design, and masculinity on men's motivation to perform the testicular self-exam. J Appl Commun Res 2000;28(2):91–116.

# 3 Terrorism and Political Socialization: Young Adults' Perspectives on the Anniversary of 9/11

## Edward M. Horowitz and Johan Wanstrom

William Schneider argues that in the aftermath of 9/11 Americans are facing enormous challenges overcoming political socialization biases from the Islamic world.[1] These biases stem from, among other things, new political challenges that followed the 9/11 attacks. While these political challenges affect the United States as a nation on a macro level, we believe it is particularly important to understand how young adults are coping with these political challenges, as they experience terrorism and the first war of their lifetime. During adolescence and young adulthood, individuals begin to make greater cognitive sense of the world around them and try to determine their place in society. In addition, it is the period when young adults' political socialization becomes more manifested. They begin to form political attitudes and to develop important patterns of civic participation.[2,3]

The American public has never faced an act of aggression on the continent with the magnitude and severity of the 9/11 attacks, and in their aftermath, traditional socialization institutions, such as schools and families, were limited in their abilities to deal with the tragedy and its subsequent political problems. Under these circumstances, young adults, like the rest of the population, are dependent on information and interpretations of terrorism presented in the media. This information tends to focus on direct events, while often lacking any contextual information. Young adults have to make sense of the limited information presented to them in the media. As a result, they risk being misinformed. For example, we found in our study that 68 percent of the undergraduate students in our sample incorrectly believed that a majority of the 9/11 terrorists were from Afghanistan or Iraq. (They were actually from Saudi Arabia.)

Not only do young adults gain political knowledge and attitudes from parents, school, and the media, but from their historical and social environment as well.[4,5] Research has found that the historical context in which young people live affects their development.[6,7] As they finish college and enter the "real world," today's young adults may be on their way to becoming "the 9/11 generation," as they are forever marked by terrorism and its concurring effects on their sociopolitical environment.

> The political environment on college campuses appears to have changed dramatically since the terrorist attacks of 9/11. Something different is occurring when young adults on college campuses are suddenly expressing interest in politics; wearing U.S. flag lapel pins and red, white, and blue ribbons; and attending memorial rallies and "teach-ins" by the thousands. This is a distinct change in the political culture of young adults that could affect their political socialization in a variety of ways. As a University of Michigan graduate student explains it, the events of 9/11 have changed the ways these students define themselves: "Our generation, as long as we've had an identity, was known as the generation that had it easy. We had no crisis, no Vietnam, no Martin Luther King, no JFK. We've got it now. When we have kids and grandkids, we'll tell them we lived through the roaring 90s, when all we cared about was the number one movie or how many copies an album sold. This is where it changes" (p. 51).[8]

This chapter examines the reactions and responses of young adults to the ongoing U.S. war on terrorism on the anniversary of 9/11. What kind of knowledge do young adults have about the 9/11 terrorists and the historical role of the United States in the Middle East? One year after the 9/11 attacks, do young adults express satisfaction with the U.S. war on terrorism? Are they emotionally affected by the heavy media coverage that occurred on the anniversary of 9/11, and the ongoing media coverage of the war on terrorism? In what ways does patriotism affect their political attitudes?

## THE ROLE OF THE MEDIA

The ways in which young adults think about and understand terrorism is influenced to some degree by the way that terrorism is reported by the media. Research during the 1980s found that television network newscasts reported on hundreds of acts of terrorism, but focused very little attention on political or socioeconomic explanations.[9,10] Instead, these newscasts covered terrorism in an episodic frame. According to Iyengar, episodic news coverage uses case-study examples or event-oriented reports to depict the news as concrete instances (e.g., terrorists attack U.S. soldiers on patrol in Iraq).[11] Episodic framing is the predominant frame used in television news, and leads individuals to make individualistic judgments, rather than societal, when pinning responsibility for actions reported in the news.[11] For example, an individualistic judgment of a terrorist act might be that the terrorists were simply crazy or extremists who think that violent acts will solve their problems.

In contrast, news may be presented with a thematic frame.[11] A thematic frame presents issues within a more abstract framework by including much greater background information, and explaining overall outcomes and general conditions in the context of the situation (e.g., explaining the social or political grievances of a terrorist organization). This type of news coverage has the opposite effect of episodic news coverage; viewers of thematic news tend to place responsibility on society and government, instead of individuals.

Controlled experiments conducted by Iyengar found that viewers of episodic television news are more likely to support punitive measures than social or political reform as the best way to fight terrorism.[11] In addition, Iyengar found that support for punitive measures against terrorism is correlated with conservative political ideology. Supporting Iyengar's earlier findings and extending them across media, Eckstein found that in the first month following the Oklahoma City bombings of 1995, and the month following the attacks of 9/11, newspaper coverage was more episodic than thematic.[12] In addition, Eckstein found newspaper coverage of the two attacks to be heavily focused on the victims, not the perpetrators.

## PUBLIC RESPONSES TO THE 9/11 ATTACKS

The terrorist attacks on 9/11 created a number of specific responses among the American public. Hassan and Cainkar both describe how Arab-Americans suddenly became a distinct group in American society.[13,14] Because Arab-Americans are officially classified as Anglo-Americans in the U.S. census report, there is no official data on their numbers in the United States. However, in the post-9/11 period, the FBI and other investigative organizations quickly found a way to treat differently those whom they classified as Arabs, particularly by focusing criminal investigations on them.

Members of the public in 2001 and 2002 were constantly surveyed on their attitudes toward Arab-Americans. Between 31 and 38 percent of the U.S. public reported that they were more suspicious toward people of Arab descent after 9/11.[15] In addition, 37 to 45 percent was in favor of singling out Arab-Americans for special scrutiny at airport checkpoints.[16] However, in the post-9/11 period, the overall attitude toward Muslim-Americans (some Arabs are Christians) did not dramatically decline. Surveys by the Pew Research Center even showed that the percentage of Americans with a "very favorable" or "mostly favorable" opinion about Muslim-Americans actually increased by 16 percent from March to November 2001.[17]

Kathleen Moore surveyed Americans on their attitudes toward restrictions of civil liberties and found that they generally did not find it more acceptable to apply limitations only to Muslim-Americans.[18] Between 15 and 45 percent of those polled "strongly" supported some of the measures specified in the USA Patriot Act,* but only when it came to "increased wiretapping" did respondents show a willingness to restrict Muslim-Americans at a higher rate than other groups. Moore argues that these numbers may not be accurate and suggests the possibility of a social desirability effect.[18] President Bush communicated strong support for the Muslim-American community after the 9/11 attacks, and it was generally considered politically incorrect to publicly display negative emotions toward the Muslim community.

However, Ahmad claims that racial violence was still common in the aftermath of 9/11,[19] and Hassan argues that the FBI and other governmental agencies forcefully, but quietly, acted against the Arab-Muslim community.[13] It is hard to imagine that journalists were totally unaware of the actions against the Muslim community, but the generally sensitive climate after the terrorist attacks and the carefully framed messages from political leaders may have created an environment that

---

*The USA Patriot Act was passed by Congress and signed by President George W. Bush within six weeks of the terrorist attacks of 9/11. USA Patriot is an acronym for "Uniting and Strengthening America by Providing Appropriate Tools Required to Intercept and Obstruct Terrorism." The Patriot Act expanded the powers of law enforcement to fight terrorism both domestically and abroad. It allows the government to monitor, among other things, individual e-mail, medical records, library accounts, financial records, and telephone calls. Supporters of the measure have argued that it increases the government's ability to fight terrorism, while critics have called it an infringement on civil liberties and freedoms.

discouraged investigations by the national media into these problems. Americans generally want to leave racial problems behind and move forward toward more inclusive values.[20] The attacks of 9/11 appear to have tested the progress of inclusiveness in America; the public wished to appear to be inclusive, but the attacks elicited emotions that challenged these values. Pettigrew, for example, argues that since 9/11, Americans have acted on fear, in response to a collective threat, just as Israelis and Arabs do.[21] Terrorist violence has resulted in a tense situation in which all three groups are violating their fundamental norms and values. We therefore have entered into a negative cycle of revenge and retaliation that may be hard to break.

Since 9/11, researchers and pollsters have focused their attention on understanding the opinions and attitudes of the American public toward anti-terrorism measures, civil liberties, and Muslim-Americans. There has unfortunately been little research, however, that examines the opinions and attitudes of young adults on these issues. Yet young adults are experiencing the changing political landscape in dramatic ways, particularly as they are on the military front lines of the new and ongoing war on terrorism. While previous literature has examined the ways in which young adults seek revenge after terrorist attacks,[22] and how young adults themselves become terrorists,[23] there is little research examining the cognitive attitudes of young adults in the post-9/11 period. Just as the socialization of previous generations was shaped by the political and socioeconomic conditions of the Great Depression,[6] or the end of communism,[5] this "9/11 generation" may well be shaped by the U.S. war on terrorism.

## RESEARCH QUESTIONS AND METHODOLOGY

The unique economic and sociohistorical conditions resulting from the 9/11 terrorist attacks and the ongoing war on terrorism appear to have affected the political socialization of young adults. These conditions are different from those under which prior political socialization research has taken place. The specific goal of this study is to identify and explain how young adults are being affected by these conditions in two areas of cognition: political knowledge and political attitudes.

RQ1: How knowledgeable are young adults about the 9/11 terrorists and the historical role of the United States in the Middle East?
RQ2: Are young adults satisfied with the way the U.S. government is fighting the war on terrorism?

RQ3: Do young adults support investigating Arab college students for potential terrorist activity?

## Sample

Data for the present study are from two surveys conducted among college students in an introductory communication class at the University of Oklahoma. The first survey was administered on September 12 and 13, 2002, immediately after the one-year anniversary of 9/11. The second survey was administered on September 10 to 14, 2003, at the second anniversary of 9/11. Surveys were administered on these dates to coincide with the heavy media coverage of commemorations of the 9/11 anniversary,[24,25] although there was less intense media coverage for the second anniversary than the first. The 2002 sample consists of 532 respondents, 54 percent male and 46 percent female; and the 2003 sample consists of 296 respondents. Although this is not a random sample, this fact does not limit our ability to determine with confidence the relationships among our variables of interest. Generalization of descriptive statistics to the general population, however, should be done with some caution.

## Measurement of Independent Variables

This study used several groups of independent variables: demographic information (gender, age, religiousness); political interest and ideology; attention to media reports about 9/11 and the war on terrorism; interpersonal discussion of 9/11 and the war on terrorism; political knowledge; and emotions felt when reading about or watching news coverage of the 9/11 anniversary.

### Measures of Young Adult Demographics

The mean age of the young adults in our study is 19.8 years. As the survey was conducted in Oklahoma, the "buckle" of the Bible Belt, and given the historical relationship between the Christian Right and the conservative movement, religiousness was measured on a ten-point scale (M = 6.7).

### Measure of Political Interest and Participation

Political interest is a three-item index comprised of items measuring interest in national and international politics, and the war on terrorism. Political ideology is measured on a seven-point scale from "very liberal" to "very conservative" (M = 4.3).

## Measure of Mass Media Exposure

News of 9/11 and the war on terrorism is a three-item additive index of attention paid to the war on terrorism and the 9/11 anniversary in newspapers, and attention paid to news coverage and documentaries of the 9/11 anniversary on television.

## Measure of Interpersonal Discussion

Discussion of 9/11 and the war on terrorism is a four-item additive index measuring frequency of discussion of national and international news and politics with friends and parents.

## Measure of Patriotism

Patriotism is a three-item additive index of feelings of love for country, pride in the land, and in being an American.

## Measure of Knowledge

Six items were used to measure general political knowledge and specific knowledge of the events of 9/11. The first type of knowledge, political knowledge, measures respondents' ability to identify the chief justice of the U.S. Supreme Court, the political party that controls the U.S. House of Representatives, and the leader of the Palestinians. The second type of knowledge, 9/11 knowledge, measures respondents' ability to identify the locations where the planes crashed on 9/11, the leader of al Qaeda, and the mayor of New York City during the 9/11 attacks.

## Measure of Emotions

Affect was measured in four areas: fear, anger, sadness, and suspicion. Each of these is a three-item additive index measuring emotions felt when reading or watching recent news coverage commemorating the anniversary of 9/11. Fearful is a three-item additive index of ten-point scales measured from "a little of this feeling" to "a lot of this feeling" of fearful, afraid, and sad. Angry is a three-item additive index of angry, irritated, and annoyed. Sad is a three-item additive index of sad, dreary, and dismal. Suspicious is a three-item additive index of suspicion, distrust, and caution.

## Measure of Dependent Variables

Two dependent variables of cognitive political attitudes were measured from the 2002 survey data. Support for investigating Arab college students is a ten-point scale (from "strongly disagree" to "strongly agree") measuring support for law-enforcement agencies to focus investigations specifically on college students who are Arab or of Middle Eastern descent to see if they are involved in potential terrorist activities (M = 4.2). Satisfaction with the war on terrorism is a ten-point scale (from "not at all satisfied" to "very satisfied") measuring support for the way the U.S. government is fighting the war on terrorism (M = 6.3). In addition, knowledge of U.S. involvement in the Middle East was measured from the 2003 survey data by five questions measuring respondents' ability to correctly identify the country of origin of the 9/11 terrorist hijackers and demonstrate knowledge of U.S. political allies and international affairs in the Middle East.

## POLITICAL ATTITUDES AT THE ONE-YEAR ANNIVERSARY OF 9/11

Results found that young adults who are more religious, indicate a strong interest in politics, and are politically conservative express greater support for the way the U.S. government is fighting the war on terrorism (table 3.1). There is no significant difference in support for the war on terrorism between males and females, or between younger and older college students. Young adults who paid a lot of attention to news coverage of the 9/11 anniversary and the war on terrorism also indicated support for the war on terrorism. They also discuss these events more than those who do not support the war on terrorism. In addition, supporters of the war on terrorism are highly patriotic. However, those expressing great support for the war have neither political knowledge nor knowledge of the events of 9/11. Instead, they tend to feel a wide range of strong emotions when reading or watching recent news coverage commemorating the anniversary of 9/11, expressing fear and sadness, as well as suspicion.

More male young adults than females agree that law-enforcement agencies should be specifically focusing their investigations on college students who are Arab or of Middle Eastern descent (table 3.1). Similar to those supporting the war on terrorism, those who support investigations of Arab students are more religious, indicate a strong interest in politics, and are politically conservative. Support for investigating Arab college students is also significantly correlated with communication measures: paying attention to media coverage of the anniversary of 9/11 and the war on terrorism, and discussing these events with parents and friends. However, students supporting such investigations pay less attention to the media than those who support

Table 3.1
Factors Correlated with Support for Investigating Arab College Students
and Satisfaction with the War on Terrorism

|  | Satisfaction with the War on Terrorism | Support for Investigating Arab College Students |
|---|---|---|
| Gender (male) | .07 | .11* |
| Age | .01 | .02 |
| Religiousness | .19** | .13** |
| Political interest | .15** | .14** |
| Ideology (conservative) | .31** | .24** |
| Attention to news of 9/11 and the war on terrorism | .31** | .17** |
| Discussion of 9/11 and the war on terrorism | .16** | .16** |
| Patriotism | .40** | .15** |
| Political knowledge | .02 | .09 |
| 9/11 knowledge | .03 | .01 |
| Fear | .12* | .06 |
| Anger | .05 | .19** |
| Sadness | .14** | .08 |
| Suspicion | .13** | .17** |

N = 532
* = p < .05
** = p < .01

the war (.17 vs. .31). While support for these types of investigations is correlated with patriotism (.15), this is less than half as strong as the patriotism of those who express satisfaction with the war on terrorism (.40). Like students who support the war on terrorism, those who support investigating Arab college students have neither political knowledge nor knowledge of the events of 9/11. Students who support investigating Arab students are suspicious, but unlike those who support the war on terrorism, neither fearful nor sad. The distinctive difference in emotions between the two political attitudes is that students expressing support for investigating Arab students are angry, the only emotional dimension that was not correlated with support for the war on terrorism.

## POLITICAL KNOWLEDGE AT THE TWO-YEAR ANNIVERSARY OF 9/11

On the days immediately surrounding the two-year anniversary of the 9/11 attacks, we asked 361 undergraduate students five questions about their knowledge of American involvement in the Middle East. Like the

2002 survey respondents, these were students taking an introductory class in communication, with a broad representation of all students from all the colleges at the university campus. Young people generally possess less political knowledge than other adults,[26,27] but one should also keep in mind that these undergraduates are supposed to represent the educational upper half of the young people in the state. One would therefore expect this subset of young people to be politically socialized and to demonstrate some basic knowledge of international politics.

Most students (87 percent) knew that Islam is the main religion in the Middle East, but only a minority of the students knew the answers to the other questions (table 3.2). Just less than half (49 percent) knew that Israel controls the area that the Palestinians consider to be their homeland. The conflict between the Israelis and the Palestinians is one major source for the hostility toward America in the region. However, that hostility is not because America controls the Palestinian homeland, but because of U.S. support for Israel. Four percent of the students appeared to have tried to put *a* and *b* together, concluding that the United States controls all controversial areas in the Middle East in which terrorists might be active. Only 30 percent of the students correctly listed Israel as America's closest ally in the Middle East. Some answered Saudi Arabia (which is not totally incorrect, as Saudi Arabia has long been a close ally of the United States), but a majority of the students either left the question blank or indicated countries like Iran or Pakistan.

Another major cause of controversy in the Middle East is U.S. oil dependency. Fewer than one-third (30 percent) of the students knew that Saudi Arabia exports more oil to America than any other country in the region (table 3.2). Once again, many students appeared to draw a direct link to America's involvement in Iraq. A majority of the students in the study (51 percent) stated that Iraq was the Middle East country exporting the most oil to the United States. A small percentage (8 percent) listed Kuwait, the country at the center of the war fought by the United States in 1990 and 1991.

The clearest example of how students tried to make sense of U.S. actions in the Middle East was found in the answers to what country most of the 9/11 terrorists came from. Nearly half (45 percent) of the students thought that they were from Afghanistan, while another 23 percent thought they were from Iraq (table 3.2). In other words, more than two-thirds of the students thought that terrorists came from the two Middle Eastern countries that the United States has invaded as a part of the "War on Terrorism." One student even answered that most of the hijackers came from Afghanistan, but traveled through Iraq on the way

Table 3.2
Undergraduate Students' Responses to Questions about
the United States and the Middle East

| Question | Answer | Percent of Those Responding |
|---|---|---|
| What is the most common religion in the Middle East? | Islam | 87* |
| | Wrong/other | 13 |
| The area that the Palestinians consider to be their homeland is now controlled by what country? | Israel | 49* |
| | United States | 4 |
| | Wrong/other | 47 |
| Which Middle Eastern country exports the most oil to the United States? | Iraq | 51 |
| | Saudi Arabia | 30* |
| | Kuwait | 8 |
| | Wrong/other | 11 |
| Which country is generally considered to be the United States's strongest ally in the Middle East? | Israel | 30* |
| | Wrong/other | 70 |
| From what country did a majority of the 9/11 hijackers, as well as Osama bin Laden, come from? | Afghanistan | 45 |
| | Iraq | 23 |
| | Saudi Arabia | 15* |
| | Wrong/other | 17 |

* Correct answer

to the United States. Only 15 percent of the students knew that the majority of the 9/11 hijackers came from Saudi Arabia.

## DISCUSSION

Walter Lippmann, one of America's most influential journalists and philosophers of the twentieth century, once said, "The best government will be the one which governs the least and requires, therefore, the least training and experience in the art of governing. The best education for democracy will be the one which trains, disciplines, and teaches the least" (p. 75).[28]

Lippmann represents a school of democratic thought that advocates limited political socialization. Lippmann even argued that too much cultivation into the political arena could have negative effects on democracy, since it could create an environment in which collective political decisions reach into the private sphere. Almond and Verba, in their classic analysis of western democracies, argue that the role of citizens in a democracy is one of "potentially active citizens," with the political elite doing most of the governing and the rest of the public playing a passive supportive role unless they find the governing elite unacceptable.[29]

Benjamin Barber[30] calls this a "weak democracy" and instead promotes what he calls a "strong democracy" where citizens play an active deliberating role in the political policy making.

The American public has traditionally played a passive role in politics, especially foreign affairs. The United States (other than Hawaii) has not been attacked by any foreign political group or government in almost 200 years. Historically, foreign affairs seldom had a strong, direct effect on the daily life of ordinary Americans; the threat of a possible nuclear war and the oil shortages of the 1970s had perhaps the most impact. As a result, there was little need for any political socialization regarding foreign affairs or conditions in foreign countries. A (silent) majority of the public, even during the dark days of the Vietnam War, followed the lead of the Oval Office and political and military leaders. Military conflicts and terrorist attacks that took place abroad gave Americans no real incentive to explore their contexts. Violence was generally too far away to have a major impact on Americans.

The terrorist attacks on 9/11 may have changed this situation. Foreign terrorists were suddenly killing civilian Americans in the middle of New York City, Washington, DC, and in the countryside of Pennsylvania. Foreign affairs were now more than distant considerations; they were suddenly real and affecting many aspects of the American life. However, a major problem was that the educational system had not prepared Americans for this new reality. Educational institutions in the 1950s and 1960s tried to prepare young Americans for nuclear attacks, but (thankfully) such attacks never happened. The 1995 Oklahoma City bombing introduced the American public to terrorism on U.S. soil, but the source of that act turned out to be domestic, rather then international. The international terrorists struck before the American educational system had addressed the question of how to understand and respond to international terrorism. Louise Cainkar, for example, describes how "years of Arab activists' efforts to find receptive hosts and funders for such events (education about Islam) suddenly bore fruit after 9/11, often sponsored by institutions that had closed their doors to Arabs in the past" (p. 224).[14]

Like our educational institutions, parents did not know how to handle the 9/11 attacks, since nothing like them had ever happened in the America that they knew. Therefore, the political socialization of youth and young adults regarding international terrorism was left to the media—which constitute an institution that tends to present spectacular and horrific stories. As Iyengar demonstrated in his research on episodic and thematic news coverage, the media generally pay little attention to the contextual elements that set the stage for these same stories of international terrorism.[11] Media were generally effective in describing the horror and emotions resulting from terrorism, but gave the public few opportunities for understanding the context of terrorism in the international arena.

This disconnect between media coverage and political understanding seems to be reflected in the results from our sample of young adults on the first anniversary of 9/11. When examining the factors correlated with satisfaction with the war on terrorism, the role of media seems to be important, although other factors are correlated as well, particularly patriotism and the emotions of fear, sadness, and suspicion. The item with the highest correlation with satisfaction with the war on terrorism is patriotism—more so than media exposure. This suggests that young adults' evaluation of the war on terrorism is based not on an assessment, informed by media coverage, of how the war is progressing, but on patriotic feelings such as love of country (or support for the troops), as well as conservative political ideology. It may be that for these young adults, the media's functions of surveillance and reporting the news are less important than a patriotic and political allegiance to the policies and actions of President George W. Bush. Moreover, their satisfaction with the war on terrorism is not connected to any political or 9/11 knowledge. For these young adults, the role of the media in their political socialization about the war on terrorism is subordinate to their patriotic and ideological feelings—the power of the heart rather than the mind. This may help to explain the correlation of other emotional feelings: fear, sadness, and suspicion.

A somewhat different picture emerges of young adults who support investigating Arab college students on campus. The students who support such investigations tend to use the media much less than those who support the war (.17 vs. .31). Significantly, they are also much less patriotic (.15 vs. .40), suggesting that such support may be based more on reasoned decision-making than ideology. Is their support for such investigations based on a clear understanding of the political events surrounding 9/11 and America's debate over civil liberties? It seems unlikely; there is no correlation between support for such investigations and political or 9/11 knowledge. Rather than cognitive decisions, it is again emotions that appear to be important in explaining such support. While young adults who are suspicious support both the war and investigations of Arab college students, only young adults who are angry (.19) support such investigations. Thus, support for investigating Arab college students appears to be related to anger over 9/11 attacks, rather than a careful consideration of how such investigations might affect civil liberties. Therefore, it seems that emotions play important roles in explaining these two political attitudes among young adults.

Of all the emotions[31] correlated with these political attitudes, we remain troubled by the role that anger plays in support for investigating Arab college students. These young adults express anger when reading news of 9/11 or watching television coverage of its anniversary, yet have little knowledge of the events of 9/11 and limited general political knowledge. If they have no knowledge of 9/11 or their political world, then what exactly is making them angry? The fact that anger is not associated with knowledge could be explained with Weiner's 1985 attribution theory. The first part of attribution theory implies that we often attribute our individual achievements or success to internal attributes—for example, we believe we did well on an exam because we are smart or clever, not because of the excellent teaching of our professor. The second part of attribution theory, however, argues that we attribute disappointment and failure to external attributions: We did poorly on the exam because there was no review sheet and the professor is terrible, not because of our failure to study. Anger is then directed toward those individuals who are thought to be responsible for our own failures—in this example, the bad professor.

Attribution theory suggests that young adults who are angry about the events of 9/11 may want to attribute responsibility for the terrorist attacks to the closest and most available target. That anger then manifests itself in their support for investigating Arab college students. Results indicated that these young adults also have little knowledge of the events of 9/11 and limited political knowledge. Of course, how can they understand the events of 9/11 in any broader context if they do not receive any information from mass media about America's role in the world?

In addition, these individuals may also see 9/11 as an isolated, "controllable" event caused solely by al Qaeda terrorists whose actions could have been prevented by stronger law enforcement and airport security. For these individuals the events of 9/11 are not connected to any systematic geopolitical or socioeconomic problems that exist in the Arab world and often manifest themselves in hatred of the United States. According to attribution theory,[31] when bad events occur individuals often attribute blame to external agents. For the events of 9/11 this blame would be directed toward individuals belonging to an "axis of evil"[32,33] who should have been prevented in the first place from getting on an airplane. In contrast, the systematic problems in the Arab world that feed hatred of the United States are hard to control and not easily solved. This lack of control would set up the essential condition for anger: someone else is to blame for a controllable event. These young adults therefore appear to be directing their anger at the closest and most available target—other college students who are Muslim or of Arab descent.

Zaller presents a picture of American politics in which citizens lack an interest in political affairs and instead trust that media will check on the political leaders.[34] Media, on the other hand, are primarily interested in stories that are easy to comprehend, and the primary interest of politicians seems not the content of ideas (which is generally left to the experts), but the framing and reception of the ideas. The end result of these roles is a situation in which no institution effectively checks on the politicians; media will only report on what is considered spectacular, and political leaders are "safe" as long as their communicated ideas are not regarded as spectacular in a negative way.

What this means in the context of the aftermath of 9/11 is that the American public generally will accept whatever political leaders decide as long as the communication from politicians does not create controversy. The public possesses relatively little knowledge about international events and conditions in foreign countries, but the events of 9/11 have shown that they now have more invested in international affairs. The public therefore may tend to demand actions from their political leaders without possessing the knowledge necessary to evaluate these actions.

In the fall of 2003, we were beginning to see the effects of this situation. President George W. Bush had led military invasions into both Afghanistan and Iraq, and large numbers of the American public believed that the 9/11 terrorists came from these two countries. This lack of knowledge enabled the Republican Party to run political ads criticizing their opponents for "attacking the president for attacking the terrorists." Many democratic presidential candidates took offense to these ads. General Wesley Clark, for instance, responded, saying, "I am not attacking the president because he is attacking terrorists. I'm attacking him because he's not attacking terrorists."[35]

This situation exemplifies the problems of political socialization in a new era of global politics in which international terrorism plays a major role. Yet many questions still remain about young adults and political socialization in this era: Is the best democracy still the one that requires the least education? Should members of the general public maintain a passive role in the political process, even if international events and foreign conditions clearly have an enormous impact on their lives? What do poll numbers that express the public's support for politicians and their foreign policies really mean when the public lacks fundamental knowledge about the situations that the policies are supposed to address? These questions must be addressed as we discuss the need for political socialization in the post-9/11 era. Henry Grioux, for example, argues that we are focusing too much attention on a physical war on terrorism that may end up creating more terrorists abroad, and at the same time we are failing to give our own students the knowledge necessary to effectively approach the challenges of 9/11.[36] We are not attempting to provide answers to all the questions above, but the events of 9/11 should at least motivate a comprehensive debate about the political socialization of American youth in a new era of international relations.

Future research in this area should examine two distinct areas. First, research should determine whether young adults' post-9/11 attitudes remain consistent, or change over time. How will continuing events in a newly liberated Iraq affect their attitudes and emotions? Will their anger, so evident in our sample, diminish over time or remain strong? As this cohort of young adults mature, will they understand the events of 9/11 differently? Will younger generations be affected by a legacy of 9/11, or will the attacks become something only experienced through their history books? Continuing research in political socialization within a post-9/11 framework will help to answer these questions.

Future research should also examine the concept of civic education and what it means to be a civically educated and politically literate citizen in a post-9/11 world. Researchers need to more closely scrutinize what types of knowledge—not only about the United States, but also about the rest of the world—young adults need in order to participate as active citizens in society. With limited international knowledge and a narrow global perspective, many young adults will continue to struggle to effectively participate in debates that increasingly are affected by worldwide events and conditions. Researchers must further study both formal and informal civic education to better understand what types of programs are most effective and useful for young adults. By continuing to analyze these important issues, we will be better able to help our young citizens understand the complexities of an ever-changing and increasingly complex post-9/11 world.

## NOTES

1. Schneider W. Political pulse—a survey in the Islamic world underscores the enormity of America's challenges. Natl J 2002;34:734–39.

2. Jennings MK, Niemi RG. Generations and politics. Princeton, NJ: Princeton University Press; 1981.

3. Mcleod JM, Eveland WP Jr, Horowitz EM. Learning to live in a democracy: the interdependence of family, schools, and media. Proceedings of the Association for Education in Journalism and Mass Communication, annual convention; 1995 Aug; Washington, DC.

4. Flanagan CA, Sherrod LR. Youth political development: an introduction. J Soc Issues 1998;54:447–56.

5. Horowitz EM. Political socialization in post-communist Poland: knowledge and attitudes of young adults. Proceedings of the Association for Education in Journalism and Mass Communication, International Communication Division, annual convention; 2001; Washington, DC.

6. Elder GH Jr. Children of the Great Depression: social change in life experience. Chicago: University of Chicago Press; 1974.

7. Macek P, Flanagan C, Gallay L, Kostron L, Botecheva L, Csapo B. Post-communist societies in times of transition: perceptions of change among adolescents in Central and Eastern Europe. J Soc Issues 1998;54:547–61.

8. Kantrowitz B, Naughton K. Generation 9/11. Newsweek 2001 Nov 12; 47–56.

9. Altheide DL. Format and symbol in television coverage of terrorism in the United States and Great Britain. Int Stud Q 1987;31:161–76.

10. Paletz D, Ayanian J, Fozzard P. Terrorism on television news: the IRA, the FALN, and the Red Brigades. In: Adams W, editor. Television coverage of international affairs. Norwood, NJ: Ablex; 1982.

11. Iyengar S. Is anyone responsible: how television frames political issues. Chicago: University of Chicago Press; 1991.

12. Eckstein J. When the terrorist is American: analyzing news frames of the September 11, 2001 attacks and the 1995 Oklahoma City bombing. Proceedings of the Association for Education in Journalism, Mass Communication and Society Division, annual convention; 2003; Kansas City, MO.

13. Hassan SD. Arabs, race, and the post-September 11 national security state. Middle East Rep 2002;224:16–21.

14. Cainkar L. No longer invisible: Arab and Muslim exclusion after September 11. Middle East Rep 2002;224:22–9.

15. ABC News. Survey data. As cited in American Public Opinion on the War on Terrorism. (November 1, 2002). (p. 69). Available from: www.aei.org/ps/psfront.htm. Accessed November 28, 2003.

16. Zogby. (2002). Survey data. As cited in American public opinion on the war on terrorism. November 1, 2002. p. 70. Available from: www.aei.org/ps/psfront.htm. Accessed November 28, 2003.

17. Pew Research Center. (2000–2001). Survey data. As cited in American Public Opinion on the War on Terrorism. (November 1, 2002). (p. 69). Available from: www.aei.org/ps/psfront.htm. Accessed November 28, 2003.

18. Moore K. A part of US or apart from US? Post-September 11 attitudes towards Muslims and civil liberties. Middle East Rep 2002;224:32–5.

19. Ahmad M. Homeland insecurities: racial violence the day after September 11. Soc Text 2002;20:101–15.

20. Terkel S. Race: how Blacks and Whites think and feel about the American obsession. New York: Anchor; 1993.

21. Pettigrew TF. Peoples under threat: Americans, Arabs, and Israelis. Peace Conflict J Peace Psychol 2003;9:69–90.

22. Errante A. Where in the world do children learn "bloody revenge"? Cults of terror and counter-terror and the implication for child socialization. Globalisation Soc Educ 2003;1:131–52.

23. Wikan U. "My son—a terrorist?" (he was such a gentle boy). Anthropological Q 2002;75:117–28.

24. James C. TV searches for distinction as September 11 programs begin. NY Times 2002 Sep 3.

25. James C. Television's special day of pain and comfort. NY Times 2002 Sep 6.

26. Carpini MX. Gen.com: youth, civic engagement, and the new information environment. Pol Commun 2000;17:341–9.

27. McDevitt M, Chaffee S. Closing gaps in political communication and knowledge. Commun Res 2000;27:259–92.

28. Lippmann W. The public philosophy. 3rd ed. London: Transaction; 1995.

29. Almond GA, Verba S. The civic culture: political attitudes and democracy in five nations. Princeton, NJ: Princeton University Press; 1963.

30. Barber BA. Passion for democracy. American essays. Princeton, NJ: Princeton University Press; 1998.

31. Heider F. The psychology of interpersonal relations. New York: John Wiley; 1958.

32. Bennis P. Before and after: U.S. foreign policy and the September 11th crisis. New York: Olive Branch Books; 2003.

33. Pena CV. Axis of evil: threat or chimera? Mediterr Q 2002;13(3):40–57.

34. Zaller JR. The nature and origins of mass opinion. Cambridge, UK: Cambridge University Press; 1991.

35. Democrats pound GOP campaign ad; they say it questions patriotism of war critics. CNN online 2003 November 23. Available from: www.cnn.com.

36. Giroux HA. The abandoned generation. democracy beyond the culture of fear. New York: Palgrave Macmillan; 2003.

# 4 The Intersection of Terrorism, Interpersonal Communication, and Health

*Jennifer A. H. Becker and Sharlene Thompson*

The terrorist attacks of September 11, 2001, affected not only the intended targets, but also our nation and world. The impact of this terrorist event was forceful and widespread, as the unfolding horror was broadcast live into living rooms, coffee shops, offices, and classrooms. Hoffner, Fujioka, Ibrahim, and Ye observe, "The attacks caused massive destruction and loss of human life within a few hours. Many Americans felt personally involved because they had relatives, friends, or acquaintances who were in New York or Washington DC, or on an airplane during the time of the attacks" (p. 229).[1] The immediate impacts of this event were highly visible, from families losing loved ones, to tightened security, and reconstruction of buildings. Beyond these visible, immediate impacts, the terrorist attacks have yielded some largely unnoticed, yet formidable effects, such as those on relationships and psychosocial health. As Milliken, Leavitt, Murdock, Orman, Ritchie, and Hoge argue, "These longer term social and psychological effects of chemical or biological attack, real or suspected, [are] as damaging as the acute effects and possibly more so" (p. 53).[2] Emerging research findings support this claim. For example, in interviews with 1,009 New Yorkers, DeLisi and others found that severe symptoms due to the attacks were less than expected.[3] However, DeLisi and others and other researchers have yet to systematically theorize about and empirically investigate the less visible—yet important—impacts of these attacks on victims' interpersonal relationships and psychosocial health.

## TERRORISM DEFINED

Terrorism is a socially constructed phenomenon. The meanings of terrorism are socially and culturally situated, such that various people perceive it differently. Terrorism carries a distinct communicative element, as it communicates messages rich with meaning to large sets of audiences.[4] Thus, one definition of terrorism is violence toward a large group of people intended not only to physically harm victims but to further victimize through fear, anxiety, and uneasiness. Tuman further explains that "terror succeeds because it creates a sense of fear—a fear and dread of the unknown" (p. xvii).[4]

Terrorism is achieved through threat- and violence-based messages to multiple target audiences, making communication inherent in the act of terrorism.[4] One target audience is the object of the violence, and other audiences may be the targets of the message (e.g., the targets of influence). The communication processes contextualized by acts of terrorism are highly transactional among multiple parties. Tuman states, "These audiences in turn communicate with one another, individually, and/or collectively, directly and indirectly, as part of the greater loop that can also feed back to the terrorist" (p. 22).[4] He argues that terrorism essentially is persuasion, with the terrorist's goal being to persuade target audience(s) that they should be fearful, reconsider an issue, or take uncharacteristic action.

In looking at the impact of the terrorist attacks of September 11, 2001, much research has focused at the levels of society and the individual psyche. Previous research has conceptualized both the society and the individual person as systems, with respective groups of elements that interact and function together for the whole. Clearly, these two systems have been impacted by terrorism. Terrorism has changed the way societies operate and the way individuals think and feel. However, terrorist attacks and their aftermath also appear to have a profound influence on relational communication and psychosocial health. Simply put, terrorism affects the way individuals talk with their families and friends and how they develop relationships with others who were also victimized.[5] Therefore, to fully understand the effects of terrorism, we must consider the societal, individual, *and* relational systems, which are components of a larger communication system.[6] To achieve this objective, an explanation of General Systems Theory (GST) is in order.

## A SYSTEMS APPROACH TO UNDERSTANDING TERRORISM

Why utilize a systems approach to understanding terrorism? A systems approach clarifies the relationships between components in a system. In order to understand a system, its components must be defined, and the interplay and hierarchy among these components explicated. Given the societal, individual, and relational levels of communication, a systems approach appears to be well suited for capturing and integrating the multifaceted ways in which terrorism affects communication.

GST is a theoretical framework that was formalized by Bertalanffy.[7] Essentially, GST conceives of a given phenomenon as both a whole and interrelated parts. A system is a set of interactive, interdependent elements that function for the overall objective of the whole.[6] A system can be a tangible entity, such as a society, with groups such as families, businesses, and institutions; or it can be perceptible yet nonphysical, such as a taxonomy of communication processes and outcomes. Systems are hierarchically ordered, with each larger system influencing the smaller components (i.e., subsystems) they subsume.[8] Thus, the societal system encapsulates the relational system, which further encompasses the individual system.

A system is defined by a set of elements that typically interact with each other regularly and in patterned ways over time. Thus, when an event affects one subsystem, a chain reaction may occur as that subsystem influences, and is in turn influenced by, other subsystems. For example, when terrorism affects the individual, the altered individual then changes subsequent interactions and functioning of relationships, and even the larger society. The characteristics of the elements and the patterns of interactions between them define the quality of the interaction and functioning. Unfortunately, sometimes these characteristics and patterns draw out less adaptive, dysfunctional aspects of elements (e.g., psychosocial health problems such as anxiety disorders).

Systems are defined by their boundaries, the regions at their outside edges that act as filters for inputs and outputs.[6] Boundaries can be physical or symbolic. For example, the walls and doors of a building may define the physical boundaries of a couple's home, but the oft-unspoken rules of how communication occurs (e.g., who talks to whom, how, when, and where) define the symbolic boundaries of the relational system. Such relational dyads manage their communication boundaries through self-disclosure.[9] Specifically, couples manage personal information through rules, and through the intersection of boundary structures, which are characterized by the permeability of the boundaries, levels of privacy, and other factors. Given their varied rules and boundary structures, some dyads self-disclose openly and without inhibition, whereas others display well-guarded privacy. Boundaries define systems from the environments in which they are embedded, which are characterized by physical, spatial, temporal, and symbolic conditions.

GST is appropriate for studying human communication events.[6] System thinking accounts for the complexity of human communication, given that there is no absolute beginning or end to communication, and multiple antecedents are also consequences. GST is especially well suited for theorizing about communication as it relates to terrorism because it takes into account the interactive relationships between and among systems, allowing for greater integration of multiple parts and more accurate representation of real-life processes and outcomes.

Systems approaches to studying human phenomena, including communication, developed in large part as a reaction against perceived limitations of the linear-causal model.[10] In reality, human communication is rarely unidirectional. As an example, terrorists almost always desire some type of response from their targets, whether directly from individual or governmental targets, or indirectly through public response.[4] Most communication—including communication stimulated by terrorist attacks—allows for feedback, which stimulates further communication. Thus, GST recognizes that patterns of influence between systems are frequently bidirectional.

Given the focus of previous research on individual and societal systems as they relate to terrorism, perhaps it is not surprising that comparatively little study has been advanced on the intermediary relational system within the context of terrorism. A systems approach bolsters the focus on the relational system, or communication between at least two communicators who orient toward each other and yield meaningful influence on one another's behavior, usually in face-to-face interaction.[11]

## RATIONALE

Indeed, there is an appalling absence of scholarly research examining how terrorism is linked to interpersonal communication, particularly among those who are not terrorists but the sufferers of terrorism. There are two primary types of victims of terrorism—those who are the targets of violence, against whom harm and death are plotted; and those who are targets of influence, who are not specifically besieged, yet are traumatized to varying degrees. Some research exists on targets of violence (e.g., Milliken et al.[2]), but comparably less research has been produced on targets of influence. There is some research on how parents should communicate about terrorism to their children (e.g., Cohen[12]), yet relatively little scientific advancement on how adults communicate with each other in light of terrorist events.

This is not to say that scholars fail to recognize the existence of the social dimension of terrorism. Instead, they tend to focus on psychosocial processes and effects at a broad, conceptual level (cf. Moghaddam & Marsella[13]), as opposed to more intimate, fine-grained analyses of actual interchanges between people. Most scholars imply that a sense of belongingness and community is beneficial to mitigating the harm of terrorism and that a holistic perspective aids in our understanding of responses to terrorism (cf. Danieli, Engdahl, & Schlenger[14]), yet relatively few have examined the actual processes and effects that occur as two people engage in meaningful communication in response to terrorism.

However, people outside of academe have recognized and called for satisfaction of the intense need for communicating with family, friends, colleagues, and close others. For example, following the September 11, 2001, attacks, the Compassion Center and service centers provided social and other forms of support to people in need (Levant, Barbanel, & DeLeon[15]). Advertisements in New York subways bore messages such as "Heroes talk" and "Speaking to family and friends can be helpful."[15] Even governmental leaders were called upon to communicate, when Congressman Jim McDermott, a psychiatrist, advised his colleagues to go home to their constituencies and discuss the events and consequences of terrorism.[16]

Clearly, terrorism disrupts the social order. It can debilitate victims' thoughts and emotions with anxiety, fear, uncertainty, and lack of predictability.[17] It is not surprising then, that terrorism appears to have unique impacts on interpersonal communication.

## THE IMPACTS OF TERRORISM ON INTERPERSONAL COMMUNICATION

Following September 11, 2001, people seemed especially motivated to communicate with others. Mehl and Pennebaker captured snippets of 11 participants' conversations at regular intervals for 10 days from September 11, 2001.[18] They found a spike in the number of phone calls on September 11 and 12, with most of the calls pertaining to the attacks. Although participants initially interacted with groups of people and talked on the telephone on September 11 and 12, over the next eight days, there was a significant increase in the relative amount of time spent with one person. Although findings from the study are exploratory, they seem to reveal a tendency to engage in face-to-face interpersonal communication following terrorism.[18]

When individuals have been traumatized by terrorism, they often have strong preferences for whom they will communicate with about their experiences and views. Those who have been affected firsthand often seek out others with similar experiences.[2] Others rely on intimates, family, and friends to self-disclose and receive support. By turning to close others, individuals can achieve an array of basic and interpersonal needs. Supportive interpersonal communication can enhance feelings of security and safety, in part because it connects individuals to a larger social, ideological, political, or religious group.[19]

Individuals who have been traumatized by terrorism (as well as individuals reaching out to others who have been traumatized) sometimes perform simple, yet out-of-the-ordinary acts of kindness. Following a terrorist event, life loses its routine, its feeling of ordinariness, and its sense of normalcy. Even mundane daily practices such as riding a train home are different, and such differences appear to alert people to the humanity of others and lead them to communicate in atypical ways. Psychologist Laura Barbanel recounts, "On a ride home on a crowded 'F' train, the only one going to Brooklyn in those first days [following September 11, 2001], I saw people make room for one another and give directions to passengers who were unfamiliar with this subway line with an attitude of concern rarely demonstrated in the city" (p. 273).[15] Communication among strangers on a train is typically aloof and impersonal communication—anything but interpersonal—yet following a terrorism event, strangers may swiftly become intimates. Terrorism not only changes individuals' perceptions, thoughts, and emotions, but also how they relate to others.

Supportive interpersonal communication can facilitate sense-making, thereby allowing individuals to understand and transform the meaning and significance of a terrorist event. For example, Barbanel recounts how she counseled a young woman who had defied security guards' instructions to remain in the World Trade Center after the attacks. The woman escaped but was unable to resume activities and showed symptoms of acute stress reaction. Barbanel narrates, "I pointed out her resourcefulness in saving herself. She stared at me in silence and after a moment said, 'Thank you.' This simple recognition of her own active engagement in her flight to safety diminished her sense of helplessness and helped to reduce her symptoms."[15] By communicating with Barbanel in an open and supportive way, the woman was able to constructively reinterpret her experience and regain psychosocial health.

The need to make sense of one's experiences seems to reflect an innate drive. Niederhoffer and Pennebaker suggest that when individuals experience trauma, the world is no longer as they once knew it, and they feel disconnected from their world.[20] Trauma, including trauma derived from terrorism, motivates victims to find meaning in the traumatic event and to restore a sense of order, control, and predictability. An essential step to regaining connection to the social world is self-disclosure through talking or writing. As Barbanel's story exemplifies, the meaningful (co-)construction of one's account can yield psychosocial health benefits.

The benefits of disclosure about traumatic events appear to be achieved through three interrelated processes.[20,21] The first pertains to inhibition of thoughts and feelings about a traumatic event. Inhibition poses long-term, low-level stress to the autonomic and central nervous systems, a condition that diminishes health. Individuals who inhibit expression of traumatic events are at increased risk for major and minor health problems. In contrast, expression of thoughts and feelings reduces stress, which improves health. The second process pertains to sense-making. Individuals who engage in verbal expression appear to experience cognitive changes that facilitate reasoning and insight, as compared to individuals who engage in nonverbal expression (e.g., exercise). The cognitive changes associated with verbal expression are linked to improved psychosocial health. The third process concerns the edification of social support networks. Maintaining and developing supportive interpersonal relationships enhances feelings of connection to one's social world—connections that may become vulnerable following an act of terrorism.

Although disclosure provides long-term benefits to psychosocial health, individuals who communicate their troubled thoughts and feelings are likely to experience distress as they disclose them.[20] Nevertheless, people seem driven to disclose very intense, negative thoughts and feelings regarding traumatic events.

Of course, individuals have varying abilities to verbally communicate the complexity of their trauma.[2] Some individuals may not be conscious of the psychological impacts of terrorism. Some remnants of the terrorist attack may reside in implicit memory, rather than in explicit memory, which prohibits reflection.[22] Lack of conscious awareness can obstruct individuals' capacity to engage in interpersonal communication, particularly about the trauma. Other individuals are naturally reticent or may feel restricted by cultural norms that thwart self-disclosure about traumatic experiences.

## Maintaining Trauma through Communication

Of course, not all interpersonal communication is beneficial. Communication may serve to increase or extend a victim's distress and prevent the victim from resuming normal functioning. For example, repeatedly narrating one's experiences—and hence "reliving" the events of a terrorist attack—may be detrimental, depending on whether the self-disclosure is therapeutic.[22]

The need to communicate with others following terrorism can be likened to a magnetic pull, drawing victims together as they share their thoughts and feelings. During this self-disclosure process, individuals may experience emotional contagion, an affective process that involves an emotional response parallel to another person's emotions.[23] Following acts of terrorism, certain sentiments commonly are shared and appear to be "contagious."[17] For example, Kulic narrates how "Paul," a member of a support group he facilitated, was especially angry and "spread" his anger to other members of the group. "Paul served as the catalyst and release valve for other members' own rage" (p. 197),[24] Kulic says, in describing the apparent emotional contagion that occurred in the group setting. Thus, interpersonal communication following terrorism may provoke and sustain certain emotions, although communication that is therapeutic may transform and channel emotions into healthy outlets and facilitate improved psychosocial health.

Those who engage in "too much" interpersonal communication about traumatic events risk negative consequences. For example, trauma workers (including but not limited to therapists, emergency-response workers, health and caregiving professionals, and even lawyers) who have extensive interaction with victims of terrorism are particularly vulnerable to emotional contagion. Extensive emotional contagion is associated with compassion fatigue, also known as secondary traumatic stress disorder (STSD), which is the equivalent of post-traumatic stress disorder (PTSD).[25] Compassion fatigue is a "cost of caring" and communicating with those in need.[25]

## Overcoming Terror through Communication

Terrorism is probably the most frightening for targets of violence and their immediate contacts. The trauma of terrorism may manifest itself in behavioral health problems, which can be addressed, in part, by comprehensive outreach, support, and care systems. For example, following September 11, 2002, a plan called "Operation Solace" was implemented to address behavioral health problems anticipated to occur primarily among Pentagon employees located in the national capitol region affected by the terrorist attack.[2] The plan called for behavioral health care upon request, "therapy by walking around" to each office and desk in the workplace, and telephone contact. Given that the terrorist attacks occurred in a work context for Pentagon employees, Operation Solace was designed to address issues within the very context in which they originated. In this way, the program may have restricted the effects of terrorism to the work environment and may have mitigated negative effects on workers' relationships with family and friends. Additionally, Milliken and others suggest the relational system of workers' lives may have been less stressed and better able to buffer the effects of terrorism on other aspects of workers' lives.

An advantage of developing and implementing a proactive plan to address behavioral health issues is that problems can be alleviated before they mushroom into more perilous predicaments. The trauma following events such as September 11, 2001, was life changing, yielding influence on every aspect of people's lives and relationships. Unfortunately, as Sheehy observes, "the tendency is for people accustomed to being healthy and highly functioning to wait, following a severe trauma, until their marriages are falling apart, their jobs are in peril, or they can barely manage to get dressed in the morning, before they seek professional help" (p. 329).[26] Through communication campaigns such as Operation Solace, individuals can overcome obstacles to regain psychosocial health.

## Relational Closeness

Events of great magnitude, such as the September 11, 2001, attacks and the Oklahoma City bombing, often trigger people to investigate and reprioritize their values and then to strategize plans to reify these values in their daily activities.[2] People sometimes comment on "finding the good in evil" in their quest to finder a deeper, positive meaning and to reframe the terror they have witnessed. Often, people vow to put their loved ones first in their lives. Thus, terrorism can motivate individuals to "pull together" and to enhance relational closeness.

Relational closeness can also be increased unwittingly, as the result of "pulling together" in time of need. Identifying with a larger familial, work, or community group can promote pro-social behaviors that enhance feelings of care, concern, and connection. The processes of relationship building also influence the larger societal systems. Much of the news coverage following September 11, 2001, focused on how this terrorist event brought people together and how this was a positive outcome, particularly for New Yorkers. Fifty-seven percent of Americans and 59 percent of New Yorkers believe that the terrorist attacks and outcomes of September 11, 2001, have brought people closer together.[27] In this way, terrorism can facilitate long-lasting cohesion that aids in the healing process.

## THE IMPACTS OF TERRORISM ON PSYCHOSOCIAL HEALTH

Crises such as terrorist attacks are characterized by uncertainty and intense emotional responses.[28] After a terrorist event, people experience emotions such as shock, grief, anxiety, and fear for their mortality and of an uncertain future. They come together and express these emotions to close relational partners and in some circumstances, even to strangers. Not surprisingly, terrorism disrupts communication practices at the individual, relational, and societal levels, which are closely related to psychosocial health.

As scholars have begun to study the interrelationships between the physical, mental, and social domains of the biopsychosocial model of health,[29] they have recognized that some mental-health problems are closely linked to distressed relationships and troubled interpersonal communication in general.[30] Such mental health problems are better characterized as psychosocial problems, a distinction that emphasizes the importance of interpersonal communication and socialization as contributing factors to the psychopathology. Psychosocial problems include PTSD, major depressive disorder, bipolar disorder, social anxiety disorders, loneliness, personality disorders, somatoform disorders, and addictions to drugs and alcohol.[30] Individuals affected by these psychosocial problems communicate more negatively and less effectively, which may further damage interpersonal processes and relationships. Unfortunately, negative interactions with others may, in turn, diminish psychosocial health.

The terrorist attacks of September 11, 2001, appear to have led to several different psychosocial problems, including anxiety, depression, and PTSD,[31] as well as somatoform disorders.[32] After terrorist attacks, individuals may come to hospitals with medically unexplained physical symptoms, and psychological stress may exacerbate existing psychological and physical conditions.[32] Susser, Herman, and Aaron write, "The psychological damage caused by the attacks of September 11 mirrored the physical destruction and showed that protecting the public's mental health must be a component of the national defense" (p. 1).[33]

## Factors That Diminish Psychosocial Health

Given that a main objective of terrorists is to inflict terror to achieve political, religious, or financial goals, terrorism often influences the psychosocial health of its targets of violence, targets of influence, and the larger population.[31] Mental health problems were pronounced among individuals who were exposed to the September 11, 2001, attacks, particularly immediately afterward.[1] Such individuals were more upset and had more intense feelings of emotional distress compared to those who learned of the attacks after some time had passed. There appear to be sex differences in emotional distress, such that women were more upset, sad, and fearful, whereas men expressed more anger. Additionally, there is an association between emotion and diffusion of information, such that the stronger a person's emotion, the more likely they are to interpersonally diffuse information as a coping mechanism. Thus, emotional responses at the individual level seem connected to the need to communicate with relational partners to manage distress. Thus, in order to understand psychosocial health, we must consider multiple elements of the larger system.

Brown, Bocarena, and Basil have also examined the diffusion of information after September 11, 2001.[34] They focused on information from the media, which can be considered an element of the societal system. Brown and others found that the visual information presented on television (as compared to nonvisual media and interpersonal interactions) has the greatest impact on individuals' views, beliefs, and emotions about the terrorist attacks of September 11, 2001. Further, Ahern and others investigated the relationship between psychosocial health and viewing frequency of images of people jumping and/or falling from the twin towers of the World Trade Center in New York City.[35] Viewing frequency of negative images is strongly related to PTSD and depression,[35,36] a finding suggesting that heavy viewing of traumatic events (such as watching people plummet to their death) can lead to psychopathology. Viewing television coverage of September 11, 2001, appears to heighten individuals' emotional involvement, which is related to a stronger need for interpersonal connections.[28] Increased social support and coviewing of television are recommended as coping strategies to improve psychosocial health.

Why have some people experienced more emotional distress following September 11, 2001? One factor appears to be geographical proximity to the locations of terrorist attacks. Schlenger and others report a direct relationship between proximity to New York City and PTSD symptoms following September 11, 2001.[37] However, even university students 600 miles from New York City showed PTSD symptoms and depression, with women disproportionately affected.[38] Additionally, people who were socially and psychologically closer to primary victims (e.g., those who died) reported more emotional distress.[39] The relapse rate for recovering alcoholics increased dramatically following September 11, 2001.[40] Cardenas and others, also found increases in drug and alcohol use.[38] Finally, those who were highly educated and married reported lower levels of PTSD symptoms. Married individuals generally have more social support, which further suggests that interpersonal relationships may buffer the trauma of terrorism.

There are specific predictors of PTSD symptoms among victims of terror. Tucker, Pfefferbaum, Nixon, and Dickson examined what factors lead to PTSD symptoms for Oklahoma City–bombing survivors and victims six months after the bombing.[41] Findings indicated that injury, feeling nervous or afraid, and reporting that counseling helped were highly associated with PTSD symptoms.

### Improving Psychosocial Health through Social Support

Social support is central to the recovery and healing processes following trauma.[24] Social support essentially is achieved through transactional communication, with individuals giving and receiving support through interpersonal communication.[42] A vast body of evidence has demonstrated that social support affects mental and physical well-being. Conversations about stresses (ranging from minor daily hassles to life-changing events such as terrorism) "can help or hinder individual efforts at managing everyday stresses and health crises."[42] Enacted support, which refers to what dyads do and/or say to help one another negotiate difficult situations and/or stresses, may mediate the potential for PTSD and depression. For example, the participants who were married in the Cardenas and others study appear to have benefited from increased enacted support through the co-viewing of television coverage of terrorist attacks.[38]

Although social support is beneficial, some targets of terrorism tend to isolate themselves.[43] Indeed, a ruminative, passive coping style may prolong depression,[44] which suggests that victims who segregate themselves and repeatedly mull over the causes, meanings, and consequences of their depressive symptoms are at risk for deteriorating psychosocial health. In contrast, a problem-solving, active coping style is directly associated with greater satisfaction with health care and less substance abuse.[45] Adults who are securely attached to their partners appear to be more likely to seek social support and thus have more flexible and adaptive ways of coping with stress.[46] Social support is both a protective factor that buffers incurred stress and a means to enhance coping and improve psychosocial health.

Emotional distress appears to mediate the relationship between perceived social support and healthy outcomes for victims of terrorism. Wentzel and McNamara found that emotional distress was a mediator between perceived support from peers and prosocial outcomes for sixth graders, such that those who are more accepted by peers have less distress and thus more prosocial behaviors.[47] Victims of terror who perceive and have strong social support may have less emotional distress, and, therefore, have healthier outcomes.

### Improving Psychosocial Health through Self-Disclosure

A specific activity of social support is self-disclosure through oral or written communication to another person. Pennebaker and his colleagues have amassed a considerable body of evidence supporting the multifaceted health benefits of self-disclosure.[21] Compared to individuals who disclose about superficial topics, individuals who disclose about traumatic experiences show significant drops in physician visits, increased immune functioning, improved mood, and behavioral changes such as improved grades among students, lower absenteeism among university personnel, and other improvements. These benefits have been found consistently among various populations.

Although the simple act of self-disclosure about a traumatic event appears to provide some benefit, greater improvements are found to the degree that individuals use more positive-emotion words and a moderate amount of negative-emotion words.[20] Words that suggest causal inferences (e.g., because, reason) and insight (e.g., realize, understand) are predictive of the greatest improvements, presumably because they are indicative of sense-making.[22]

### IMPLICATIONS

The immediate and visible effects of terrorism are devastating and inflict large-scale pain and suffering. However, scholars must be cautious to avoid narrowly focusing on these immediate, outward, and highly visible effects, at the expense of more long-term, inward, and subtle, yet significant effects. As has been shown, terrorism influences interpersonal relationships and psychosocial health.

Although previous theory and research on terrorism has privileged the societal and individual systems, this chapter highlights the relational system, or the system that encompasses two individuals who orient toward each other and yield mutual influence. An individual's psychosocial health is intimately related to his or her interpersonal communication and relationships, which like the societal and individual systems, can be shaken by acts of terrorism. Future terrorism researchers would be well advised to employ the systems metaphor, particularly in exploring relationships between the relational and societal systems and subsystems. Additionally, future research on how relational dyads manage their communication boundaries of self-disclosure following terrorism would be enlightening and useful for practitioners and scholars.

As discussed, the effects of terrorism extend to targets of violence and targets of influence, both of which can suffer trauma. These individuals are susceptible to PTSD and other psychosocial health problems. As they disclose their experiences to others, emotional contagion may occur, and excessive emotional contagion may lead to secondary traumatic stress disorder among trauma workers and even family and friends of victims.[25]

Of course, interpersonal communication produces positive benefits for many individuals affected by terrorism. Supportive interpersonal communication can enhance feelings of security and comfort and facilitate the sense-making process. Targets of terrorism are well served by communication with close others that "reconnects" them to their social world and restores a sense of predictability.[20] Because self-disclosure is associated with a number of health benefits, targets of terrorism should communicate as many positive emotions as possible, a moderate amount of negative emotions, and inferences and insights that allow for meaningful construction and closure of the traumatic event. However, individuals dealing with psychosocial health problems should observe the advice of their health care providers.

Following the terrorist attacks of September 11, 2001, many individuals have been diagnosed with psychosocial problems such anxiety, depression, and PTSD,[31] as well as somatoform disorders.[32] Individuals affected by these psychosocial problems communicate more negatively and less effectively, which may lead to the deterioration or termination of interpersonal relationships. Unfortunately, negative interactions with others may, in turn, diminish psychosocial health. Psychosocial health problems were more pronounced among those who were exposed to the attacks as they occurred[1] and those who viewed images of people jumping and/or falling to their death.[35] Factors associated with heightened emotional distress include geographical proximity to the locations of the attacks,[37,38] social and psychological closeness to primary victims,[39] previous addiction to drugs and/or alcohol,[40] lower education levels, and being unmarried. PTSD symptoms were associated with injury, feeling nervous or afraid, and reporting that counseling helped.[41]

Social support, which is enacted through communication, is central to the recovery and healing processes following trauma.[24] Research on social support has consistently documented positive effects on physical and psychosocial health. Compared to those with a problem-solving, active coping style, individuals with a ruminative, passive coping style are at greater risk for deteriorated health. Practitioners should encourage clients to engage in active problem solving and to reach out to their social support network to buffer stress and enhance health.

Thus, the relational system is profoundly impacted by terrorism, although these impacts often are less immediate and visible. An examination of how terrorism affects the relational system and psychosocial health, put simply, reveals that the way we relate to others affects our health, and vice versa. These simple conclusions are consistent with the biopsychosocial model,[29] yet not nearly as profound as the actual processes and outcomes, as played out in the lives of millions affected by the trauma of terrorism.

## NOTES

1. Hoffner C, Fujioka Y, Ibrahimm A, Ye J. Emotion and coping with terror. In: Greenberg BS, editor. Communication and terrorism: public and media responses to 9/11. Creskill, NJ: Hampton Press; 2002. p. 229–44.

2. Milliken CS, Leavitt WT, Murdock P, Orman DT, Ritchie EC, Hoge CW. Principles guiding implementation of the Operational Solace plan: "pieces of PIES," therapy by walking around, and care management. Mil Med [Suppl 9] 2002;167:48–57.

3. DeLisi LE, Maurizio A, Yost M, Papparozzi CF, Fulchino C, Katz CL, et al. A survey of New Yorkers after the Sept. 11, 2001, terrorist attacks. Am J Psychiatry 2003;160:780–3.

4. Tuman JS. Communicating terror: the rhetorical dimensions of terrorism. Thousand Oaks, CA: Sage; 2003.

5. Cox GR. Surviving terrorism, international and personal. Illn Crisis Loss 2001;9:272–83.

6. Ruben BD. General system theory: an approach to human communication. In: Budd R, Ruben B, editors. Approaches to human communication. Rochelle Park, NJ: Hayden Books; 1972. p. 120–44.

7. Bertalanffy L von. An outline of general systems theory. Br J Philos Sci 1950;1:134–65.

8. Miller K. Organizational communication: approaches and processes. Belmont, CA: Wadsworth; 1999.

9. Petronio S. The boundaries of privacy: praxis of everyday life. In: Petronio S, editor. Balancing the secrets of private disclosures. Mahwah, NJ: Lawrence Erlbaum; 2000. p. 37–49.

10. Polkinghorne D. Methodology for the human sciences: systems of inquiry. Albany, NY: State University of New York Press; 1983.

11. Knapp ML, Daly JA, Albada KF, Miller GR. Background and current trends in the study of interpersonal communication. In: Knapp ML, Daly JA, editors. Handbook of interpersonal communication. 3rd ed. Thousand Oaks, CA: Sage; 2002. p. 3–20.

12. Cohen JA. Practice parameters for the assessment and treatment of children and adolescents with post-traumatic stress disorder. J Am Acad Child Adolesc Psychiatry [Suppl] 1998;37(10):4S–26S.

13. Moghaddam FM, Marsella AJ. Introduction. In: Moghaddam FM, Marsella AJ, editors. Understanding terrorism: psychosocial roots, consequences, and interventions. Washington, DC: American Psychological Association; 2004. p. 3–7.

14. Danieli Y, Engdahl B, Schlenger WE. The psychological aftermath of terrorism. In: Moghaddam FM, Marsella AJ, editors. Understanding terrorism: psychosocial roots, consequences, and interventions. Washington, DC: American Psychological Association; 2004. p. 223–46.

15. Levant RF, Barbanel L, DeLeon PH. Psychology's response to terrorism. In: Moghaddam FM, Marsella AJ, editors. Understanding terrorism: psychosocial roots, consequences, and interventions. Washington, DC: American Psychological Association; 2004. p. 265–82.

16. The psychiatrist in the House feels the nation's trauma. NY Times 2001 October 1;Sect. A:16.

17. Weigert AJ. Terrorism, identity, and public order: a perspective from Goffman. Identity: Int J Theory Res 2003;3:93–113.

18. Mehl MR, Pennebaker JW. The social dynamics of a cultural upheaval: social interactions surrounding September 11, 2001. Psychol Sci 2003;14:579–85.

19. Staub E. Understanding and responding to group violence: genocide, mass killing, and terrorism. In: Moghaddam FM, Marsella AJ, editors. Understanding terrorism: psychosocial roots, consequences, and interventions. Washington, DC: American Psychological Association; 2004. p. 151–68.

20. Niederhoffer KG, Pennebaker JW. Sharing one's story: on the benefits of writing or talking about emotional experience. In: Snyder CR, Lopez SJ, editors. Handbook of positive psychology. London: Oxford University; 2002. p. 573–83.

21. Pennebaker JW. Writing about emotional experiences as a therapeutic process. Psychol Sci 1997;8:162–6.

22. Siegel DJ. Memory, trauma, and psychotherapy: a cognitive science view. J Psychother Prac Res 1995;4:93–112.

23. Miller KI, Stiff JB, Ellis BH. Communication and empathy as precursors to burnout among human service workers. Commun Monogr 1988;55:250–65.

24. Kulic KR. An account of group work with family members of 9/11. J Spec Group Work 2003;28:195–8.

25. Figley CR. Compassion fatigue as secondary traumatic stress disorder: an overview. In: Figley CR, editor. Compassion fatigue: coping with secondary traumatic stress disorder in those who treat the traumatized. New York: Brunner/Mazel; 1995. p. 1–20.

26. Sheehy G. Middletown America: one town's passage from trauma to hope. New York: Random House; 2003.

27. The Children's Health Fund. 2002, August. The nations children still feeling effects of terrorist attacks, according to children's health fund. Marist poll: however anniversary events will be helpful to their children parents say. Available from: www.childrenshealthfund.org. Accessed September 13, 2003.

28. Step MM, Finucane MO, Horvath CW. Emotional involvement in the attacks. In: Greenberg BS, editor. Communication and terrorism: public and media responses to 9/11. Creskill, NJ: Hampton Press; 2002. p. 261–74.

29. Engel GL. The need for a new medical model: a challenge for biomedicine. Sci 1977;196:129–36.

30. Segrin C. Interpersonal processes in psychological problems. New York: Guilford; 2001.

31. Taintor Z. Assessing mental health needs. In: Levy B, Sidel V, editors. Terrorism and public health: a balanced approach to strengthening systems and protecting people. Oxford: Oxford University Press; 2003. p. 49–68.

32. Lacy TJ, Benedek DM. Terrorism and weapons of mass destruction: managing the behavioral reaction in primary care. South Med J 2003;96:394–9.

33. Susser ES, Herman DB, Aaron B. Combating the terror of terrorism. Sci Am 2002;287(2):1–7.

34. Brown WJ, Bocarena M, Basil M. Fear, grief, and sympathy responses to the attacks. In: Greenberg BS, editor. Communication and terrorism: public and media responses to 9/11. Creskill, NJ: Hampton Press; 2002. p. 245–60.

35. Ahern J, Galea S, Resnick H, Kilpatrick D, Bucuvalas M, Gold J, et al. Television images and psychological symptoms after the September 11 terrorist attacks. Psychiatry 2002;65:289–300.

36. Saylor CF, Cowart BL, Lipovsky JA, Jackson C, Finch AJ Jr. Media exposure to September 11. Am Behav Sci 2003;46:1622–42.

37. Schlenger WE, Caddell JM, Ebert L, Jordan BK, Rourke KM, Wilson D, et al. Psychological reactions to terrorist attacks: findings from the national study of Americans' reactions to September 11. JAMA 2002;288:581–8.

38. Cardenas J, Williams K, Wilson JP, Fanouraki G, Singh A. PSTD, major depressive symptoms, and substance abuse following September 11, 2001, in a midwestern university population. Int J Emerg Ment Health 2003;5:15–28.

39. Chen H, Chung H, Chen T, Fang L, Chen J. Brief report: the emotional distress in a community after the terrorist attack on the world trade center. Community Ment Health J 2003;39:157–65.

40. Zywiak WH, Stout RL, Trefry WB, LaGrutta JE, Lawson CC, Khan N, et. al. Subst Abuse 2003;24:123–8.

41. Tucker P, Pfefferbaum B, Nixon SJ, Dickson W. Predictors of post-traumatic stress symptoms in Oklahoma City: exposure, social support, peri-traumatic responses. J Behav Health Serv Res 2000;27:406–16.

42. Albrecht TL, Goldsmith DJ. Social support, social networks, and health. In: Thompson T, Dorsey AM, Miller KI, Parrott R, editors. Handbook of health communication. Mahwah, NJ: Lawrence Erlbaum; 2003. p. 263–84.

43. Kluger J, Dorfman A, Gorman C, Horowitz J, Park A, Ellin H, et. al. Attack on the spirit. Time 2001 Sep 24;158:1–4.

44. Nolen-Hoeksema S. Responses to depression and their effects on the duration of depressive episodes. J Abnorm Psychol 1991;100:569–82.

45. Leslie MB, Stein JA, Rotheram-Borus MJ. The impact of coping strategies, personal relationships, and emotional distress on health-related outcomes of parents living with HIV or AIDS. J Soc Personal Relationships 2002;19:45–66.

46. Ognibene TC, Collins NL. Adult attachment styles, perceived social support and coping strategies. J Soc Personal Relationships 1998;15:323–45.

47. Wentzel KR, McNamara Interpersonal relationships, emotional distress, and prosocial behavior in middle school. J Early Adolescence 1999;19:114–25.

# 5 Communication Ethics in the Wake of Terrorism

*Shannon A. Bowen*

Terrorist organizations seek legitimacy through media coverage of their acts. When an act of terror occurs, often overlooked ethical components are present in how the media communicate about the act, and therefore convey legitimacy to perpetrators of violence. This topic is further complicated when one considers that the media not only have the power to convey legitimacy, but with their choice of what to cover and how to cover it, actually to set the public agenda and influence opinion about that agenda. Fan and Brosius write, "It has been shown that the mass media have *profound* impacts both in forming the public agenda ... and in influencing opinion related to that agenda" (p. 163; emphasis added).[1] Add to this bold concept the idea that media frames interpret how audience members define and understand problems, the inherent meanings conveyed through labels, and the social construction of reality that takes place through communication, and a picture emerges of the tremendous ethical responsibility of communicators, particularly the mass media. Further explorations of how the media set the public agenda, such as cognitive priming and issue salience, reinforce the idea that communication confers legitimacy, and are discussed in this chapter. This chapter will review communication theories relevant to terrorism, offer systematic ways to analyze the ethics of communicating in the wake of a terrorist act, and conclude with suggestions for a normative course of action for those who communicate about terrorism.

## TERRORIST ACTS AS PSEUDOEVENTS

A seminal scholar in the field offers this definition of terrorism: "An anxiety-inspiring method of repeated violent action, employed by (semi-) clandestine individual, group, or state actors, for idiosyncratic, criminal or political reasons" (p. 70).[2] Terrorist acts can be thought of as means of conveying messages to groups within the public through the mass media. To be sure, terrorist acts have purposes other than generating media coverage. Terrorists seek out economic targets to create financial loss,[3] civil targets to generate fear in opponents by creating mayhem,[4] and sacred targets to enact religious warfare.[5,6] Paletz and Vinson argue that terrorist acts are carried out primarily to affect people other than the immediate victims.[7] Terrorist events are real acts of violence and warfare. However, in light of today's information society, terrorist acts can also be conceptualized as pseudoevents.

Pseudoevents are activities designed to gain news coverage and attention for a cause or issue.[8] Gaining this type of attention is congruent with the perspective on terrorism offered by Ramakrishna and Tan: "It is fundamentally an asymmetric method by which a weaker actor seeks to obtain its ends by breaking the will of a stronger power" (p. 9).[9] Terrorists use violence as a pseudoevent to gain notoriety and legitimacy through media coverage of their acts. For the purpose of this discussion, a terrorist act can be studied, independent from its other consequences, as a strategic pseudoevent seeking communication.

Terrorists use radical acts of violence as tools of communication: They communicate their goals, beliefs, and objectives through acts of overt aggression. The message conveyed by terrorism can be as diverse as political dissidence to one of hatred, rage, and mass murder. These pseudoevents create a cycle in which media report terrorist acts, and terrorists commit atrocities in order to garner media attention. The terrorist act as a pseudoevent is used to convey a message to a larger public—a divisive message that serves to reinforce the ideology of those sympathetic to the terrorist cause, or to create fear in all those seen as a "generalized other"[10] by the terrorist group.

Applying the models of public relations[9,11] reveals that the communication strategies of terrorists are indeed radically asymmetrical. This type of asymmetrical activity is imbalanced in favor of the terrorist group because no response is sought or welcomed from the opposing side of the issue. The terrorist act as a pseudoevent is based on an asymmetrical worldview[12] that holds life as a "zero-sum" game,[13] in which there are clear winners and losers and collaboration or compromise is unacceptable. Other characteristics of an asymmetrical worldview[13] evident in terrorism are an internal orientation, a closed communication system, tradition, central authority, resistance to change, and to varying extents, efficiency and elitism.

Although these variables are generally applied in organizational communication, they are equally applicable to a terrorist organization when conceptualized as a radically obstructionist group.[14] The characteristics of an asymmetrical worldview reveal that terrorist organizations are relatively closed systems in terms of systems theory. However, they do need to communicate with the outside environment in order to gain notoriety for their cause, create terror in opponents, influence political policy, gain support for their cause among sympathizers, and recruit new members. This communication is almost exclusively a one-way dissemination of information. Therefore, terrorist groups employ the press agentry model of public relations, in which pseudoevents and persuasive, one-way communication are used to gain publicity for the group. Among terrorists, as in other arenas, press agentry is often carried out without regard for the truth.[8] Although the application of the term pseudoevent is unique to this chapter, Schaffert endorses the idea that "terrorists actually design their atrocities for television" (p. 68),[15] and other scholars[16,17] emphasize that a primary objective of terrorists is recognition for a group, cause, or leader. Such recognition is a precursor to legitimacy in the public arena.

Newsworthiness is accorded to terrorist acts largely due to the nature of their victims: usually a civilian population, unaware of the impending threat, and unprepared for attack. The resulting shock and disbelief create terror—and news. Pritchard and Hughes find that "murders of certain victims (e.g., children, seniors, women) are culturally deviant, and thus especially newsworthy" (p. 64).[18] The unusual nature of the attacks, their cruelty, their sheer violence, and their scale appear to be indicators of the newsworthiness of terrorists' acts. Hoffman terms the well-coordinated terrorist attacks of September 11 "spectacular" attacks,[19] and it stands to reason that the spectacular generates news coverage. Clair, MacLean, and Greenberg argue that such events traumatize not only those who experience them firsthand, but also those who view media coverage of them as well.[20] For example, recall watching the film of civilians jumping to their deaths from the burning World Trade Center on September 11, 2001: A terrorist atrocity of such magnitude shocked the world and created an unparalleled demand for communication from a multitude of sources, particularly from the news media. Furthermore, as Pangi points out, "the need for strong communication ... is particularly important immediately following the attack when a proactive communications strategy can aid recovery and rescue efforts" (p. 432).[21] A spectacular or traumatic event exacerbates the need for communication. In summary, communication plays a large role in the aftermath of terrorism, and media coverage is highly sought after, both by members of the affected public and by terrorists themselves. How the media sets the agenda regarding terrorism and its prominence in the minds of the audience also carries ethical implications. Agenda-setting theory will be reviewed and applied to terrorism so that we can evaluate the morality of communication decisions with full knowledge of their implications.

## AGENDA-SETTING THEORY

McCombs and Shaw identify what they call the "agenda-setting function of the mass media" (p. 176);[22] this theory asserts that media tell audiences what issues are important by highlighting them in coverage and placement, thereby advancing them on the public agenda. Before agenda setting was labeled as such, scholars noted the existence of the phenomenon. Lang and Lang assert that the media "force attention to certain issues" (p. 217).[23] Several researchers[22,24] have credited Cohen with the phrase that became the archetype of agenda-setting theory: "While the media may not tell us what to think, they are stunningly successful in telling us what to think about" (pp. 293–4).[25]

McCombs and Shaw's landmark study concludes that "the media appear to have exerted a considerable impact" (p. 155)[22] on what people view as issues of importance. Agenda setting is an influential theory within the mass communications discipline. More than 200 subsequent empirical studies have found agenda-setting effects,[26] including Winter and Eyal,[27] Smith,[28] Eaton,[29] and Broisus and Kepplinger.[30] Ghanem established that agenda-setting research was entering a second phase, in which the effects of the media agenda on what the public thinks has been replaced by a research focus on "how the public thinks about it" (p. 3).[31]

Agenda setting has progressed from the idea that the media suggest topics for the public agenda to the recent proposal that the media actually affect the behavior of the audience. How far-reaching are the effects of agenda setting? Do the effects stop at the prevalence of a topic, or do they include changed attitudes, values, and even behavior? Ghorpade concludes that media agenda setting had a significant influence on behavior.[32] Roberts demonstrated that the media agenda was not limited to setting the public agenda, but also influenced behavioral outcomes.[33] Issues of importance to voters were found to change over time and to mirror the media agenda, and as the respondents' agenda changed, so did their voting intention.[33] The implications of these and other recent studies[30,34-38] in agenda setting are clear: Agenda setting may exert a much more powerful force on society than was originally conceived. McCombs and Shaw reformulated the original concept of agenda setting to this new assertion: "Media not only tell us what to think about, but how to think about it, and, consequently, what to think" (p. 65).[36] If the mass media do play a role in telling audiences what to think, the ethical implications for terrorism coverage are enormous because the media can imply approval or disapproval, legitimacy or illegitimacy, and can even serve to stimulate terrorists to further activity by providing them with publicity. Before considering the ethical implications of placing terrorist acts on the media and public agendas, a few key concepts from agenda-setting research will be reviewed.

## Agenda-Setting Concepts

The stream of agenda-setting research spawned much inquiry into the communication factors that comprise an agenda-setting effect, how certain variables influence the process, and so forth. These concepts can help clarify the agenda-setting function of the mass media, and the factors that can alter the impact of mass communication upon audiences or other groups. Although many concepts have been researched, those most germane to the discussion of communicating about terrorism are images or pictorial representations, issue obtrusiveness versus cognitive priming, concrete versus abstract issues, and salience.

### Images in Agenda Setting

McCombs and Bell credit the original idea for the agenda-setting study to Lippmann's book *Public Opinion*.[39] In it, Lippmann contends that the media create a pictorial presentation of the world—"the pictures inside our heads"—rather than an objective representation of reality (p. 3).[40] Terrorism creates memorable visual representations as described by Lippmann. These images produce strong responses in most audience members: Horror, revulsion, astonishment, and intimidation are common reactions. These images convey importance and reinforce the agenda-setting function of the media, and also advance the social construction of reality surrounding the meaning and interpretation of a terrorist act.

## Issue Obtrusiveness versus Cognitive Priming

Perhaps these images of terrorism have an important impact on only those involved in terrorism, either as potential targets or as perpetrators? The concepts of issue obtrusiveness and cognitive priming address this question. Demers hypothesized that as the obtrusiveness of an issue increased, the power of the media to set the agenda was lessened.[41] In other words, Demers expected that the media had a weak or nonexistent agenda-setting effect on issues with which people had personal experience, but he found no support for that hypothesis. To the contrary, data supported the cognitive priming hypothesis, which posits that previous or personal exposure to an issue only serves to stimulate interest in media coverage of it, thus enhancing the agenda-setting effect.[41] Therefore, media coverage is a powerful agenda setter among people with some personal interest in terrorism or who have had exposure to terrorist activities in the past. The cognitive priming hypothesis partially explains the polarizing nature of media coverage in the Middle East or in Northern Ireland.

## Concrete versus Abstract Issues

Another type of research that concentrates on the issues within agenda-setting theory is the analysis of concrete versus abstract issues. A concrete issue is one that is easy to understand or visualize by an audience. An abstract issue is defined as one difficult for an audience to relate to, conceptualize, or visualize. Although the difference can be somewhat subjective, researchers use empirical pretests to assure the validity of their measurements.

Yagade and Dozier conducted a study comparing the agenda-setting effects for concrete versus abstract issues.[42] This study tested the hypothesis that the news media are able to set the public agenda about concrete events, but do not set the agenda for abstract (conceptual) issues. The hypothesis was proven to be true in that no agenda setting or a decreased agenda-setting effect was found for issues that were abstract or conceptual. A strong agenda-setting effect was found to exist for issues that were concrete, or easy to visualize. Yagade and Dozier's research might explain why terrorists often seek a target with visual impact, newsworthiness of location, or a symbolic importance. For instance, attacking the Pentagon represents a concrete stance against U.S. military power and would have much higher agenda-setting potential than attacking a nondescript apartment building in which many Americans reside.

## Issue Salience

The salience[43] of issues is often referred to in agenda-setting research. Issue salience determines what amount of prominence and penetration the issue has with the audience. Yagade and Dozier's study is significant because it illustrates a divergence of salience between concrete and abstract issues. Which issues are salient, and why, leads to further understanding of the agenda-setting power of the mass media. Wanta and Wu explore whether interpersonal communication, such as conversation, enhances the salience of issues and plays a role in agenda setting.[44] The study of interpersonal communication provides important information about the agenda-setting role of the media. By examining interpersonal communication, researchers can gauge the extent of agenda setting, its importance relative to more informal types of communication, and whether it is enhanced or offset by interpersonal communication. Wanta and Wu find that frequency of discussion was the single largest predictor of issue salience. Specifically, the researchers found that positive interpersonal communication enhanced the agenda-setting effect of the media, and negative, or contrary interpersonal communication interfered with agenda setting.[44] In short, depending on its content, conversation with opinion leaders[45] and within a personal reference groups[46-48] can either reinforce or negate agenda setting.

The research on salience, concrete and abstract issues, cognitive priming, and Lippmann's concept of images all show that agenda setting by the media is a powerful[49] and multifaceted phenomenon. The media's ability to confer importance and legitimacy to terrorists, and to influence how people think about terrorist acts, implies a tremendous ethical responsibility.

## AGENDA-SETTING THEORY AND TERRORIST ACTS

Once a terrorist act is placed on the media agenda, a level of legitimacy is conferred as the act is evaluated as newsworthy. Prestige-press reporting, and the ensuing coverage by smaller media outlets, perpetuates the status of the act as an item on the news agenda. Media coverage reports real-world activities, but also enacts a social construction of reality[50] in which the terrorist's messages of fear are conveyed to a larger public through the mass media. Agenda-setting theory[22] and the social construction of reality[50] work in tandem to explain how issues rise to prominence, how credibility is conveyed through the media, and how mediating variables such as interpersonal communication socially construct the meanings around the issue, based on societal norms and the interpretations of that culture. In essence, terrorists use a pseudo-event to garner media attention, the media convey importance and legitimacy by covering the event (and concepts surrounding the event such as issue and responsibility frames), the event gains salience among audience members, opinion leaders interpret the meaning of the terrorist act,[45] members of the public discuss the event, and some of them might perpetuate the news cycle by seeking further information[51,52] about the terrorist act. An agenda is created, solidified, used to construct social meaning, and then potentially perpetuated. Terrorist events are sometimes perpetuated on the media agenda to the point of causing a change in public policy.[53]

Although agenda-setting theory is not without weaknesses, and is open to criticisms,[54,55] it has clearly found acceptance in the discipline[36] through its explanatory power. Scholars of terrorism appear to recognize the agenda-setting effect of the media. For instance, Schaffert contends that "the public's perception of terrorism can likely be influenced by the media's use of terms and labels, with a significant result being the possible acceptance as legitimate politicians of terrorists guilty of heinous crimes" (p. 64).[15] The literature on terrorism is replete with assertions and findings that terrorists use their violent actions (pseudo-events) to gain access to the media agenda, in an attempt to legitimize their cause.[56-59] Nacos concludes that news does contribute significantly to "increasing respectability and legitimacy" (p. 73)[53] for terrorist groups. One way that the news media is responsible for lending legitimacy to terrorist violence is through framing.

## FRAMING

Framing theory can help us to understand how messages about terrorism can convey attitudes, ideas, power, and legitimacy. Framing can legitimize a certain interpretation of events, or can emphasize certain aspects of the event that lead to a conclusion congruent with the framer's ideology. Frames create a perspective for thinking about topics covered in the news.[60] Entman explains framing as the defining of problems: "To frame is to *select some aspects of a perceived reality and make them more salient in the communicating context, in such a way as to promote a particular problem definition, causal interpretation, moral evaluation, and/or treatment recommendation* for the item described" (p. 52; emphasis in original).[61]

All of these aspects of framing are important in communicating about terrorism, but the aspect of moral evaluation is particularly vital. How media communicate about a terrorist act, the labels chosen, and the terms used in reporting the incident can convey innumerable moral interpretations of the act. The moral aspect of framing is revealed in the "valencing of information" in which information is conveyed in either a positive or negative light.[62] Rhetorical and thematic structures[62] can indicate support or disapproval (valence) for the information being relayed, and in terms of broadcast media, nonverbal cues can add to the communication context.

Communicators' own social constructions of reality are often the first interpretive frames that filter information in deciding how it is relayed. Scholarly inquiry bears out this assertion: Researchers found that media perceptions of the level of deviance associated with a group are related to how the issue is framed.[63,64] For terrorist activities of spectacular or traumatizing magnitude, specific frames of the act can emerge in the media. For example, Lule found that four frames emerged in the four weeks following the September 11 terrorist attacks: "The end of innocence (everything has changed), the victims (we might have been), the heroes (amid the horror), [and] the foreboding future (as horrible as it is to imagine)" (p. 280).[65] Although event-specific frames often emerge, there are typical types of framing[65] that are likely to appear when the media report terrorist acts: issue framing and responsibility framing.

## Issue Framing

According to Fine, issue framing addresses how cues used to present an issue affect how that issue is perceived.[66] Terrorist acts are usually subject to issue framing in which disputing parties "vie for their preferred definition of a problem or situation to prevail."[62] Moghadam illustrates this concept, reporting that some Islamic scholars argue that suicide bombings are a legitimate act, and "consistently use the terms *shaheed* and *istishhad* (martyrdom) when referring to suicide attackers" (p. 70).[67] Issue-framing strategies by terrorist organizations frame suicide bombers as participants in "jihad bi al saif (holy war by means of the sword)"[67] rather than as murderers of innocents, as suicide bombers are sometimes framed in the West. Iyengar found that issue framing was prominent in legitimizing terrorists' actions because the study showed that many viewers inculcated issue frames describing terrorists' grievances as the cause for violence.[68]

## Responsibility Framing

When a terrorist group claims responsibility for a particular event, the media uses responsibility framing to report the information. Responsibility framing attributes causes of events[68] and might also convey legitimacy and power to the terrorist group. Responsibility framing is an ideal opportunity for the terrorist organization to seek legitimacy in terms of the labels applied and the reasons that explain their action. If these attributes were not desirable, terrorist groups would not be eager to claim responsibility for their actions.

By combining agenda-setting theory with framing theory in this chapter, understanding is gained of how the media spotlight certain events as important, placing them on the public agenda, and how communicators contextualize those messages through framing. Researchers argue that a combination of agenda setting and framing provides a better explanation of media effects than either theory alone. The two theories together allow a comprehensive explanation of effects, because they can encompass the "nuances of coverage within the issue, in addition to the sheer amount of coverage" (p. 205).[69] Making professional communicators aware of the power and impact of the mass media, as indicated by both agenda setting and framing, would help foster serious ethical deliberation about the nature and content of media coverage, and could serve to make that coverage more ethically responsible.

Communicating in the mass media about the reasons (issue framing) and responsibility (responsibility framing) for an act requires a high level of ethical sensitivity and deliberation. Communicators should consider carefully the frames applied to terrorist acts in light of the ethical course of action. Is it the ethically responsible course of action to relay issue frames to a broader audience? Are responsibility frames appropriate, or will they serve the goals of the terrorists, thereby rewarding and encouraging violence? Research shows that not only do the frames affect audience perceptions, but also the words that are chosen convey meanings. The labels applied to terrorists also figure into the ethical analysis of what to communicate in the wake of terrorism.

## LABELING TERRORISTS: ACTIVISTS OR MURDERERS?

Can L. A. Grunig's definition of activist publics be extended to include terrorist organizations?[70] She writes: "An activist public is a group of two or more individuals who organize in order to influence another public or publics through action that may include education, compromise, persuasion, pressure tactics, or force" (p. 504).[70] The extreme activities of pressure tactics and force are used by activists. However, it should be emphasized that terrorist groups, by the nature of their deadly and illegal actions, can be argued to constitute groups of criminal perpetrators. However, are the terrorist organizations then *illegitimate* activist groups? Similar to activist organizations, terrorist organizations, according to Kozlow, are generally comprised of leaders, active terrorists, active supporters, and passive supporters—who might provide financial support and can potentially be mobilized to provide logistical support.[17] However, terrorist organizations have key differences from activist organizations, and this perspective shows that terror groups are not illegitimate activists, but are better conceptualized as rogue militant organizations.

Disparity between activism and terrorism is evidenced when examining each type of group's mode of communication. Terrorist organizations rely on propagandistic techniques of communication that reach far beyond simple persuasion. Fear and intimidation are primary external communication tactics, often with the intent to harm those who receive the communication. Legitimate activist groups often rely on public-relations models of press agentry and two-way asymmetrical communication, but without the intent of harming those who receive the message—rather, activists intend to persuade others to view their issue as meritorious. Propagandistic strategies, as used by terrorist groups, are derived from a social science paradigm based on the psychology of persuasion, fear, authority, coercion, extortion, or indoctrination. These approaches are used by terrorist groups in both internal and external communication, but internal communication is likely to have the added components from combat psychiatry of manipulation, affirmation, discipline, and support.[71] Public-relations strategies, as used by activist groups, are derived from an entirely different disciplinary background: that of objective communication based in journalism, and that of rhetoric grounded in arguing one's perspective with the ultimate motive of discovering truth. Activism communicates to persuade, educate, or enact social change. Terrorism on the other hand, communicates to gain concession and hegemony through terror, using any means that will achieve the desired outcome, and without concern for objectivity or truth.

Intention is another factor that distinguishes activism from terrorism. Activist organizations might intend to cause harm to an organization, but it is normally harm of a financial nature as caused by boycotts. Activists usually do not intend to cause violent physical harm to people, whether or not they are employed by the target organization. Terrorists intend to cause harm of a violent nature: primarily physical harm, but also financial harm as a secondary consequence is welcomed by the terrorist group.[72] Terrorist targets are normally civilians or bystanders, rather than those employed by a particular organization. Therefore, activism and terrorism are separated by the concept of Kantian intention discussed later in this chapter. The intention of the activist group is to cause nonviolent harm, generally financial, to an organization, leading to change; morally this can be determined to be well-intentioned action. The intention of the terrorist group is to cause violent harm to random individuals; this motive fails deontological tests of morally good intention and therefore can never be justified as moral. The motive for communication shows substantial and enduring ideological differences between terrorism and activism that reveal they are *not* simply varying extremes on the same continuum, but are opposites in communication purpose, intention, and ideology.

Ethical dilemmas arise when media distinguish between groups that are legitimate activist organizations, those that are terror organizations, and those that are unknown—about which accurate information is not forthcoming or readily available. The ethical distinction arises when media representatives label these groups as either terrorists, activists, freedom fighters, insurgents, rebels, protesters, revolutionaries, guerillas, or dissidents. Each term is laden with the ethical values associated with the word. Therein lies the legitimacy conveyed in a label.[73] We can further understand the power conveyed by labels by looking at the symbolic interactionist school of sociology,[74,75] the social construction of meaning theory from that tradition,[76] and its subtheory of labeling.[46]

## SYMBOLIC INTERACTIONISM AND CONSTRUCTING THE MEANING OF TERRORISM

Mead's symbolic interactionist perspective (as named by Blumer[77]) emphasizes that shared meanings are created through interaction among social actors.[10,78] These shared meanings define the norms of society. Berger and Luckman call this process the social construction of reality.[50] Yerby elaborated their theory: "Social constructionists explore how reality is intersubjectively created through communication" (p. 347).[79] Giddens reasoned, "we create society at the same time as we are created by it" (p. 11).[80] Communication, in the form of language, symbols, and semiotics, is the primary means through which we create our social reality.[81]

Cooley expounds that humans define themselves as they speculate others might see them, as if they were social actors on a stage, presenting the self to others.[82,83] Mead adds the conceptions of the spontaneous self; the reflective self derived from interaction, and the generalized other as a nonspecific, abstract audience.[84] Social actors define reality through their communication in interactions with others, and through a speculative conversation with the generalized other. From the symbolic interactionist viewpoint, crime is defined by reference to meanings encoded in what people communicate to one another.[73,85] The stigma[86] of being labeled a terrorist conveys illegitimacy and disapproval for behavior that is illegal and outside the norms of society. Contrast the terms "terrorist" and "insurgent"; the latter conveys a greater sense of legitimacy because insurgents are seen as those dedicated to a cause but not necessarily engaged in overtly violent or murderous activities.

Acts defying what society defines as normal are then labeled according to their severity as deviant, criminal, vile, and so forth. The labels carry implied meanings and values[73] that give social actors cues as to the level of the transgression against societal norms. These encoded cues are decoded by message receivers to help evaluate the meaning of the message, and the subject's legitimacy or illegitimacy is established. As Tuman explains, "definitions and labels create possibilities for empowering people, causes, issues, and movements—or taking power away from the same" (p. 33).[59] Terrorists view their interaction with the world in an in-group versus outsider[73] status, constructing a reality in which acts of aggression and violence earn rewards. Moghadam reports that these motivations for terrorists include an elevation in social status after death, admiration, gifts, and monetary benefits to family, revenge, conferral of dignity gained through martyrdom, and "the expectation of sexual benefits" in the afterlife (p. 73).[67] The social construction of reality for the terrorist organization includes reinforcing the in-group versus outsider status through the use of closed, asymmetrical, authoritarian communication,[12] as discussed earlier in this chapter. This type of communication and social construction allows the group to operate as a cohesive, deviant subculture.[73,87] A reality is socially constructed, in which using violence, terror, mass murder, and other extreme transgressions of norms are "proper" methods through which a terrorist group can communicate messages to others.[59]

Scholars of a rhetorical perspective[88-91] in communication agree with sociologists that the terms applied to issues, groups, and events can carry many perspectives and meanings. Heath, for instance, reasons that "perspectives are not only embedded in claims that advocates make, but also in the key terms (especially god and devil terms) that are current at any moment in a society" (p. 53).[89] Word choice used to communicate information in the wake of a terrorist act is a crucial consideration for the ethical communicator. Messages conveyed through violence and subsequent claims of responsibility can be latent with terms that imply legitimacy. The ethical choice of what word is used to describe events by terrorists is an aspect of communication that is little discussed, but should be attended to rigorously. Communicators must evaluate not only what words should be used, but also whether they want to send the message to terrorist groups that violence is a legitimate method of gaining media attention and sending messages to the public. Approaches from moral philosophy can help to analyze these ethical decisions regarding communicating about terrorists acts.

## MORAL PHILOSOPHY AND ETHICAL ANALYSIS

There are two broad approaches in moral philosophy to making ethical choices: consequentialism and nonconsequentialism. Consequentialism determines an ethical course of action based on the outcome of a decision. Nonconsequentialism determines an ethical course independently of outcome, instead basing the decision on moral principles. There are several philosophical schools within each of these two approaches to moral reasoning. However, the most well-known form of analysis from each school of thought is reviewed here: utilitarianism and deontology.

### Utilitarian Analysis

The consequentialist approach to moral philosophy argues that actions are neither good nor bad in and of themselves, but are defined as such by their consequences. The utilitarian analysis of a moral dilemma seeks the decision with the greatest good consequences and the least harmful consequences. To make an ethical decision, one must carefully weigh the potential alternatives with regard to the likely consequences of each. In utilitarianism, that which is ethical is defined as that which produces "the greatest good for the greatest number of people."[92] Although utilitarians argue over whether the utilitarian test should be act specific (act utilitarianism) or applied to entire classes or types of actions (rule utilitarianism),[93] they agree that the anticipated consequences of a decision should determine the moral worth of the action. Maximizing good for the greater number is thought to be ethical because it serves the majority and accentuates good in the long term, so it is seen as benefiting society or serving the collective good. In applying these principles to communication, the maxim becomes: What are the consequences of this communication? What information must be communicated (or withheld) in order to serve the greater good for the greatest number of people?

The utilitarian maxim allows the communicator to evaluate the morality of a decision based on the number of people affected, so that the communication can serve the public good by benefiting the majority. However, utilitarianism is not without its weaknesses, such as the difficulty and fallibility of predicting future consequences of decisions. Utilitarianism quantifies people into numbers in which "more is better" rather than a system based on justice,[93] and can be used to privilege one group in society over another when misapplied. If the decision-maker is careful to guard against these problems, utilitarianism can be applied to situations in order to understand the consequences of a decision and to arrive at a conclusion of what the theory defines as the ethical course of action.

Applying a utilitarian analysis to the communication issues following an act of terror is a revealing way to analyze the situation. Exactly what should be communicated in order to serve the greater good? One can create various decision alternatives as possible responses to the issue: Communicate all that is known about the crisis, talk about the terrorist group, discover the motives of the terrorist act, interview the family or supporters of the terrorist and survivors of the act, and so on. The analysis will depend on the specific situation and the goals of the communication. For instance, the public-relations person for a hospital treating survivors of a terrorist act would likely talk about the number of victims and the nature of their injuries rather than motivations (issue frames) for the terrorist act. Although these types of communication also hold ethical implications and can be subjected to moral analyses, communication by the news media is the primary focus herein because of the potential the media holds for legitimizing terrorist activities, placing the terrorist group on the media agenda, and conveying the frames to publics that terrorists seek with their pseudoevents.

Legitimacy is the goal of many terrorist acts, and that legitimacy can be conferred through recognition by a major media outlet. Kozlow contends that "groups that are attempting to gain recognition generally execute spectacular attacks that attract a significant amount of media attention" (p. 22).[17] Should this attention be given to them by the media? In conducting a utilitarian analysis, media representative (reporters, editors, photographers, anchors, and commentators) must decide the potential consequences of communicating various perspectives and facts about this act. Various alternatives from full coverage of all that is known to minimal coverage or no coverage must be evaluated. Are there security risks to the public if certain information is not made known? Have there been threats to other targets or ethnic groups, and will warning them serve to save lives or incite a panic? Which communication alternative will produce the greater good for the greatest number of people? Consider that withholding information is often a way to serve the greater good, as in the case of military intelligence, and the utilitarian calculation increases in complexity.

When terrorists claim responsibility for the act, should the media report the name of the terrorist organization, thereby conveying legitimacy? Or should they use anonymous language, such as "a terrorist group claimed responsibility?" A name is a label[73] that is often laden with values[86] and holds the power to convey legitimacy.[94] Giving the terrorist group a voice in the public sphere[95] implies that violence earns them a legitimate role in the dialogue, the right to weigh in on an issue, or the ability to influence public policy and the political process through violence. Is this a message that should be sent? Although the terrorist group clearly impugns the norms of society with acts of fear, intimidation, and violence, the media (intentionally or unintentionally) might confer a legitimate role in the public opinion process to the group by naming them and relaying the terrorists' issue-framing message to millions. What are the potential consequences of sending such a message? In the application of a utilitarian analysis, a case can be made that the greater good for the greater number is served by not naming the particular terrorist organization perpetrating an act. Perhaps the terrorist act would be less satisfying and attractive if the group and its cause remained nameless in the mass media. Reporters could provide the basic facts of the event but could also refuse to provide a responsibility frame, or add the violent group to the media agenda.

Would it serve the greater good to discuss the reasons behind the terrorist attack, either as commentary by experts or as claimed by the terrorists themselves? These issue and responsibility frames are common once a terrorist act is placed on the media agenda, but commonality does not mean that one can bypass a moral analysis of what *should* be communicated. The media representative must analyze the number of people potentially served by the knowledge versus the number potentially served by refusing to relay the knowledge. Could refusing to state the issue frame claimed by the terrorist group as the cause of the attack serve to delegitimize the act? Would this refusal by the mass media illustrate the illegitimacy of using acts of violence as pseudoevents? Would acts of terror decline in number or severity if terrorists saw fewer benefits in terms of media coverage and notoriety? Refusing to place the terrorist group on the media agenda could serve the greater good by providing basic factual information but not providing the media attention that such groups seek with their violence.

Bandura (as cited in Nacos) argues that without widespread publicity, terrorists would be able to achieve none of their aims.[53] Other scholars (Jenkins, as cited in Nacos,[53] p. 75; Paletz & Boiney[56]) argue that the targets of a terrorist act are those watching, rather than those injured or killed. Based on this premise, a utilitarian argument could conclude that it is in the interest of the greater good of society to report simple facts of terrorist atrocities without names, responsibility frames, issue frames, or legitimizing the group. Paletz and Boiney, along with other scholars, advocate this position as voluntarily "thinning the information made public concerning a terrorist act" (p. 14),[56] thereby denying terrorists the reward they seek. A utilitarian analysis could conclude that by framing terrorism as a despicable, criminal act of violence, its legitimacy and power are undermined, therefore serving the greater good of society.

What about the "right to know" that so many people hold dear? A utilitarian analysis could also conclude, depending on the specific case, that the public's right to know constitutes the compelling greater good. In that case, revealing all that is known about the terrorist act and responsible group is arguably the ethically correct course of action. However, this analysis closely resembles current thinking about terrorism coverage among the media, for which ever-increasing spectacular or traumatic pseudoevents are crafted by terrorists to garner attention, and then to stay on the media agenda. Therefore, an inconsistency is created in the utilitarian analysis, because *perpetuating* acts of terror by proliferate media coverage, thereby serving the interests of a small number of terrorists, is not in the interest of the greater good of society, a much larger group than the terrorists. This contradiction reveals that the media must serve the greater good of the greatest number by carefully analyzing communication about terrorist acts so as not to serve the needs of terror organizations and a small number of people who thrive on hate, fear, and destruction.

## Deontological Analysis

The second major approach to moral decision-making is a nonconsequential analysis of a situation using standards of duty, rights, or justice as universal moral principles that should guide behavior. What is ethical is determined by following these universal principles, rather than by the predicted outcome of the decision. Consequences are not ignored in this type of analysis, but they are not used as the basis for determining what is an ethical action. Moral principle defines what is an ethical course of action, and that action is ethical without allowing consequences to influence or impinge upon the application of the moral principle. The most common and arguably most comprehensive form of nonconsequential analysis comes from deontological philosophy. Deontology was developed by Immanuel Kant (1724–1804) as a means of overcoming the need to accurately predict future consequences, as in utilitarianism, and as a method of rigorous and rational judgment based on metaphysics. Kant believed that the rational will was the source of ethical judgment,[96] and designed a philosophical approach that relied on rational autonomy, equality, and duty to uphold moral norms.[96-99]

A deontological approach contains several requirements for making a moral decision, before its decision test, the categorical imperative, can be applied. The decision maker must be an autonomous moral agent, meaning that she or he is not making the decision based on prudential self-interest, greed, fear of negative repercussions, group pressure, or other factors that could bias the decision. The analysis must be one that is as objective as possible, and autonomy is necessary to allow neutrality. Autonomy implies that the moral agent has the freedom to choose among alternatives based on a rational analysis. Freedom to chose among alternatives is necessary because "ought" implies "can."[100]

A decision cannot be moral if it is self-serving or made from a nonautonomous vantage, so decisional autonomy for the communicator is absolutely necessary. In conjunction, the decision-maker must be rational and apply reason to a moral dilemma. Gert explains that Kant considered rationality and impartiality interrelated, and his argument was influential in linking these concepts across philosophy.[101] Rationality is vital in deontology, because Kant argued that our ability to reason as rational beings obligates each of us to uphold our moral duty.[102] Therefore, it is the moral obligation of the communicator to analyze the ethics of communication about terrorist acts from a rational and autonomous standpoint. Decisions cannot be morally worthy if they are made in response to pressure, greed, self-interest, fear, prejudice, or other influences that bias analysis.

Deontology determines the universal moral principles that should guide decision-making by testing the various decision alternatives under consideration with Kant's categorical imperative in the form of three decision tests: the decision must "be capable of being consistently universalized, must respect the dignity of persons, and must be acceptable to rational beings."[93] All three-decision tests should be applied in the analysis of a dilemma, and an action should pass all three tests in order to be considered moral.[93]

The first test of the categorical imperative reads: "Act only on that maxim through which you can at the same time will that it should become a universal law" (p. 88).[103] The categorical imperative holds that if you are not confident in making the alternative under consideration a timeless, universal law for all similar situations, then the decision is flawed. If you are confident that the solution would be fair in all future situations of a similar nature, then the decision has moral worth because it is universally applicable to all people (equality) including the decision-maker (reversibility). If the action passes this test, then it is consistently universalizeable. The categorical imperative is based on the freedom, autonomy, and rationality of people.[99,102] It is the ultimate norm of moral behavior because it is grounded in universal applicability and equality. When applied to communication about terrorism, this test means that all rational and autonomous communicators would arrive at the same conclusion as the decision-maker. It also means that the decision-maker would feel comfortable applying that decision as a universal law to be followed by all others as the morally correct course of action. In other words, "what is right for one is right for all."[104] Paton agrees: "To judge our own actions by the same universal standard we apply to the actions of others is an essential condition of morality" (p. 73).[105]

The second decision test of Kant's categorical imperative obligates the moral agent to treat the self and others with dignity and respect, never as a means to an end but as ends in themselves.[103] This law of dignity and respect obligates communicators to consider the needs of those on all sides of an issue with regard to maintaining their respect and dignity. It commands that people should never be used as a means to achieve selfish purposes, but should be accorded the respect due to rational moral agents. For instance, if a media representative believes that showing the gruesome injury caused by a terrorist's bomb would increase audience attention and ratings and therefore decides to broadcast the footage, s/he has treated the injured person as a means to achieve an end. This example would clearly fail the second test of the categorical imperative because it does not maintain the dignity and respect of those involved. Perhaps the injured person would consent to appear on film if respectfully asked. While that does not necessarily mean the other decision tests of the categorical imperative could be passed, the dignity and respect of others, as well as the self-respect of the communicator, would be maintained.

The final decision test of Kant's categorical imperative tests whether the decision could harmonize with an ideal "kingdom of ends" (p. 80),[103] in which all rational moral agents act from a basis of good will.

Kant argues that "if our conduct as free agents is to have moral goodness, it must proceed solely from a good will" (p. 18).[106] The decision maker should proceed only from a basis of pure moral intention. The good will is the only thing that Kant determined could "be called good without qualification" (p. 154),[107] and he illustrated how other positive attributes could be corrupted when not supported by a morally good will. If the decision passes the test of arising from good intention, then it is judged to be morally worthy.

The intention of the media is generally to provide accurate information about newsworthy events. The issues of agenda setting, framing (issue and responsibility frames as well as valence), providing legitimacy through labels, and the social construction of reality raise deeper ethical concerns about the intention of the communication. These factors should be rigorously examined before deciding how and what to communicate about terrorist actions. The moral principles of universality, dignity and respect, and intention must be addressed with respect to the media's social construction of reality, to be sure that the communication is ethical. Iyengar's research on responsibility framing discusses the weakening of accountability that can arise from showing violence, harm, or pain of victims without representing any type of punishment for terrorists. The decoupling of violence from punishment makes it appear that the perpetrators are not held responsible for their actions.[108] His frame can be damaging because it conveys a lack of moral accountability, or even provides encouragement to other terrorists.

The intentions of those seeking to use the media as a conduit of information should be carefully examined. Terrorists' intentions are well-known, specifically with regard to terrorists seeking to place their groups, issues, and acts on the media agenda. Kozlow explains, "The most common terrorist objectives include recognition, provocation, coercion, insurgency support, and intimidation" (p. 22).[17] Terrorists eagerly seek recognition in the media, even to competing against one another visibility. For instance, Moghadam reports that Hamas "claimed responsibility for some 43 percent of all suicide attacks perpetrated against Israelis" between October 2000 and June 2002, inflicting "over twice as many Israeli casualties as did Fatah" (p. 79).[67] His research illustrates that terrorist groups are eager to claim responsibility for bombings and intentionally use the agenda-setting effect to establish a consistent presence in the news. Is this intention morally worthy? Using death, violence, and random acts of terror to generate media coverage clearly fails the deontological tests of universality, dignity and respect, and intention (a goodwill). Intentions of terrorist groups to use pseudoevents to relay messages of hate through the media should be carefully considered in ethical analyses by media representatives. If intentions are not based on goodwill, the act is immoral.

Hoffman concludes that "terrorism is fundamentally a form of psychological warfare ... designed to have profound psychological repercussions on a target audience" (p. 313).[19] Placing terrorist activities on the media agenda serves to spread awareness of a terror threat, even if it is an inadvertent effect. Often, the threat of terrorism is enough to induce fear and reaction. Brown maintains that the threat of terrorist activity is being eagerly used by cable news organizations to maintain and generate viewership based on fear.[109] Should media participate in the "psychological warfare"—even inadvertently—by helping to instill terror and achieve terrorist objectives? Communicators should rigorously analyze their own intention, as well as those of terrorists, with regard to communication about the terrorist act in regard to Kant's standard of the morally goodwill.

Could a moral agent with good intentions communicate about terrorists in order to expose their criminal and deviant acts? One could certainly conclude that such an intent would be good. However, the moral decision-maker must also consider what is known about the potential legitimizing factors of that communication, the agenda-setting and framing effects of the media, and the social construction of reality through communication and labeling. Although a media exposé of the terrorist group as perpetrators of criminal violence could meet the deontological test of good intention, it may not be morally applicable to every other similar situation as a universal law. Moreover, would such an exposé maintain the dignity and respect of others, including the group that is the subject of terrorist violence? These deontological tests are difficult to meet, and indicate that judicious communication about terrorists is warranted as the morally worthy course of action. Further, one must consider the intention behind the press agentry strategy of the terrorist group with regard to generating media coverage. Tuman clarifies the strategy and the intention behind terrorism: "terrorism inspires anxiety but does so with repeated acts of violence (as opposed to singular or random acts of violence). It is 'employed,' suggesting an intentional, strategic use, as opposed to a serendipitous, unintentional, or mistaken use. Terrorism applies to those who target civilians or even military targets purposely, but does not apply to accidental violence" (p. 32).[59]

Tuman argues, in other words, that terrorism is an intentional and strategic attempt to inspire anxiety by threatening others through communication about violent acts. Clearly, this intention fails the Kantian test of action arising from a morally goodwill. Therefore, it appears that there is "no such thing as bad publicity" for a terrorist organization.

## IMPLICATIONS AND CONCLUSIONS

Professional communicators must realize that communication is not innocuous, but laden with values, meanings, and legitimacy in the social construction of the world. It is absolutely vital that communicators conduct a moral analysis of communicating about terrorism before deciding what and how to communicate about a specific terrorist act. The traditional role of news media is to provide complete coverage of a news topic[110] in an ethical manner.[104] The ethical responsibility associated with communicating about terrorism adds a new level of complexity to the journalistic role because of the far-reaching implications of agenda-setting, framing, labeling, and legitimizing. Communicators are now called to move from the role of reporters of information to the role of critical and ethical evaluators of that information. In the case of terrorism, communicators must not only decide how to communicate, but also what should be communicated to fulfill moral responsibility. These decisions must be analyzed in terms of moral philosophy or the risk of spurious, biased, or self-serving decisions is grave.

A vital dimension of this ethical responsibility is the ability to be critical of terrorist pseudoevents, sorting newsworthy facts from symbolic messages, values, and issue or responsibility frames that terrorists convey through the act. If something is to be placed on the media agenda, the communicator has the duty of engaging in the analysis of what should be communicated, in addition to the traditional analysis of what to communicate. Heath supports this perspective and explains the role of communicator as critic: "The critic engages the rhetorical act at key points, especially those where meanings become important to the quality of relationships and to the wisdom of policies and actions" (p. 38).[111] As discussed in framing theory, communicators are responsible for making a moral evaluation of the information regarding how it should be conveyed. Making informed judgments about when to communicate about a terrorist act and what to say in order to prevent the conferral of legitimacy is a difficult task, requiring wise assessment of the ethical implications of the communication and an astute understanding of the impact of mass communication in society.

The "critical role" of the communicator must be based on thorough and rigorous analysis as presented in moral philosophy rather than on a "gut instinct" approach to decision-making that can introduce bias. Giddens demands that "critique *must* be based on analysis" (p. 22; emphasis added).[112] The analysis must be conducted from a rational and autonomous standpoint. In utilitarian terms, one must ask: Is reporting the detail of the terrorist event worth the likely conferral of legitimacy to a terrorist organization that comes from even well intended media coverage? Lazarsfeld and Merton maintain that "this status function thus enters into organized social action by *legitimizing* selected policies, persons, and groups which receive the support of mass media" (p. 16; emphasis added).[94] The utilitarian analysis would decide the greater good for the greater number of people by evaluating various communication options and weighing each against creating harm or serving the interests of terrorists with the communication. A utilitarian analysis seeks to promote good and minimize harm, and any communication in the wake of terrorism should meet that standard in order to be deemed ethical.

In a deontological analysis, one must ask if the potential legitimacy conveyed by certain approaches to the communication is the morally right thing to do with regard to the obligations of universality, dignity and respect, and intention. Communicators must exercise the rational autonomy called for in a Kantian analysis. Further, the rational and autonomous decision-maker must be free to carry out the morally right course of action. What approach to communication in the wake of a terrorist act would serve as something that could be supported as a universal law and would be understood by all other rational decision-makers? What communication would maintain the dignity and respect of persons, and is based on a goodwill? Only communication alternatives meeting all of these deontological tests would be deemed ethical.

Denying terrorists the media attention they seek might be the most ethical response to their pseudoevents. Terrorist acts will, unfortunately, continue to occur as real events of hate, murder, and vengeance. However, taking these events out of the realm of pseudoevents is within the power of the media, if rational judgment finds that communication about the act would serve the terrorist goal of perpetuating fear. A fine line must be drawn between reporting factual events to an audience ("A car bomb exploded today in Dublin, killing seven.") and lending labels, meaning, issue frames, and ultimately legitimacy to the event ("The IRA said the bomb was a protest in response to ...").

Despite arguments regarding the publics' right to know, research from many disciplines reviewed here clearly indicates that communication in the wake of terrorism runs the risk of lending legitimacy to the terrorist group, the violent act, and the ideology supporting violence. The mass media are in danger of allowing themselves to become publicists for the terrorist cause of hatred and violence against innocent others as a legitimate means of expressing ideology. Therefore, the public must rely on the moral judgment of communicators regarding terrorism. Explaining the choice of reporting a terrorist act without identifying the group who claimed responsibility might be difficult, but it could also serve as a potent example of the watchdog function and the positive social role of the media.

After reviewing research on the worldviews and motivations of terrorists, agenda-setting theory, framing, labeling theory, the social construction of reality, utilitarianism, and deontology, this chapter must make the undoubtedly controversial determination that the ethical response to terrorist acts is to communicate spartanly about them, in abstract terms, and in ways that are not likely to legitimize the group or event. Many other scholars studying terrorism have arrived at this conclusion through varied means of analysis.[15,56,113-115] Although an ethical analysis could conclude that communicating detail is the moral response in an exceptional situation, communicators must still be careful not to convey legitimacy to the violence through issue frames, responsibility frames, and labels applied in the story. Terrorists want to inspire terror. By refusing to allow terrorist organizations to use their acts as pseudoevents to gain media coverage and legitimacy, the ethical tests of both utilitarianism and deontology are met. Conducting a thorough ethical analysis and communicating judiciously and carefully about the terrorist act—in ways that do not help to meet terrorist goals—is an ethically sound response. Reasoned, critical, and spartan communication that does not legitimize is the ethical response to unethical terrorist acts.

## NOTES

1. Fan DP, Brosius H-B. Predictions of the public agenda from television coverage. J Broadcasting Electron Media 1994;38(2):163–78.

2. Schmid AP. Political terrorism: a research guide to concepts, theories, databases, and literature. New Brunswick, NJ: Transaction Press; 1983.

3. Hargie O, Dickson D, Nelson S. Working together in a divided society: a study of intergroup communication in the Northern Ireland workplace. J Bus Tech Commun 2003;17(3):285–318.

4. Bok S. Mayhem: violence as public entertainment. Reading, MA: Addison-Wesley; 1998.

5. Haddad S. Islam and U.S. foreign policy toward the Middle East: an analysis of survey data. Peace Conflict: J Peace Psychol 2002;8(4):323–41.

6. Moghadam A. Palestinian suicide terrorism in the second intifada: motivations and organizational aspects. Stud Confl Terrorism 2003;26:65–92.

7. Paletz DL, Vinson CD. Introduction. In: Paletz DL, Schmid AP, editors. Terrorism and the media. Newbury Park, CA: Sage; 1992. p. 1–5.

8. Grunig JE, Hunt T. Managing public relations. New York: Holt, Rinehart and Winston; 1984.

9. Ramakrishna K, Tan A. The new terrorism: diagnosis and prescriptions. In: Tan A, Ramakrishna K, editors. The new terrorism: anatomy, trends, and counter-strategies. New York: Eastern Universities Press; 2002. p. 3–29.

10. Mead GH. Mind, self, and society from the standpoint of a social behaviorist. Chicago: University of Chicago Press; 1934.

11. Grunig JE, Grunig LA. Models of public relations and communication. In: Grunig JE, editor. Excellence in public relations and communication management. Hillsdale, NJ: Lawrence Erlbaum; 1992. p. 285–325.

12. Grunig JE, White J. The effect of worldviews on public relations theory and practice. In: Grunig JE, editor. Excellence in public relations and communication management. Hillsdale, NJ: Lawrence Erlbaum; 1992. p. 31–64.

13. Murphy P. The limits of symmetry: a game theory aproach to symmetric and asymmetric public relations. In: Grunig JE Grunig LA editors. Public relations research annual. Hillsdale, NJ: Lawrence Erlbaum; 1991. p. 115–132. (vol 3).

14. Murphy P, Dee J. DuPont and Greenpeace: the dynamics of conflict between corporations and activist groups. J Public Relations Res 1992; 4(1):3–20.

15. Schaffert RW. Media coverage and political terrorists: a quantitative analysis. Westport, CT: Praeger; 1992.

16. Hewitt C. Public's perspectives. In: Paletz DL, Schmid AP, editors. Terrorism and the media. Newbury Park, CA: Sage; 1992. p. 170–207.

17. Kozlow C. Counter terrorism. Alexandria, VA: Jane's Information Group; 2000.

18. Pritchard D, Hughes KD. Patterns of deviance in crime news. J Commun 1997;47(3):49–67.

19. Hoffman B. Rethinking terrorism and counterterrorism since 9/11. Stud Confl Terrorism 2002;25:303–16.

20. Clair JA, MacLean TL, Greenberg DM. Teaching through traumatic events: uncovering the choices of management educators as they responded to September 11th. Acad Manag Learn Educ 2002;1(1):38–54.

21. Pangi R. Consequence management in the 1995 sarin attacks on the Japanese subway system. Stud Confl Terrorism 2002;25:421–48.

22. McCombs ME, Shaw DL. The agenda-setting function of mass media. Public Opin Q 1972;36(2):176–87.

23. Lang K, Lang GE. The mass media and voting. In: Burdick E, Brodbeck A, editors. American voting behavior. Glencoe, IL: Free Press; 1959. p. 217–35.

24. Glasser TL, Salmon CT, editors. Public opinion and the communication of consent. New York: Guilford; 1995.

25. Cohen BC. The press and foreign policy. Princeton, NJ: Princeton University Press; 1963.

26. Rogers EM, Dearing JW, Bregman D. The anatomy of agenda-setting research. J Commun 1993;43(2):68–84.

27. Winter JP, Eyal CH. Agenda-setting for the civil rights issue. Public Opin Q 1981;45:376–83.

28. Smith K. Newspaper coverage and public concern about community issues. J Monogr 1987;101.

29. Eaton H. Agenda-setting with biweekly data on content of three national media. J Q 1989;66:942–8.

30. Brosius HB, Keplinger HM. The agenda-setting function of television news: static and dynamic views. Commun Res 1990;17:182–211.

31. Ghanem S. Filling in the tapestry: the second level of agenda-setting. In: McCombs M, Shaw DL, Weaver D, editors. Communication and democracy: exploring the intellectual frontiers in agenda-setting theory. Mahwah, NJ: Lawrence Erlbaum; 1997. p. 155–67.

32. Ghorpade S. Political spots: setting the agenda for voter decisions. Paper presented at the meeting of the Association for Education in Journalism and Mass Communication; 1985 Aug 3; Memphis, TN.

33. Roberts MS. Predicting voting behavior via the agenda setting tradition. J Q 1992;69(4):878–92.

34. Dearing JW, Rogers EM. Agenda setting. Thousand Oaks, CA: Sage; 1996.

35. Kosicki GM. Problems and oportunities in agenda-setting research. J Commun 1993;43(2):100–27.

36. McCombs ME, Shaw DL. The evolution of agenda-setting research: twenty-five years in the marketplace of ideas. J Commun 1993;43(2): 58–67.

37. McCombs ME, Shaw DL, Weaver D, editors. Communication and democracy: exploring the intellectual frontiers in agenda-setting theory. Mahwah, NJ: Lawrence Erlbaum; 1997.

38. Takeshita T. Exploring the media's roles in defining reality: from issue agenda-setting to attribute agenda-setting. In: McCombs M, Shaw DL, Weaver D, editors. Communication and democracy: exploring the intellectual frontiers in agenda-setting theory. Mahwah, NJ: Lawrence Erlbaum; 1997. p. 15–27.

39. McCombs ME, Bell T. The agenda-setting role of mass communication. In: Salwen MB, Stacks DW, editors. An integrated aproach to communication theory and research. Mahwah, NJ: Lawrence Erlbaum; 1996. p. 93–110.

40. Lipmann W. Public opinion. New York: Macmillan; 1922.

41. Demers D. Issue obtrusiveness and the agenda setting effects of national network news. Commun Res 1989;16(6):793–812.

42. Yagade A, David D. The media agenda-setting effect of concrete versus abstract issues. J Q 1990;67(1):3–10.

43. Iyengar S, Peters MD, Kinder DR. Experimental demonstrations of the "not-so-minimal" consequences of television news programs. Am Pol Sci Rev 1982;76(4):848–58.

44. Wanta W, Wu YC. Interpersonal communication and the agenda setting process. J Q 1992;69(4):847–55.

45. Katz E, Lazarsfeld PF. Between media and mass/the part played by people/the two-step flow of communication. In: Katz E, Lazarsfeld PF, editors. Personal influence: the part played by people in the flow of mass communications. Glencoe, IL: Free Press; 1955. p. 15–42.

46. Becker HS. Cases, causes, conjunctures, stories, and imagery. In: Ragin CC, Becker HS, editors. What is a case? exploring the foundations of social inquiry. Cambridge: Cambridge University Press; 1992. p. 205–16.

47. Becker HS. How I learned what a crock was. In: Hertz R, Imber JB, editors. Studying elites using qualitative methods. Thousand Oaks, CA: Sage; 1995. p. 124–30.

48. Weber M. The theory of social and economic organization. New York: Free Press; 1957.

49. Weaver D, Elliot SN. Who sets the agenda for the media? a study of local agenda building. J Q 1985 Spring;62:87–94.

50. Berger PL, Luckmann T. The social construction of reality: a treatise in the sociology of knowledge. New York: Freeman; 1966.

51. Grunig JE. Defining publics in public relations: the case of a suburban hospital. J Q 1978;55:109–18.

52. Grunig JE. Communication behaviors and attitudes of environmental publics: two studies. J Monogr 1983;81.

53. Nacos BL. Terrorism and the media: from the Iran hostage crisis to the world trade center bombing. New York: Columbia University Press; 1994.

54. Gurevitch M, Bennett T, Curran J, Woollacott J, editors. Culture, society and the media. New York: Routledge; 1988.

55. McQuail D. Mass communication theory: an introduction. Thousand Oaks, CA: Sage; 1994.

56. Paletz DL, Boiney J. Researchers' perspectives. In: Paletz DL, Schmid AP, editors. Terrorism and the media. Newbury Park, CA: Sage; 1992. p. 6–28.

57. Schmid AP. Goals and objectives of international terrorism. In: Slater RO, Stohl M, editors. Current perspectives on international terrorism. New York: St. Martin's; 1988. p. 47–87.

58. Schmid AP, De Graff J. Violence as communication: insurgent terrorism and the Western news media. Beverly Hills, CA: Sage; 1982.

59. Tuman JS. Communicating terror: the rhetorical dimensions of terrorism. Thousand Oaks, CA: Sage; 2003.

60. McCombs M, Danielian L, Wanta W. Issues in the news and the public agenda: the agenda setting tradition. In: Glasser TL, Salmon CT, editors. Public opinion and the communication of consent. New York: Guilford; 1995. p. 281–300.

61. Entman RM. Framing: toward a clarification of a fractured paradigm. J Commun 1993;43(4):51–8.

62. Hallahan K. Seven models of framing: implications for public relations. J Public Relations Res 1999;11(3):205–42.

63. McLeod DM, Detenber BH. Framing effects of television news coverage of social protest. J Commun 1999;49(3):3–23.

64. Shoemaker PJ. Media treatment of deviant political groups. J Q 1984; 61(1):66–75.

65. Lule J. Myth and terror on the editorial page: the New York Times responds to September 11, 2001. J Mass Commun Q 2002;79(2):275–93.

66. Fine TS. The impact of issue framing on public opinion: toward affirmative action programs. Soc Sci J 1992;29(3):323–35.

67. Moghadam A. Palestinian suicide terrorism in the second intifada: motivations and organizational aspects. Stud Confl Terrorism 2003;26:65–92.

68. Iyengar S. Is anyone responsible? Chicago: University of Chicago Press; 1991.

69. Jasperson AE, Shah DA, Watts M, Faber R, Fan DP. Framing the public agenda: media effects on the importance of the federal budget deficit. Pol Commun 1998;15(2):205–25.

70. Grunig LA. Activism: how it limits the effectiveness of organizations and how excellent public relations departments respond. In: Grunig JE, editor. Excellence in public relations and communication management. Hillsdale, NJ: Lawrence Erlbaum; 1992. p. 503–30.

71. Daniels AK. The philosophy of combat psychiatry. In: Rubington E, Weinberg MS, editors. Deviance: the interactionist perspective. 5th ed. New York: Macmillan; 1987.

72. Lake A. 6 nightmares: real threats in a dangerous world and how America can met them. New York: Little, Brown & Company; 2000.

73. Becker HS. Outsiders: studies in the sociology of deviance. New York: Free Press; 1963.

74. Mead GH. Social consciousness and the consciousness of meaning. Psychol Bull 1910;7:397–405.

75. Park RE. Human communities. Glencoe, IL: The Free Press; 1952.

76. Collins R. Three sociological traditions. New York: Oxford University Press; 1985.

77. Blumer M. The Chicago school of sociology: institutionalization, diversity, and the rise of sociological research. Chicago: University of Chicago Press; 1984.

78. Mead GH. The social self. J Philos Psycho Sci Methods 1913;10: 374–80.

79. Yerby J. Family systems theory reconsidered: integrating social construction theory and dialectical process. Commun Theory 1995;5(4): 339–65.

80. Giddens A. Sociology: a brief but critical introduction. 2nd ed. New York: Harcourt Brace Jovanovich; 1987.

81. Pierce CS. Philosophical writings of Pierce. New York: Dover; 1955.

82. Cooley CH. Human nature and the social order. 1964 ed. New York: Schocken; 1902.

83. Goffman E. The presentation of self in everyday life. Garden City, NY: Doubleday; 1959.

84. Mead GH. The philosophy of the act. Chicago: University of Chicago Press; 1938.

85. Goffman E. Encounters: two studies in the sociology of interaction. Indianapolis: Bobbs-Merrill; 1961.

86. Goffman E. Stigma: notes on the management of spoiled identity. Englewood Cliffs, NJ: Prentice-Hall; 1963.

87. Simmons JL. The nature of deviant subcultures. In: Rubington E, Weinberg MS, editors. Deviance: the interactionist perspective. 5th ed. New York: Macmillan; 1987. p. 206–7

88. Cheney G, Vibbert SL. Corporate discourse: public relations and issue management. In: Jablin FM, Putnam LL, Roberts KH, Porter LW, editors. Handbook of organizational communication: an interdisciplinary perspective. Newbury Park, CA: Sage; 1987. p. 165–94.

89. Heath RL. A rhetorical enactment rationale for public relations: the good organization communicating well. In: Heath RL, editor. Handbook of public relations. Thousand Oaks, CA: Sage; 2001. p. 31–50.

90. Toth EL. The case for pluralistic studies of public relations: rhetorical, critical, and systems perspectives. In: Toth EL, Heath RL, editors. Rhetorical and critical aproaches to public relations. Hillsdale, NJ: Lawrence Erlbaum; 1992. p. 3–16.

91. Vaughn MA. Organizational identification strategies and values in high technology industries: a rhetorical-organizational aproach to the analysis of socialization processes in corporate discourse. J Public Relations Res 1997;9(2):119–39.

92. Mill JS. Utilitarianism. New York: The Liberal Arts Press; 1861/1957.

93. De George RT. Business ethics. 5th ed. Englewood Cliffs, NJ: Prentice Hall; 1999.

94. Lazarsfeld PF, Merton RK. Mass communication, popular taste and organized social action. In: Marris P, Thornham S, editors. Media studies: a reader. Edinburgh: Edinburgh University Press; 1948/1996. p. 14–23.

95. Habermas J. Legitimation crisis. McCarthy T, translator. Boston: Beacon Press; 1975.

96. Sullivan RJ. Immanuel Kant's moral theory. Cambridge: Cambridge University Press; 1989.

97. Bowen SA. A theory of ethical issues management: contributions of Kantian deontology to public relations' ethics and decision making. Unpublished doctoral dissertation. College Park, MD:University of Maryland; 2000.

98. Bowen SA. Elite executives in issues management: the role of ethical paradigms in decision making. J Public Aff 2002;2(4):270–83.

99. Bowen SA. Expansion of ethics as the tenth generic principle of public relations excellence: a Kantian theory and model for managing ethical issues. J Public Relations Res 2004;16(1):65–92.

100. Baron MW. Kantian ethics almost without apology. Ithaca, NY: Cornell University Press; 1995.

101. Gert B. Morality: its nature and justification. New York: Oxford University Press; 1998.

102. Sullivan RJ. An introduction to Kant's ethics. New York: Cambridge University Press; 1994.

103. Kant I. Groundwork of the metaphysic of morals. Paton HJ, translator. New York: Harper & Row; 1964.

104. Christians CG, Fackler M, Rotzoll KB. Media ethics: cases and moral reasoning. White Plains, NY: Longman; 1995.

105. Paton HJ. The categorical imperative: a study in Kant's moral philosophy. New York: Harper & Row; 1967.

106. Kant I. Lectures on ethics. Infield L, translator. Indianapolis, IN: Hackett Publishing; 1963.

107. Kant I. Metaphysical foundations of morals. Friedrich CJ, translator. In: Friedrich CJ, editor. The philosophy of Kant: Immanuel Kant's moral and political writings. New York: The Modern Library; 1993. p. 154–229.

108. Iyengar S. Framing responsibility for political issues. Annals Am Academy 1996;546(July):59–70.

109. Brown H. Terror threat logo is useless information. Media Ethics 2003;14(2):1–16.

110. Day LA. Ethics in media communications: cases and controversies. 2nd ed. Belmont, CA: Wadsworth Publishing Company; 1997.

111. Heath RL. In: Toth EL, Heath RL, editors. Rhetorical and critical approaches to public relations. Hillsdale, NJ: Lawrence Erlbaum; 1992. p. 37–61.

112. Giddens A. Sociology: a brief but critical introduction. 2nd ed. New York: Harcourt Brace Jovanovich; 1987.

113. Frey BS. Fighting political terrorism by refusing recognition. J Public Policy 1987;7(2):179–88.

114. Hacker FJ. Crusaders, criminals, and crazies: terror and terrorism in our time. New York: W. W. Norton; 1976.

115. Scanlon J. The hostage taker, the terrorist, the media: partners in public crime. In: Walters LM, Wilkins L, Walters T, editors. Bad tidings: communication and catastrophe. Hillsdale, NJ: Lawrence Erlbaum Associates; 1989. p. 115–30.

# 6 Using Binary Language to Sell the War in Afghanistan

## Michael Ryan and Les Switzer

Political terrorism is by design chaotic, irrational, ferocious, inhumane, and unpredictable. The continuing suicide bombings in Israel, the 2003 bombings of United Nations and International Red Cross headquarters in Baghdad, the bombings and burnings of black churches, the murder of a doctor who performed abortions, and the vandalism of sport-utility vehicles in America often seem to have no rational explanations—except to the terrorists.

Other kinds of terrorism—such as sexual terrorism[1,2] and other forms of abuse;[3,4] racial terrorism and hate crimes;[5,6] electronic terrorism, or "cyberstalking";[7] criminal violence;[8] and the assault on the earth's resources by "environmental" or "ecological" terrorists[9]—are more ambiguous, often hidden, and sometimes controversial. Nevertheless, they share the characteristics (e.g., irrationality) of political terrorism.

Many options are open to those victimized by terrorist attacks, and responsible news media in free societies help governments, groups, and individuals explore and refine the potential responses. This chapter explores the seeds of terrorism, media and violence, real-world frames, and frames and binary language. It reports a case study of U.S. media coverage of the war against terrorism between September 11, 2001, and October 8, 2001, when the United States attacked Afghanistan. Two questions guide this research:

- Did media endorse or oppose the use of violence as part of the U.S. response to the September 11 attacks?
- Did media (1) rely on binary oppositions or (2) explore the semantic space between the extremes as they framed potential U.S. responses?

## SEEDS OF TERRORISM

Sophisticated terrorists use violence and threats that seem irrational precisely because they cannot win military, legal, cultural, personal, environmental, or electoral victories. Thus, terrorism is often associated with the tactics of the powerless. Acts of terrorism are often committed because terrorists perceive they have no other choices, terrorism being the last resort of the powerless.

"Terrorism" has become a formulaic term of abuse that discourages, if not deadens, any rational discussion or debate and encourages what has been called (by the powerless) state-sponsored terrorism.[10] In the immediate aftermath of the September 11, 2001, attacks, the word was used to demonize anyone who defied the social order. Any "recognized state," challenged by separatists or insurgents within its borders, could label its opponents "terrorists." Since the United States could not be criticized "for doing whatever it deems necessary in its war on terrorism, no one should criticize whatever [other countries] now do to suppress their own terrorists" (p. C:1).[11]

The powerless, in the context of the current war against terrorism, are overwhelmingly Muslim.[12] The United States listed thirty-three groups as "foreign terrorist organizations" in 2002, and almost all were Muslim groups based in the Middle East.[13]

Scholars have identified several kinds of terrorism, but there is no universally accepted definition of terrorism because the word has no intrinsic meaning. The Organization of the Islamic Conference, a fifty-seven-member grouping that has sought to counter a perceived "defamation campaign" against Muslim religion and culture following the September 11 attacks, could not produce a definition. The world's biggest Islamic body reiterated that Islam rejects aggression and values "peace, tolerance, and respect," but it left the job of defining "terrorism" to the United Nations. A proposed United Nations conference to define terrorism, however, has not been convened because it is opposed by the United States.[14]

The different *kinds* of terrorism typically have similar goals. "Terrorism is a tactic or technique by means of which a violent act or the threat thereof is used for the prime purpose of creating overwhelming fear for coercive purposes" (p. 3), according to the National Advisory Committee on Criminal Justice Standards and Goals.[15] Terrorists frequently hope:

- to convey the propaganda of the deed and to create extreme fear among their target group;

- to mobilize wider support for their cause among the general population and international opinion by emphasizing such themes as the righteousness of their cause and the inevitability of their victory;
- to frustrate and disrupt the response of the government and security forces, for example, by suggesting that all their practical antiterrorist measures are inherently tyrannical and counterproductive or an unnecessary overreaction;
- to mobilize, incite, and boost their constituency of actual and potential supporters and in so doing to increase recruitment, raise more funds, and inspire further attacks (p. 30–31).[16]

## MEDIA AND VIOLENCE

Framing is a critical construct in the world of terrorism, for the frames that ultimately predominate determine how incidents are reported and perceived. Terrorists understand quite well that they cannot achieve their objectives if the media do not report, widely and continuously, terroristic threats and acts, and if the media do not frame violence in ways that maximize feelings of foreboding and spectacle.[17,18]

But terrorists also know the media must frame their violence as persuasive rhetorical statements, for this frame helps the terrorists gain maximum exposure to, and acceptance of, their goals.[19] That is, terrorists' violent acts are seen by them as persuasive "essays," in which they convince others that their grievances are real, and their proposed solutions are reasonable. It is difficult for terrorists to achieve their goals when the media frame their violence consistently, and *only*, as, for example, crimes against human decency, while ignoring the terrorists' grievances. In such cases, terrorists often respond with escalated violence.

Terrorism "achieves its goal not through its acts but through the response to its acts" (p. 19).[20] Terrorists seldom "win" in societies in which the media are not allowed to report terrorist actions.[21] They have more success in societies in which media are free to give meaning to violent attacks and threats. Critics of media coverage of terrorism frequently argue that "by devoting extraordinary broadcast time and column inches to even minor violence and elevating them to the level of spectacular reality show, the mass media, especially television, play into the hands of terrorists" (p. 194).[22]

Park Dietz puts the case more strongly: "Terrorists use news organizations as their advertising agencies, recruiting them into providing intense coverage to increase the societal impact of an attack. Terrorists use sensational and innovative methods of attack, select high-profile targets, submit prepared messages directly to news organizations, and even attack the news organizations themselves to boost coverage."[23]

Knowledgeable terrorists understand what editors want. They know journalists value conflict, timeliness, oddity, proximity, prominence, and consequence. Their violent acts and threats reflect most of these values. Their statements even contain the element of prominence when they manage to murder a prominent abortion doctor, United Nations official, Spanish ambassador, Red Cross worker, or U.S. colonel. "Terrorists engage in recurrent rhetorical forms that force the media to provide the access without which terrorism could not fulfill its objectives" (p. 14).[19]

Some are so sophisticated, they are choreographers of terror: "These new transnational gunmen are, in fact, television producers constructing a package so spectacular, so violent, so compelling that the networks, acting as executives, supplying the cameramen and the audience, cannot refuse the offer. Given a script with an uncertain ending, live actors—the terrorists, the victims, the security forces, the innocent bystanders—and a skilled director who choreographs the unfolding incident for maximum impact, television is helpless" (p. 50).[18]

Terrorists try to generate fear among large numbers of ordinary citizens in hopes those fearful men and women will change the ways they live, and accept, or even demand, repressive measures. As terrorist-inspired fear increases, for instance, pregnant women may avoid abortion clinics, United Nations personnel may leave a country in which they are not safe, consumers may stop buying sport-utility vehicles or building homes in the "wrong" places, or a government may impose repressive measures that deny some individuals their civil rights.[24,25]

All of this, of course, is part of the larger rhetorical statement. The violence is part of an effort to have grievances, and their potential solutions, addressed.

Terrorists enjoy little success when their violent actions fail to elicit the kinds of responses they seek. "Terrorism wins only if you respond to it in the way that the terrorists want you to. . . . If you choose not to respond at all, or else to respond in a way different from that which they desire, they will fail to achieve their objectives. The important point is that the choice is yours. That is the ultimate weakness of terrorism as a strategy" (p. 23).[20] The weakness is apparent, however, only when the media refuse to play the game.

The media, in fact, have several options in framing the potential responses to terrorist attacks and to the threat of terror. At one extreme, a frame may exclude all information about a terrorist attack—there is simply no narrative, or story, because there is no frame on which to hang the narrative. At the other extreme, a frame may include essentially all details about a terrorist attack, and the narrative elevates the act to spectacle. One example occurred in the summer of 2000, when armed terrorists held hostages on the island of Jolo in the Southern Philippines. International journalists beamed to audiences around the world images of suffering hostages. "The hostage drama on Jolo was not reality television of the *Survivor* variety, but brutal real life drama." Very little was excluded from the frame, and "the lines between news and entertainment were often blurred" (p. 78).[22]

The best responses, of course, probably lie within the extremes— within the semantic space that frequently is ignored as potential responses are framed.

## REAL-WORLD FRAMES

Media professionals and critics learned long ago that too many bits float by on the information stream for writers to attend to all of them.[26] Indeed, they can attend to very few bits. They weave those that seem relevant, interesting, and important into frames, and then they construct on this foundation the narratives that readers and viewers find compelling and useful.[27] The facts reported by the media have no intrinsic meaning. "They take on their meaning by being embedded in a frame or story line that organizes them and gives them coherence" (p. 157).[28]

The social realities that writers frame, of course, invariably omit useful (and not so useful) facts and opinions.[28-31] Opinions or facts that do not support a writer's frame typically are left on the cutting room floor or in a writer's notes. They are dismissed as naïve, irrelevant, unimportant, uninteresting, or, in the case of a war against terrorism, "unpatriotic."

Discarded information bits do not disappear, but they are ignored. Framing helps to create social continuity, and that is important. "The problem is that the same power that forces the present to 'make sense' leaves its representation of society incomplete" (p. 135).[32] This process tends to lead to the exclusion, not the inclusion, of ideas, options, and marginalized individuals and groups.

The process also can lead to false assumptions about, and misreadings of, important facts and issues, problems, opinions, and alternatives. Indeed, one reason for misunderstandings of political issues "lies in the dubious ways we classify news stories about public policy into discrete and autonomous spheres and so foster false beliefs about the causes of problems and the consequences of governmental actions. The prevailing classification schemes obscure the close links among developments that are routinely categorized into separate domains" (p. 232).[29]

"Media frames, largely unspoken and unacknowledged, organize the world both for journalists who report [on] it and, in some important degree, for us who rely on their reports" (p. 7).[33] There are thousands of individuals writers, but "media frames" are accepted and used by virtually all of them. Feminists are framed differently from non-feminists;[34] war is framed as sanitized theater;[35-37] Arabs are framed as uncivilized, violent, and ignorant;[38] motorcycle gangs are framed as outlaws.[39] Media frames—especially mainstream media frames—seldom permit alternatives.

Media frames are influenced by the rhetorical strategies of governmental, ideological, and political elites.[40] News is an important site of contention in this process because anxious readers and viewers look to the news media when they need help making sense of the senseless, finding answers to complex and agonizing questions, and deciding what behavior is appropriate or inappropriate in difficult situations.[41] News is important also because it often repeats an "approved" narrative constantly, which is critical if a frame is to continue to have persuasive power over its audience.[41]

Battles frequently rage between and among competing groups, ideologies, and institutions that want to see their frames prevail.[42,43] Although all players are important, this chapter focuses on the government and the media as frame-makers and frame-breakers during the sale of the war against terrorism. Using the war against terrorism as a context, of course, means that this chapter also focuses on political terrorism and excludes other types of terrorism.

Frames typically can be divided into four functions: They define problems and issues, determine causes, offer judgments, and suggest solutions.[44] "A single sentence may perform more than one of these four framing functions, although many sentences in a text may perform none of them. And a frame in any particular text may not necessarily include all four functions" (p. 52).[27]

A frame-maker selects bits of information and incorporates them into a frame to make them more salient to others. The bits are embedded in text-containing frames, "which are manifested by the presence or absence of certain keywords, stock phrases, stereotyped images, sources of information, and sentences that provide thematically reinforcing clusters of facts or judgments" (p. 52).[27]

## FRAMES AND BINARY LANGUAGE

The perspective on language adopted in this article was outlined initially by the Swiss-French scholar, Ferdinand de Saussure (1857–1913), the founding father, as it were, of structural linguistics, which is now widely recognized as essential in the process of communicating the modern condition.[45]

Two aspects of de Saussure's argument seem particularly compelling for mass media practices in the late-modern era. First, de Saussure suggests that language is not a spontaneous act, nor is it some kind of natural law. Language is, rather, given meaning by human beings, who constitute a language community. Words are meaningless unless the language community assigns them values. Second, de Saussure argues that words are assigned meaning in terms of their opposition to other words. The widespread use of dichotomies in language, along with the apparent need to see the world in terms of oppositions, suggests that they fulfill a deeply felt social need.

Binary language expresses one's experiences: Dichotomies are conceptual maps of meaning that help human beings make sense of the world. The development of modern industrial culture in the West was facilitated by binary signs. Where these dichotomies are naturalized, they can become dominant ideological discourses, even in a democratic society.

While this argument has been challenged in the cultural transformation that is moving society inexorably toward a postmodern epoch, it does explain how people perceive social reality. The world of binary signs reemerges again and again during periods of real or perceived crises to dominate the discourse of the cultural—especially the political—order.

Thus, news is an unending stream of information bits (events, problems, issues, individuals), which are constantly divided into opposing categories and groups.[31] Many cultures have created and maintained binary worlds in which women are not equal to men,[46] minorities are granted fewer rights than dominant majorities,[38] and "outsiders" are treated with suspicion.[33,39]

Binary opposites often are used to describe violent acts. Government officials, for example, used words that were judgmental, inflammatory, and sensational in describing the perpetrators of 127 incidents of political violence from 1980 to 1985.[47] The official sources favored descriptive characterizations (e.g., cowards, criminals, murderers) to nominal characterizations (e.g., hijackers, attackers, gunmen). Witnesses and media personnel tended to use the more neutral terms.

Two competing metaframes often are employed to explain violent conflicts.[48,49] Powerful antagonists seek to maintain order by using the law-and-order frame to maintain the status quo. "The major focus of this frame is the need to respond to a *threat* being posed by some upstart and the justification for using force to stop that threat and maintain order." The weaker antagonist typically employs an injustice and defiance frame that promotes "a particular grievance against a more powerful antagonist and includes a call for the oppressed to confront the more powerful enemy" (p. 141).[49]

The mass media employed language, image, and story narratives to demonize Saddam Hussein in the 1991 Persian Gulf War and to frame the military effort as a defensive response to aggression by Iraq. "It was a story told within the limits of a good versus evil dynamic, as Kuwait was rescued from an evil dictator and 'democracy' was restored in the region. Violence was safely packaged in formats that were palatable to home audiences, thereby shielding them from the harsh realities of death and destruction which might have encouraged awkward questions to be asked about the factors behind the conflict" (p. 26).[35]

The Danish newspaper, *Politiken*, analyzed the British press' war coverage (figure 6.1) and concluded that journalists had declared war in the Persian Gulf.

The binary view of social reality is most apparent when groups compete to create the dominant frame. "They do this by talking across each other, not by dialogue. Dialogue means that when one side raises a subject, the other side addresses it. When there is true dialogue, stakeholders bring facts to each other's attention and debate the value of these facts" (p. 110–1).[50]

In a binary world, controversies are not resolved because combatants are unwilling to move away from their partisan positions, and the way they frame problems and issues reflects these positions. The semantic space between two binary oppositions is not always visited as journalists construct social reality.

## FRAMING THE WAR: A CASE STUDY

This case study seeks to determine whether the news media (1) endorsed or opposed the use of violence as part of the U.S. response to the September 11 attacks, and (2) relied on binary oppositions or explored the semantic space between the extremes to frame the potential U.S. responses. This section focuses on contextual issues and war coverage.

| The Allies have: | The Iraqis have: |
|---|---|
| Army, navy, and air force | A war machine |
| Guidelines for journalists | Censorship |
| Briefings to the press | Propaganda |
| **The Allies:** | **The Iraqis:** |
| Eliminate | Kill |
| Neutralize | Kill |
| Hold on | Bury themselves in holes |
| Conduct precision bombings | Fire wildly at anything |
| **The Allied soldiers are:** | **The Iraqi soldiers are:** |
| Professional | Brainwashed |
| Cautious | Cowardly |
| Full of courage | Cannon fodder |
| Loyal | Blindly obeying |
| Brave | Fanatic |
| **The Allied missiles:** | **The Iraqi missiles:** |
| Do extensive damage | Cause civilian casualties |
| **George Bush [senior] is:** | **Saddam Hussein is:** |
| Resolute | Intractable |
| Balanced | Mad |

**Figure 6.1**
**Binary Signs Used in Framing the 1991 Iraq War**

Source: *Politiken's* findings are summarized in War of words, *In These Times* 1991;15(12):5.

## Contextual Issues

The context within which media and government responded to the political violence of September 11 was not unknown to those who launched the attacks. Political terrorism was common in the United States and around the world long before September 11, and the news media were inclined to report extensively about terrorist activities—frequently elevating them to the level of spectacle.

Brigitte Nacos, for example, reports that "when more blood is spilled in instances of political violence, more printer's ink and air time are devoted to those events by the mass media" (p. 84).[22] In 2000, "terrorism was more frequently discussed on TV and radio news broadcasts than all or some of the four important domestic policy issues [health insurance, Medicare, poverty, and Social Security]" (p. 85).[22]

Terrorists know that two factors influencing U.S. news coverage of terrorism are government behavior and public attitudes. As Paul Pillar notes, "Combating international terrorism is—now, as at times in the past—a major objective of the United States. There is broad support for this effort within different branches of government, across the political spectrum, and among the American public" (p. 1).[51] Indeed, a Chicago Council on Foreign Relations poll mentioned terrorism more often than any other issue as a threat to U.S. interests.[52]

The seeming irrationality of terrorism is one reason why so many Americans support counterterrorism activities. "This consensus for counterterrorism is made possible by the nature and clarity of the counterterrorism mission, which involves the prevention of malicious and sometimes lethal harm against innocent and unsuspecting people. Saving innocent lives is about as noncontroversial as issues of public policy ever get" (p. 1–2).[51]

U.S. responses to terrorist acts have varied widely. More than 2,400 terrorist actions were aimed at American citizens and interests from 1983 to 1998.[53] In almost every case, the preferred counterterrorism response was law enforcement. The government used military force in only three incidents: "the 1986 Libyan bombing of a West German discotheque; the 1993 Iraqi attempt to assassinate former President Bush in Kuwait; and the 1998 bombing of two U.S. embassies in East Africa by [Osama] bin Laden operatives" (p. 85).[53]

Five kinds of responses to terrorism had been used by the time of the September 11 attacks, and the media and the government could have argued for any or all of them. The options were (1) to use political and diplomatic pressure, including censure, travel restrictions, and the breaking off of diplomatic relations; (2) to employ economic pressure, including trade embargoes, reduced investments, withdrawal of aid, and seizure of assets; (3) to use military strikes; (4) to launch covert operations against the terrorists; and (5) to engage law-enforcement personnel to pursue terrorists.[53] These options, of course, are not mutually exclusive.

Not insignificant was the fact that the United States was led at this crucial time by a president who had little experience in foreign affairs, who was trying to cope with the job and get his administration organized, and whose primary constituency consisted of ultra-conservative voters.[54] One such follower, Ann Coulter, said of the U.S. response: "We should invade their countries, kill their leaders and convert them to Christianity."[55] While the president may not have endorsed such an extreme position, much of his constituency did.

## Marketing Violence

A troubling aspect of media coverage of terrorism is the relationship between news coverage and the need of media organizations, particularly commercial broadcast networks, to make money. Certainly, the label "War Against Terrorism" is catchy, and its repeated display helps a news medium claim it has aligned itself with public opinion. It is not profitable to raise uncomfortable questions when public opinion seems to be resolute in favor of vengeance.

"The irony is that in seeking to grab the attention of audiences, program makers are actually fostering very negative attitudes towards the developing world and other international issues and in the long run will reduce audience interest" (p. 185).[56] When broadcast journalism is driven by audience ratings "most reporting . . . is reduced to a simplistic version of often complex realities, a process that is compounded by the absence of any credible and comparable alternative global news service" (p. 211–2).[57]

Some scholars suggest that the media's drive to boost ratings has changed journalism. A study examining Swedish media coverage of the September 11 attacks and the war in Afghanistan, for example, indicates that journalistic content was compromised in the competition for audiences. The study characterizes much of the coverage of terrorism as "pseudo-journalism" or "postjournalism" and suggests that "the line between fact and fiction sometimes has become increasingly hard to discern" (p. 73).[58]

Both U.S. government planners and al Qaeda marketed the September 11 attacks as a media event. This "warfare model" favored the media-savvy Americans over the terrorists, at least in the short term.[59] U.S. media were already well versed in the news value of international terrorism. In their analysis of a Rand Corporation study of terrorist acts between 1968 and 1980, Gabriel Weimann and Hans-Bernd Brosius find that "deviance" was the most compelling factor in defining the significance of these events. Their research supports the so-called "contagion hypothesis," which suggests that American media—especially network television—played a significant role in the diffusion of international terrorism prior to September 11.[60]

Those who would understand the media's role in helping to frame the response to the September 11 attacks must realize that September 11 to October 8 was the most critical period during the war against terrorism. It was then that the United States faced real choices: to respond to terrorism with violence or to respond using a myriad of other methods that exclude violence (law enforcement, economic sanctions, diplomatic pressure). The news media, during any such critical period, must explore options clearly and objectively and try to help government and the people find the right path.

## War Coverage

Scholars have analyzed a variety of texts generated after the September 11 attacks, including news stories, photographs, editorials, and editorial cartoons. Much of that research focuses on content produced from September 11 to October 8, the time period for this case study.

During the initial eight hours following the September 11 attacks, the broadcast media apparently adhered to the first step in framing:[44] They tried to help define the problem by serving primarily as information sources.[61] "In fact, more than 76 percent of the stories were identified as presentation[s] of facts, whereas 19 percent of stories were primarily analytical." The media emphasized political or economic factors more than human interest factors. "Only 4 percent of the stories were framed from a human interest perspective" (p. 116).[61]

What television coverage of September 11 did *not* emphasize during the first eight hours also is significant. "Patriotism was not a visible theme in the coverage. There was no demonstrated patriotism in 96 percent of the news stories, some patriotism in 3 percent of the stories, and high patriotism in less than 1 percent. ... American values demonstrated through the use of specific words and expressions were not a frequent occurrence in the news coverage. Only 3 percent of the stories emphasized freedom/liberty" (p. 119).[61]

Carolyn Kitch, in her study of U.S. newsmagazines, found that "bearing witness and giving testimony were key to the first stage of coverage, which corresponded with what anthropologists call 'separation'—the first stage of the funeral, which is the loss of the dead and the resulting tear in the social fabric" (p. 216). [62] The newsmagazines' coverage initially expressed disbelief and shock.

The frame-makers in government and the media followed the second, third, and fourth framing steps beginning on the second day, but not precisely in the same sequences. Research suggests that some news reports proclaimed right away the cause of the terrorist attacks (Saddam Hussein, for example); some made value judgments (this is a "war" between East and West); and some suggested solutions early on (invade Iraq). The media quickly vaulted to step four (suggest a solution). For most, that solution was war, and it was framed in binary terms.

*The Enemy as Animal*

In an analysis of 242 depictions by 85 editorial cartoonists of Osama bin Laden, al Qaeda, or the Taliban, the cartoonists used multiple categories, most of which were dehumanizing—enemy as animal (29 percent), aggressor (21 percent), abstraction (12 percent), barbarian (8 percent), enemy of god (6 percent), faceless (5 percent), desecrator of women and children (4 percent), criminal (4 percent), and death (2 percent). Nine percent of depictions fell into a "humanized" category (p. 147).[63] "In the case of the current war, no longer are al Qaeda human beings, who might have a rationale for their behavior, but insects and rodents to be exterminated. . . . Dissenting views were noticeably absent in the cartoons analyzed in the present study" (p. 150).[63]

Brigitte Nacos reports that bin Laden was mentioned in 2,538 stories disseminated by ABC, NBC, CBS, CNN, NPR, the *New York Times*, and the *Washington Post*, compared to 2,446 mentions for President Bush. This is a bit unusual since bin Laden was unavailable for comment and Bush "went public at a breathtaking rate. In the twenty-six days from September 11 to October 6, President Bush made more than fifty public statements" (p. 148).[22] References to bin Laden, of course, were negative.

The quest for revenge was reflected in reader letters, columns, and photographs published by U.S. newsmagazines. *Time* and *Newsweek* "used head shots of bin Laden in which either he was in a red light or the photo was digitally changed to make him appear red, like a devil; *Newsweek* used the image, closely cropped, as its cover" (p. 217–8).[62] Bin Laden appeared in the crosshairs of a riflescope to illustrate a *U.S. News & World Report* cover story.

Bin Laden was demonized in seventy-one editorials published in the ten largest U.S. newspapers as corrupt, murderous, ruthless, cowardly, and hated. Such codes as cowardly, vicious, jealous, and extremist also were used to describe everyone who had not boarded the war train.[64]

*Choosing Sides*

It is important in any war to know who is on which side. After all, the terrorist also "interprets the world in starkly polar terms between good and evil" (p. 39). [65] Editorial writers for the ten largest U.S. newspapers used binary terms to draw the lines between "us" and "them." Eighteen asserted that "you're either with us or with the terrorists"—with ten of the editorials citing Bush as their reference. [64]

An analysis of the *New York Times'* editorials, news reports, advertisements, and columns suggests that Muslims and Arab-Americans were framed as "different" from other Americans. Frames of Muslims and Arab-Americans as "the 'Other' encourage the emergence of a specific ideological vision in the news coverage which has cultivated a climate of fear in United States citizens" (p. 3). [66]

Editorial writers in Michael Ryan's study eventually tried to isolate the "good" Arabs/Muslims/Afghans from the "bad" ones—to suggest that there are a few bad dates in every batch and that all other Arabs/Muslims/Afghans had no real grievances against the United States. Twenty-six writers said Muslims were not the enemy, and thirteen asserted that the Afghan people were not the enemy. *USA Today* used President Bush's visit to an Islamic center to make the point: "President Bush took time out of his day Monday to meet with Islamic leaders on their sacred ground. At a mosque two miles from the White House, Bush excoriated those who would intimidate and harass American Muslims, saying they 'represent the worst of humankind'" (p. A:23). [67] Nevertheless, Muslims—especially those deemed to be of "Middle Eastern" origin—continued to be isolated and targeted for persecution as a group. [68]

As they dehumanized the opposition, the media praised and made heroes of Western leaders, victims, survivors, and rescue workers. "This shift of focus from victims to heroes helped to effect a transition from death to life, and it coincided with the rhetorical shift from shock to sorrow to patriotism" (p. 219). [62]

Political leaders also were portrayed as heroes—to their benefit. "The construction of political leaders as heroes ... can legitimize the actions of those leaders and buttress their authority at critical times. The [*New York*] *Times'* portrayal of President Bush as 'a leader whom the nation could follow' offered implicit (and politically important) support for the administration's response to September 11" (p. 284). [17] President Bush elevated his own status by "attacking the 'evil' of the terrorists, using the word five times in his first statement on the September 11 terror assaults, and repeatedly portraying the conflict as a war between good and evil in which the United States was going to 'eradicate evil from the world' and 'smoke out and pursue ... evil doers, those barbaric people'" (p. 144).[54]

Editorial writers treated Bush most favorably.[64] The president was mentioned in 81 of 104 editorials, and none suggested he was wrong about any aspect of the war against terrorism. Thirty-one said he was right in his approach and decisions, and twenty-three tacitly endorsed his views by citing them without comment. Editorials applied thirty-four positive descriptors (e.g., able, bold) to the president. Seven news media outlets cited Bush 2,446 times, and nearly all citations were favorable or neutral.[22]

*Official Voices*

After September 11, the news media relied heavily on official sources, most of whom supported military strikes. Ryan reports that 66 of 90 sources cited in 104 editorials were government leaders, some elected and some not, and virtually all expressed support for military strikes. Of these sixty-six leaders, thirty-two served at one time in the U.S. government, eighteen served in Middle Eastern governments, nine served in European governments, and seven served in other governments.

The only unofficial voice cited more than twice was that of Osama bin Laden, who tried on September 24 to frame an alternative narrative—that "the allies" were attacking all of Islam and all of the Arabic world—but that story was stillborn, at least in ten newspapers' editorials.[64] Five writers did report his view, but they ridiculed it and asserted the war was not against "good" Arabs and Muslims, but against the bad ones—like bin Laden.

These editorial writers did not cite sources that would contest the official view, so they virtually ignored fundamental reasons behind the attacks. Only five sources suggested U.S. foreign policy might be culpable—either because it treated previous terrorists too gingerly or because it ignored real grievances in the Arab world. Furthermore, "what was not noted was that the dominant right-wing and Bush-administration discourses, like those of bin Laden and radical Islamists, are fundamentally Manichaean, positing a binary opposition between good and evil, us and them, civilization and barbarism. It is assumed by both sides that 'we' are the good and the 'other' is wicked, an assertion that Bush made in his incessant assurance that the 'evildoers' of the 'evil deeds' will be punished, and that the 'evil one' will be brought to justice, implicitly equating bin Laden with Satan himself" (p. 145).[54]

*America Assaulted*

Research suggests that the government and news media framed the terrorist attacks as an assault against only the United States. This practice "precluded other sorts of framing such as 'an attack on the West' which might have appeared had we seen the spontaneous street demonstrations of shocked and saddened people in Berlin, Copenhagen, Paris, London, and other parts of the world. The 'world' part of the WTC accounted for over 1,000 now missing 'foreigners,' and the functions of many of the businesses within it were emphatically global. But ours was an American story."[69] Print and electronic media used slogans such as "War on America" and "America's New War" across the United States, suggesting the attacks were a U.S. problem.[54]

Fifteen prior wars were cited in editorials in the largest newspapers to remind readers of prior military success (e.g., in World War II) or of prior failure (e.g., the Vietnam War).[64] Editorials also cited the Civil War, Korean War, and the American Revolution. Virtually all wars were used to illustrate the triumph of U.S. military might, although there were a few exceptions. The *New York Times* noted, for instance, that "the country has not forgotten the lessons they learned in Vietnam about the limits of a superpower's ability to wage war against guerrilla troops in distant lands" (p. A:34).[70]

Eight previous attacks against U.S. targets were mentioned. Three editorials reminded readers of a successful U.S. response (e.g., to the 1998 bombings of the embassies in Kenya and Tanzania), and twenty-one reminded them of an unsuccessful response (e.g., to the 2000 attack against the USS *Cole*). Most endorsed *Newsday's* sentiment: "The only way to prevent such carnage is to root out terrorist organizations that could plan and execute it. Anything else would just be the kind of ineffective, half-hearted, stop-start operations U.S. security forces have undertaken for the past two decades with abysmal results" (p. B:1).[71]

*Military Strikes*

Military strikes were assumed from the start to be part of the U.S. response. For example, "The *New York Times* . . . constructed and celebrated heroes and bolstered leaders as they responded to the crisis. It mobilized for war and warned of a foreboding future, of suffering and sacrifice to come" (p. 286).[17] Further, "ABC News broadcast eighty-six stories that contained the terms 'war' and 'terrorism,' CBS News aired ninety-six such segments, NBC News broadcast 133, CNN televised 316, and National Public Radio aired 166. The U.S. print press available in the LexisNexis archive produced a total of 5,814 articles that mentioned the two terms" (p. 146).[22]

None of the 104 editorials Ryan studied argued against or suggested alternatives to military intervention, although two did refute arguments against a military response. While twelve editorials counseled caution, few detailed the potential risks of military intervention. Of the 104 editorials, 95 did not mention potential Afghan casualties. The nine editorials that did address the issue were published primarily after September 30, when military strikes were imminent. The editorials said any civilian casualties must be minimized, but beyond that, their intent was not always clear.[64]

The justification for military strikes was assumed by seventy-six editorials, while ten noted the terrorists attacked U.S. civilians; nine said they declared war; and seven said strikes would be legitimate acts of self-defense. The New York *Daily News* stated yet another justification: "Make no mistake. The enemy will use all means to obtain those weapons [of mass destruction] and will use those weapons against us. Unless we destroy the enemy first" (p. 40).[72]

That this frame was a work in progress is suggested by Ryan's finding that the twenty-seven demands to "get" Osama bin Laden followed September 21, after evidence allegedly linked him to the terrorist attacks. Similarly, most of the fourteen demands to depose the Taliban followed September 30, after the Taliban had rejected Mr. Bush's demand to "turn over" bin Laden. The Taliban and bin Laden were essentially outside the frame before September 21.

Forty-one editorials (primarily before September 21) said an objective should be to make governments stop sheltering terrorists. Editorials mentioned this objective less frequently after it was clear that the administration would need at least some of those countries to contribute to the war against terrorism.

## CONCLUSIONS

The answer to this study's first research question—whether media endorsed or opposed the use of violence as part of the U.S. response to the September 11 attacks—is clear: The mass media unabashedly endorsed the use of U.S. violence, with little dissent and little exploration of the alternatives situated between the binary opposites.

On October 8, 2001, America declared an open-ended, violent, worldwide war against terrorism. The media partnered with the administration in creating the war frame, and the international community was not surprised when the United States announced military attacks. "In the nearly four weeks since the terror attacks of September 11th, the war metaphor had been invoked so often by media organizations and by public officials that the American public was hardly surprised when President Bush revealed the start of the military phase in what cable TV networks had long described in their on-screen banners as 'America's New War' or 'War against Terrorism'" (p. 146).[22]

The law-and-order frame was dominant to an almost unprecedented degree. It was unassailable—whether the source was government; the mass media; or educational, social, cultural, religious, and political institutions in civil society. All spoke as one, monologic voice. Those individuals or groups that endorsed and supported the injustice and defiance frame[49] were at best ignored or at worst attacked.[73-75]

The mass media generally did not even seriously examine the difficulty associated with declaring a "war against terrorism," which is so unlike a traditional war. "Unlike most wars, [counterterrorism] has neither a fixed set of enemies nor the prospect of coming to closure, be it through a 'win' or some other kind of denouement. Like the cold war, it requires long, patient, persistent effort, but unlike it, it will never conclude with the internal collapse of an opponent. There will be victories and defeats, but not big, tide-turning victories. Counterterrorism is a fight and a struggle, but it is not a campaign with a beginning and an end" (p. 217–8).[51]

### Alternatives to Military Strikes

Supporters of military frames typically cast potential responses to threats as "battles" (or "epic struggles") that must be won. "This pattern has been most apparent with U.S. policies toward state sponsors of terrorism, in which unyielding hard lines have sometimes been favored over strategies of engagement that—although they might be better suited to elicit further improvements in behavior from the states involved—are avoided as being soft on terrorism" (p. 6).[51]

The French cultural theorist, Jean Baudrillard, an exponent of postmodernism in popular culture, coined the expression "hyperreality" to convey the idea that mass media have saturated everyone's outer world, and colonized everyone's inner world, with endless commodities in the form of information, ideas, images, sounds, and other objects. The prefix "hyper" suggests that the mediated reality is "more real than real" (p. 108–9, 157–8).[76] In essence, the media framed both the September 11 attacks and the war in Afghanistan as hyperreal events.

This focus on the hyperreal typically means the media can cover only one conflict at a time, and they generally focus on only the violent phases of that one conflict. This means "the media are largely responsible for the absence of [other] conflicts from the public agenda or the policy agenda, and major conflicts (and the massive amount of human suffering that they entail) will be ignored" (p. 233).[77] The media thus help "to shift focus and funds from more cost-effective, long-term efforts directed at preventing violent conflict and rebuilding war-torn societies to short-term emergency relief" (p. 132).[78]

Had they consulted some unofficial sources, journalists might have benefited from the work of specialists inside and outside the academy. "In the terminology of systems theory," Bernhard Debatin argues, "there was a lack of exchange of information among the scientific system, the political system, and the media system" (p. 171).[79] The news media did not serve as an effective bridge between the political system and the academic/scholarly community, as they frequently do in other potential conflict situations, such as that of the political system and the medical/professional community.

The media might have learned, and reported to their audiences, for example, that it can be extraordinarily helpful to view terrorism as a kind of communicable disease. Within that context, counterterrorism "deals with threats that come in many different forms, some more virulent than others. Some of the threats are waxing; some are waning. Some are old; others are very new" (p. 218).[51] Journalists might also have discovered much about the language they use, for as Murray Edelman notes, "the connections among misleading language, public opinion, and public policy are powerful, though subtle. Language itself does not create errors in belief and in governmental action. But it can play powerfully on established prejudices, spread biases to a wider population, and make them compelling elements in formulating public policy. It does so all the more effectively because the role of language as itself a form of political action is not readily recognized" (p. 239).[29]

Some journalists allowed themselves to be used by those who wanted to stifle dissent about the military strikes. "[T]he call for patriotism and counterstrike led very quickly to a situation in which critical words were stigmatized by the government as unpatriotic and intolerable, even when they were clearly satirical" (p. 173–4).[79] Brigitte Nacos correctly notes:

As laudable as the we-are-all-in-this-together contributions of the media were in many respects, by dwelling endlessly on the outburst of patriotism and the idea of national unity without paying attention to other important matters in the political realm, the media helped to create an atmosphere in which criticism of the various crisis-related policy initiatives in Washington was mostly absent from the mass-mediated public debate. When people like Attorney General John Ashcroft questioned the patriotism of those on the right and left of the political spectrum who were critical of some aspects of his anti- and counterterrorist policy proposals, there was not a massive outcry in the media on behalf of civil liberties—most of all freedom of expression (p. 195).[22]

Conflict journalism clearly dominated during the three-week buildup to the military attacks. As in other contexts, conflict journalism focused on violence and its effects and on tangible institutions and results.[48] Localized teach-ins, socials, peace walks, petitions, rallies, and public protests across the country seeking to focus public attention on the injustice of bombing Afghanistan were essentially ignored by the mass media or rendered ineffective and counterproductive in the crusade against terrorism. Patriotic support for the military option was mandated by the media for weeks. Virtually all other alternatives were ridiculed, ignored, or otherwise marginalized—opening the window of opportunity for the Bush administration in its ongoing effort to market the war against terrorism.[80]

### Negotiating Semantic Extremes

The answer to this study's second research question—whether media relied on binary oppositions or explored the semantic space between the extremes as they framed their responses to the September 11 attacks—is equally clear. The answer is the former. Journalists most assuredly employed binary oppositions to construct the war frame. These professionals are educated to explore the semantic space between polar opposites, but they ignored this injunction in depicting social reality after September 11.

In using binary oppositions to support violence, President Bush argued: "You are either with us or with the terrorists." For him, and for the media that uncritically reported his remark, there was no middle ground. "You" could not be neutral. If "you" did not support violence as part of the U.S. response, "you" were with the terrorists.

If one lines up these binary signs in rows and columns (see figure 6.2), one has essentially established the roots of the stereotype for (non-Western) violence and (Western) nonviolence. Columns to the left provide a normative framework that the ordinary person might associate

| Terrorists | Non-terrorists | Terrorists | Non-terrorists | Terrorists | Non-terrorists |
|---|---|---|---|---|---|
| Abnormal | Normal | Fearful | Secure | Radical | Moderate |
| Aggressive | Defensive | Foreign | Domestic | Repression | Freedom |
| Apathetic | Energetic | Guilty | Innocent | Snake | Human |
| Barbaric | Civilized | Hate | Love | Stupid | Wise |
| Bin Laden | Bush | Headstrong | Deliberate | Terrorist | Insurgent |
| Brutal | Kind | Illogical | Logical | Them | Us |
| Chaos | Order | Imitation | Original | Tribal | Individual |
| Coward | Hero | Inhumane | Humane | Uneducated | Educated |
| Darkness | Light | Insect | Human | Unhealthy | Healthy |
| Death | Life | Irrational | Rational | Unjust | Just |
| Defeat | Victory | Lower | Higher | Unskilled | Skilled |
| Enemy | Ally | Murder | Preservation | Vicious | Kind |
| Evil | Good | Muslim | Christian | Violent | Peaceful |
| Exterminate | Preserve | Non-Christian | Christian | War | Peace |
| Extreme | Moderate | Poor | Rich | Warlike | Peace-loving |
| Fanatic | Tolerant | Profane | Sacred | Weak | Strong |

**Figure 6.2**
**Binary Words Used in Framing the Military Response**

with the terrorist, and columns to the right provide the normative framework that the ordinary person might associate with the nonterrorist.

This dichotomous discourse presumes a stable linguistic framework because it seeks to secure fixed, particular readings of news texts in which the meaning of nonviolence (nonterrorist) is placed in simple opposition to the meaning of violence (terrorist). This is the world in which everyday discourse about the "war against terrorism" can easily segue into "us" (civilized American Christians) versus "them" (foreign, and therefore uncivilized, Muslim terrorists)—in newspapers, on talk radio, on television, and even in the pulpit.

The binary model is condemned for fostering a false sense of stability and unity in language. Critics argue that, "we live, think and act in terms of concepts that are historically obsolete" (p. 255).[81] Society needs "a pluralism of content to reflect the diversity and complexity of the world"—a "peace journalism" that embraces the new global era (p. 58).[82]

## Shutting the Window of Opportunity

What one often refers to as "reality" or thinks of as "truth" is found not in binary signs, but in the semantic space people negotiate between these signs. Journalists are quite capable of exploring this space, but they failed in the case of the war against terrorism.

The window available to journalists to explore violence as an option was open for roughly three weeks—between September 11 and October 8, when the United States attacked Afghanistan. If journalists wanted to explore the ground between the binary extremes, they would have looked seriously at the terrorists—where they came from, what their grievances were, and why they considered political violence their final option. "Understanding the enemy is very crucial because only then can we prepare creative, reasonable, and just responses. But I think that as long as you have an image of the enemy, you can't make a distinction between reaction and responding. We *do* have to respond, and we *do* have to seek justice, but a reaction is not a response—it's unthinking" (p. 125).[83]

Journalists were most comfortable in maintaining the image of a binary world in which the choice was either "attack militarily" or "do nothing." The complexities were not addressed. Only one outcome seemed possible. Like the culture they represented, journalists essentially ignored the vast middle ground. The dominant political discourse skillfully used xenophobia, religious fervor, fear, and patriotism to market, through the media of mass communication, a "total war" to ensure the American way of life would be protected. In essence, journalists helped sell violence in the war against terrorism.

The media narrative—mirroring the Bush narrative—was all about evil, and America's crusade stance was certainly understood by the majority of Americans in the aftermath of September 11. The religious symbolism was apparent to many Americans as they attended worship services on October 8, 2001, the day the bombs fell on Afghanistan—World Communion Day. This is the one day in the calendar year when Christians throughout the world sit down together and celebrate Eucharist in a symbolic act of unity and peace.

# NOTES

1. Houston M, Kramarae C. Speaking from silence: methods of silencing and of resistance. Discourse Soc 1991;2(4):387–99.

2. Kissling EA. Street harassment: the language of sexual terrorism. Discourse Soc 1991;2(4):451–60.

3. Goddard CR, Stanley JR. Viewing the abusive parent and the abused child as captor and hostage: the application of hostage theory to the effects of child abuse. J Interpers Violence 1994;9(2):258–69.

4. Graham-Kevan N, Archer J. Intimate terrorism and common couple violence: a test of Johnson's predictions in four British samples. J Interpers Violence 2003;18(11):1247–70.

5. Husselbee LP, Elliott L. Looking beyond hate: how national and regional newspapers framed hate crimes in Jaspar, Texas, and Laramie, Wyoming. J Mass Commun Q 2002;79(4):833–52.

6. Petrosino C. Connecting the past to the future: hate crime in America. J Contemp Crim Justice 1999;15(1):22–47.

7. Spitzberg BH, Hoobler G. Cyberstalking and the technologies of interpersonal terrorism. New Media Soc 2002;4(1):71–92.

8. Criminologists have noted parallels between "the dynamics of crime and the desire to punish" and "criminal violence and the violence of the state." This is an argument against employing binary language that positions the socially inclusive "citizen" against the criminally exclusive "underclass"—a form of terrorism [e.g., Young J. Merton with energy, Katz with structure: the sociology of vindictiveness and the criminology of transgression. Theor Criminol 2003;7(3):389–414.].

9. Schwartz DM. Environmental terrorism: analyzing the concept. J Peace Res 1998;35(4):483–96.

10. The term "state terrorism" is difficult to personalize and is open to varied interpretations—especially from the U.S. perspective. Nevertheless, state terrorism is recognized as an acute form of political terrorism. It was present in the past—as in Islamic Asia's response to colonialism [e.g., Dale SF. Religious suicide in Islamic Asia: anticolonial terrorism in India, Indonesia, and the Philippines. J Confl Resolution 1998;32(1):37–59.]; in Stalin's Soviet Union [e.g., Grossman PZ. The dilemma of prisoners: choice during Stalin's great terror, 1936–38. J Confl Resolution 1994;38(1):43–55.]; and in Nazi Germany [e.g., Westermann EB. The Holocaust course at the United States Air Force Academy. Ann Am Acad Pol Soc Sci 1996 Nov;548:116–22.]. And it is present today—in countries like El Salvador [e.g., Taylor RW, Vanden HE. Defining terrorism in El Salvador: "La Matanza." Ann Am Acad Pol Soc Sci 1982 Sep;463:106–18.]; Colombia [e.g., Bibes P. Transnational organized crime and terrorism: Colombia, a case study. J Contemp Crim Justice 2001;17(3):243–58.]; Guatemala [e.g., Davenport C, Ball P. Views to a kill: exploring the implications of source

selection in the case of Guatemalan state terror, 1977–1995. J Confl Resolution 2002;46(3):427–50.]; Iran [e.g., Mozaffari M, Why the bazar rebels. J Peace Res 1991;28(4):377–91.]; and in the ongoing Israeli–Palestinian conflict. The term "state terrorism," moreover, has many other dimensions. The U.S.-imposed sanctions against Iraq after the 1990–1991 Persian Gulf War, for example, was by most accounts a disaster for the Iraqi people—and, for the victims and their Muslim sympathizers, a classic example of state terrorism. According to the United Nations, the embargo alone resulted in more than 1.2 million deaths. In the southern and central parts of Iraq, children under five were dying in 1999 at more than twice the rate they were a decade earlier [UNICEF. Iraq surveys show "humanitarian emergency." [News release]. 1999 Aug 12. Available from www.unicef.org/newsline/ 99pr29.htm. Accessed November 28, 2003.].

11. Whitbeck JV. More danger lurks if we allow U.S. to define meaning of "terrorism." Houston Chronicle 2002 Mar 17;Sect. C:1, C5.

12. Bulliet RW. Rhetoric, discourse, and the future of hope. Ann Am Acad Pol Soc Sci 2003 Jul;588:10–7.

13. U.S. Department of State. State Department adds three groups to foreign terrorist list. [News release]. 2002 March 27. Available from: usinfo.state.gov/ topical/pol/terror/02032701.htm. Accessed November 29, 2003.

14. Muslim nations fail to define terrorism: conferees absolve Palestinians of blame. Houston Chronicle 2003 Apr 3; Sect. A:19.

15. National Advisory Committee on Criminal Justice Standards and Goals. Report of the task force on disorders and terrorism. Washington DC: United States Government Printing Office; 1976.

16. Wilkinson P. Terrorism and propaganda. In: Alexander Y, Latter R, editors. Terrorism & the media: dilemmas for government, journalists & the public. Washington DC: Brassey's; 1990. p. 26–33.

17. Lule J. Myth and terror in the editorial page: The New York Times responds to September 11, 2001. J Mass Commun Q 2002;79(2):275–93.

18. Bell JB. Terrorist scripts and live-action spectaculars. Columbia J Rev 1978 May/June;17(1):47–50.

19. Dowling RE. Terrorism and the media: a rhetorical genre. J Commun 1986;36(1):12–24.

20. Fromkin D. The strategy of terrorism. In: Elliot JD, Gibson LK, editors. Contemporary terrorism: selected readings. Gaithersburg, MD: International Association of Chiefs of Police; 1978. p. 11–24.

21. Laqueur W. Terrorism makes a tremendous noise. Across Board 1978 Jan;15(1):57–67.

22. Nacos BL. Mass-mediated terrorism: the central role of the media in terrorism and counterterrorism. Lanham, MD: Rowman & Littlefield; 2002.

23. Dietz P. The media and weapons of mass hysteria. Undated. Available from: www.facsnet.org/issues/specials/terrorism/dietz.php3. Accessed November 1, 2003.

24. Dreyfus R. Domestic antiterrorism measures may endanger civil liberties. In: Young M, editor. The war on terrorism. San Diego: Greenhaven; 2003. p. 109–17.

25. Zakariah F. Freedom vs. security. In: Young M, editor. The war on terrorism. San Diego: Greenhaven; 2003. p. 118–129.

26. Tuchman G. Making news: a study in the construction of reality. New York: Free Press; 1978.

27. Entman RM. Framing: toward clarification of a fractured paradigm. J Commun 1993;43(4):51–8.

28. Gamson WA. News as framing: comments on Graber. Am Behav Sci 1989;33(2):157–61.

29. Edelman M. Contestable categories and public opinion. Pol Commun 1993;10(3):231–42.

30. Iyengar S. Framing responsibility for political issues. Ann Am Acad Pol Soc Sci 1996 Jul;546:59–70.

31. Switzer L, McNamara J, Ryan M. Critical-cultural studies in research and instruction. J Mass Commun Educ 1999;54(3):23–42.

32. Durham FD. Breaching powerful boundaries: a postmodern critique of framing. In: Reese SD, Gandy OH Jr, Grant AE, editors. Framing public life: perspectives on media and our understanding of the social world. Mahwah, NJ: Lawrence Erlbaum; 2001. p. 123–36.

33. Gitlin T. The whole world is watching: mass media in the making and unmaking of the new left. Berkeley: University of California Press; 1980.

34. Lind RA, Salo C. The framing of feminists and feminism in news and public affairs programs in U.S. electronic media. J Commun 2002;52(1):211–28.

35. Carter C, Weaver CK. Violence and the media. Buckingham, England: Open University Press; 2003.

36. Catmur WB. Theatre of war: high culture and popular entertainment in the spectacle of Kosovo. Javnost Public 2000;7(3):67–75.

37. Hrvatin SB, Trampuz M. Enjoy your enemy or how the Kosovo (media) war broke out. Javnost Public 2000;7(3):77–85.

38. Shaheen JG. Reel bad Arabs: how Hollywood vilifies a people. New York: Olive Branch; 2001.

39. Fuglsang RS. Framing the motorcycle outlaw. In: Reese SD, Gandy OH Jr, Grant AE, editors. Framing public life: perspectives on media and our understanding of the social world. Mahwah, NJ: Lawrence Erlbaum; 2001. p. 185–94.

40. Shah DV, Domke D, Wachman DB. The effects of value-framing on political judgment and reasoning. In: Reese SD, Gandy OH Jr, Grant AE, editors. Framing public life: perspectives on media and our understanding of the social world. Mahwah, NJ: Lawrence Erlbaum; 2001. p. 227–43.

41. Bird SE, Dardenne RW. Myth, chronicle, and story: exploring the narrative qualities of news. In: Carey JW, editor. Media, myths, and narratives: television and the press. Newbury Park, CA: Sage; 1988. p. 67–86.

42. Gurevitch M, Levy MR. Introduction. In: Gurevitch M, Levy MR, editors. Mass communication yearbook. Beverly Hills, CA: Sage; 1985. p. 11–22. (vol 5).

43. Norris P. Introduction. In: Norris P, editor. Women, media, and politics. New York: Oxford University Press; 1997. p. 1–18.

44. Gamson WA. Talking politics. Cambridge, England: Cambridge University Press; 1992.

45. De Saussure is very influential in various branches of critical-cultural theory—in linguistics, literary studies, social anthropology, psychology/ psychiatry, history, and in other disciplines in the human sciences [De Saussure F. Course in general linguistics. In: Bally C, Sechehaye A, editors. Harris R, translator. London: Duckworth; 1983.]. His ideas were developed and revised by various scholars—such as Claude Lèvi-Strauss (anthropology), Jacques Lacan (psychology/psychiatry), and Roland Barthes (linguistics/semiology).

46. Costain AN, Braunstein R, Berggren H. Framing the women's movement. In: Norris P, editor. Women, media, and politics. New York: University of Oxford Press; 1997. p. 205–20.

47. Picard RG, Adams PD. Characterizations of acts and perpetrators of political violence in three elite U.S. daily newspapers. In: Alali AO, Eke KK, editors. Media coverage of terrorism: methods of diffusion. Newbury Park, CA: Sage; 1991. p. 12–22.

48. Fawcett L. Why peace journalism isn't news. J Stud 2002;3(2):213–23.

49. Wolfsfeld G. Media and political conflict: news from the Middle East. Cambridge, England: Cambridge University Press; 1997.

50. Miller MM, Riechert BP. The spiral of opportunity and frame resonance: mapping the issue cycle in news and public discourse. In: Reese SD, Gandy OH Jr, Grant AE, editors. Framing public life: perspectives on media and our understanding of the social world. Mahwah, NJ: Lawrence Erlbaum; 2001. p. 107–21.

51. Pillar PR. Terrorism and U.S. foreign policy. Washington, DC: Brookings; 2001.

52. Rielly JE, editor. American public opinion and U.S. foreign policy, 1999. Chicago: Chicago Council on Foreign Relations; 1999. p. 15.

53. Malvesti ML. Explaining the United States' decision to strike back at terrorists. Terrorism Pol Violence 2001;13(2):85–106.

54. Kellner D. September 11, the media, and war fever. Telev New Media 2002;3(2):143–51.

55. Coulter A. This is war: we should invade their countries. Natl Rev Online [serial online] 2001 Sep 13: Available from: www.nationalreview.com/ coulter/coulter091301.shtml. Accessed November 28, 2003.

56. Philo G. Television news and audience understanding of war, conflict and disaster. J Stud 2002;3(2):173–86.

57. Thussu DK. Managing the media in an era of round-the-clock news: notes from India's first tele-war. J Stud 2002;3(2):203–12.

58. Nord LW, Strömbäck J. Making sense of different types of crises: a study of the Swedish media coverage of the terror attacks against the United States and the U.S. attacks in Afghanistan. Harv Int J Press Pol 2003;8(4):54–75.

59. Louw PE. The "War against Terrorism": a public relations challenge for the Pentagon. Gaz 2003;65(3):211–30.

60. Weimann G, Brosius H-B. The newsworthiness of international terrorism. Commun Res 1991;18(3):333–54.

61. Mogensen K, Lindsay L, Li X, Perkins J, Beardsley M. How TV news covered the crisis: the content of CNN, CBS, ABC, NBC and Fox. In: Greenberg BS, editor. Communication and terrorism: public and media responses to 9/11. Cresskill, NJ: Hampton; 2002. p. 101–20.

62. Kitch C. "Mourning in America": ritual, redemption, and recovery in news narrative after September 11. J Stud 2003;4(2):213–24.

63. Hart WB II, Hassencahl F. Dehumanizing the enemy in editorial cartoons. In: Greenberg BS, editor. Communication and terrorism: public and media responses to 9/11. Cresskill, NJ: Hampton; 2002. p. 137–51.

64. Ryan M. Framing the war against terrorism: U.S. newspaper editorials and military action in Afghanistan. Gaz 2004;66(5):363–82.

65. Devine PE, Rafalko RJ. On terror. Ann Am Acad Pol Soc Sci 1982 Sep;463:39–53.

66. Brennan B, Duffy M. "If a problem cannot be solved, enlarge it": an ideological critique of the "other" in Pearl Harbor and September 11 New York Times coverage. J Stud 2003;4(1):3–14.

67. Another kind of war. USA Today 2001 Sep 18; Sect. A:23.

68. The climate of paranoia that the media helped to construct has reached the point that Muslim citizens in the United States must be careful about what they say and do at school, at university, at work, in travel and recreational pursuits, and at worship. Indeed, the literature about the demonization of the non-Western "other" was growing long before the September 11 attacks, especially in academic circles. A pioneering study in support of this argument was written by Edward Said [Said EW. Orientalism. New York: Pantheon; 1978.]. Said poses dichotomous stereotypes of the "Orient" and the "Occident," both Western terms, in the nineteenth and twentieth centuries. This binary discourse positions the Oriental as "inferior" to the Occidental in every way— from religion to behavior. Orientalism is the Westerner's modus operandi for maintaining power by "dominating, restructuring and having authority over the Orient." This book helped to shape the modern understanding of state terrorism in the context of the Middle East (another Western term)—long before September 11.

69. Uricchio W. Television conventions. Telev Arch [serial online]. 2001 Sep 16. Available from: tvnews3.televisionarchive.org/tvarchive/html/article_wu1.html. Accessed November 1, 2003.

70. Mr. Bush's most important speech. The New York Times 2001 Sep 21;Sect. A:34.

71. The war against terrorism: U.S. must push for global alliance against terrorism. Newsday 2001 Sep 16;Sect. B:1.

72. Total barbarism demands total war. New York Daily News 2001 Sep 15; Sect. Editorial:40.

73. Jensen R. U.S. just as guilty of committing own violent acts. Houston Chronicle 2001 Sep 14;Sect. A:33.

74. Switzer L, Ryan M. What Christians should do: reconsider revenge. Houston Chronicle 2001 Oct 5;Sect. A:39.

75. Sontag S. Comment: Tuesday, and after. New Yorker 2001 Sep 24; 77(28):32.

76. Barker C. Cultural studies: theory and practice. Thousand Oaks, CA: Sage; 2000.

77. Hawkins V. The other side of the CNN factor: the media and conflict. J Stud 2002;3(2):225–40.

78. Jakobsen PV. Focus on the CNN effect misses the point: the real media impact on conflict management is invisible and direct. J Peace Res 2000; 37(2):131–43.

79. Debatin B. "Plane wreck with spectators": terrorism and media attention. In: Greenberg BS, editor. Communication and terrorism: public and media responses to 9/11. Cresskill, NJ: Hampton; 2002. p. 163–74.

80. Konner J. Media's patriotism provides a shield for Bush. The personal is political [serial online]. 2002 Jan 9. Available from: www.margieadam.com/action/konner.htm. Accessed November 30, 2003.

81. Beck U. The silence of words: on terror and war. Secur Dialogue 2003; 34(3):255–67.

82. Tehranian M. Peace journalism: negotiating global media ethics. Harv Int J Press Pol 2002;7(2):58–83.

83. Keen S. The new face of the enemy. In: Beliefnet, editor. From the ashes: a spiritual response to the attack on America. Emmaus, PA: Rodale; 2001. p. 122–6.

# 7  Community Right-to-Know vs. Terrorists' Exploitation of Public Information

*Robert L. Heath, David B. McKinney, and Michael J. Palenchar*

Throughout this three-volume series on community preparedness and communication response to terrorism, risk-management and communication theories play an integral role in the analysis, understanding, and improvement of communication systems. The value of an approach rooted in narrative theory and risk communication lies in its ability to assist in analysis of content and development of a community infrastructure that promotes meaning cocreation process among individuals and organizations threatened by terrorist actions. This effort to cocreate meaning may mitigate or at least respond to such crises.

Risk assessment, risk management, risk abatement, and risk communication are timeless facets of human existence. Indeed, Mary Douglas reasons that risk management and control is perhaps the most fundamental rationale humans have for creating, organizing, and maintaining society.[1] History is an ongoing drama in which people assess, communicate about, creatively prevent, and accommodate risks.[2]

Occupations are created to serve specific risk-management and control functions. Police, fire, and hazardous-material handlers, and medical-treatment personnel are among the more obvious. Within industry, operations and maintenance workers, occupational safety experts, and environmental and risk-management specialists are at the front line. However, the list can include all professions. For example, teachers prepare children to manage risks as adults. Likewise, the clergy deals with the management of risks, including creation, death, birth, eternity, and faith. In fact, risk management affects an all-encompassing range of social affiliations, including governmental and nongovernmental organizations, scientific and technical organizations, corporations, environmental groups, and private health and safety organizations.

Ancient civilizations developed many means to forecast hazards and predict the outcomes of risks. Sometimes these calculations had a scientific basis, and at other times they were steeped in mysteries beyond empirical observation. The origins of risk analysis have been traced back to at least the Babylonians in 3200 BC. Our human ancestors used rituals, myths, symbols, and metaphors to predict risks and to communicate knowledge needed to accommodate or avoid hazards.[3] They developed narratives to explain, predict, manage, and cope with a variety of risks. Some of these risks were natural, such as earthquakes and storms. Others were man-made, such as war and political strife. Most were poorly understood.

Techniques for assessing, managing, and responding to risks have matured since the time of the ancients, in some ways only a little and in others, quite substantially.[1] What Fischhoff noted twenty years ago holds true today: Much of risk management involves going beyond the available empirical data either to guess at what the facts might be or to figure out how to live with the uncertainty of the risk.[4] One can argue that throughout history, the societies, cultures, and even individual bands of people that survived did so because they were capable of managing risks.

Today, risks are great. Advances in science have led to an increase in the number of fields that require risk management and risk-communication initiatives. New fields such as biogenetics, social changes like increased travel, and industrial advances like petrochemical and other specialty chemical manufacturing, to name a few, all require risk assessment, as well as political and social discussions of risk-communication procedures. New developments, such as nanotechnology, alternate energy sources, virtual surgery, and advanced space travel, only increase the importance of sophisticated risk-management and risk-communication processes.

Since 9/11, significant thought, discussion, and planning has focused on reducing the risks of a successful terrorist attack. One of the risks that looms on the horizon is the possibility that terrorism launched against some person, organization, or state can change established risk equations. Just within the first few years of the twenty-first century, terrorism has caused wars and other socio-political-economic changes. The most obvious form of terrorism with this effect is the slaying of a head of state or other notable figure, or a high-profile attack against iconic structures, communities, gatherings, or means of mass transportation.

Sometimes death falls on a segment of a society targeted for criminal attack. Attacks against property abound. Devastating capabilities, such as weapons of mass destruction, suggest the importance of knowing, preventing, and responding to local, national, and international terrorism.

This chapter combines the experiences and insights of risk assessors, risk responders and risk communicators. It blends best practices derived from industrial experiences with a review of the academic and government literature. The chapter assumes that the dynamics of risk assessment and response are changing to focus on detecting risks, implementing appropriate measures to prevent specific risk situations from occurring in the first place, and reducing the magnitude of their consequences after they have occurred. In this context, a risk situation could be an attack on a chemical manufacturing and gasoline refinery complex, including storage facilities, transfer terminals and transportation centers, any of which might operate near residential neighborhoods. Other risk scenarios include the threat of cyberterrorism, economic espionage, and the misuse of chemical products by terrorists. At risk is the destruction of property, the disruption of an economy, and the harm, or even death, of workers and area citizens. The safety of people and their property rests on the shoulders of risk assessors, risk responders, and risk communicators. Such risks pose challenges in crisis planning and response that demanding thoughtful, ethical, and effective professional responses.

The purpose of this chapter is to draw upon the practical and strategic insights of experts on community relations, as well as academic sources, to explore some of the best practices and challenges of responsible emergency management and risk communication in an industrial setting. Professionals in security and communication are among the many who are dedicated to helping society manage risks. However subtle and debatable the principles surrounding terrorism might be, such professionals have a responsibility to protect, to the best of their ability, the lives and well-being of citizens and employees, as well as the financial health of industrial operations, and of the community as a whole. Such professionals work within constraints of law; corporate policy; community policy; and local, state, and federal policy to navigate the safest route for the groups they serve.

Terrorism poses substantial risk-management challenges to such professionals. Statistically, the worst-case scenario is least likely to happen. Plant facilities that rely on security and communications professionals are an ideal, yet difficult target of attack. Yet if such an attack were attempted, how prepared would they be to prevent, mitigate, and respond to the attack in a responsible manner? What communication and security challenges have had to be readdressed in the months following the 9/11 attack? What changes in planning, policy, and procedures have occurred? What does the future hold? These topics are not only addressed in a practical sense but also are framed in terms of narrative theory and research based on principles of risk and crisis communication.

## ORIGINS OF COMMUNITY RIGHT-TO-KNOW

Chemical manufacturing and oil refining are key elements in the American lifestyle and economy, and also critical to the nation's infrastructure. The chemical industry is a $460 billion enterprise, with more than one million workers in the United States, producing more than 70,000 different products. It is the nation's largest exporter, accounting for approximately 10 percent of U.S. exports. Chemical companies invest more in research and development than any other private business sector, accounting for one in every seven patents awarded each year in the United States.[5]

Activists and other interests have singled out such industries for criticism in the past, but in the post-9/11 atmosphere, security professionals realized that their roles had changed in both dramatic and subtle ways.[6] In the past, working with government officials, health and safety personnel, and risk management and risk communication professionals, as well as lay persons, the chemical industry developed philosophies based on the principles of community right-to-know and risk democracy that might need revisiting. They had security, but after 9/11, many felt the need to address whether those measures were sufficient to protect against a sophisticated network of terrorists who might target the industry because of its political, strategic, and symbolic importance.

The philosophy of community right-to-know began to change dramatically in the mid-1980s, after a toxic methyl isocyanate gas release in Bhopal, India, at a Union Carbide India facility, killed more than 3,800 nearby community residents and plant workers. (The exact death toll remains under debate, with some casualty estimates reaching into tens of thousands, when long-term health consequences are included.) After this incident, the U.S. government became deeply involved in chemical-related risk assessment, mitigation, and communication processes. The Bhopal tragedy, along with other energy-related crises such as Chernobyl, Love Canal, Three Mile Island, and *Exxon Valdez*, caused citizens to worry that similar risks loomed near their homes or workplaces.

Prior to these iconic events, an unconcerned public and injudicious regulatory climate was the norm. For example, before the Three Mile Island accident, concerned local residents at hearings were barred from raising questions about evacuation plans in case of an emergency. Risk assessors and hearings officials had determined that a serious accident as virtually impossible.[7] "The partial meltdown of Unit 2 in 1979, however, undermined the credibility of the organizations responsible for such probability estimates while also serving as a major catalyst in transforming a previously docile and trusting population into antinuclear activists."[7] Activists of all sorts sought to compel changes in the industry. The events in Bhopal, and at other chemical manufacturing, transportation, and storage facilities, awakened a complacent public and fueled the arguments of many community activists.

Immediately after the Union Carbide tragedy in Bhopal, Rosenblatt observed, "If the world felt especially close to Bhopal last week, it may be because the world is Bhopal, a place where the occupational hazard is modern life."[8,9] The historical realities of risk management as the essence of society became front-page and top-of-the-hour news hooks. Worries that what happened in India could happen in many communities in the United States prompted federal legislators to create the Emergency Planning and Community Right-to-Know Act of 1986, section three of the Superfund Amendments and Reauthorization Act of 1986 (SARA). This legislation mandated each state's governor to appoint members to a State Emergency Response Commission (SERC), which in turn created local emergency-planning committees (LEPCs). This act gave the Environmental Protection Agency (EPA) the power to mandate the formation of LEPCs throughout the country.

LEPCs are required to create four programs: emergency planning and response, emergency notification, right-to-know, and emissions inventory. Specifically, LEPCs were designed to plan for manufacturing-related emergencies, but they were also intended to provide information to nearby residents, government officials, industry representatives, health and safety officials, and any other concerned individuals and organizations, and to serve as a forum where such individuals and groups could voice concerns. Legislators believed SARA, along with LEPCs, would create a communication apparatus and strategic business-planning process to empower people to air concerns about risks that threaten them.

Among other outcomes, this federal initiative was intended to increase the flow of various kinds of technical information from experts to lay persons and to open channels of commentary between them. It is also likely that another motive for the legislation was to pressure industry to adopt and implement even higher standards of community and employee safety.

In response to this initiative, the chemical industry became more proactive, undertaking what it called its Responsible CAER (Community Awareness and Emergency Response) program, which will be discussed in more detail in a later section. The Responsible CAER program includes the formation of community advisory committees (CAC) (sometimes called community advisory panels). CACs are intended to serve as forums for public dialogue about risk identification, assessment, and reduction.

Research has led to mixed reviews of LEPCs' ability to communicate environmental information to citizens. Heath and Abel and Heath and Palenchar have found that proactive communication on the part of LEPCs can increase awareness of emergency-response practices among community residents.[10] Such groups add to the public's knowledge and use of emergency response practices. At the same time, Heath, Bradshaw and Lee discovered that the public lacks awareness of the existence of LEPCs and CACs. As a result, use of such organizations is low, in spite of the fact that more than two-thirds of the residents surveyed approved of their intended functions. Additionally, the study showed that these organizations played a limited role in communication activities in communities that lack local city government. Overall, their findings suggest that "a fully functioning communication infrastructure leads to a healthier community that responds to risks as manageable uncertainties. Infrastructures that can exert little control and are weak cannot be corrected simply by the creation of such committees as the LEPCs and CACs."[11]

These federal and industry initiatives raised several central issues, including how best to understand and control risks, as well as how to gain acceptance for those measures that foster the most favorable outcomes in any community of multiple, and potentially conflicting interests.[12] Industry took this as an opportunity to increase the willingness of relevant communities to support its presence, through Responsible Care. If part of the incentive of the government policy was to divide industry from community and to reduce community support for the industrial activities then that measured outcome needed to be central to the planning and operations of companies as a proactive solution to the community friction.

Risk management is not a new principle to engineers, managers, security personnel, and communication specialists. Although the term has become increasingly popular in management discussions, the concern is timeless. Sound professionals don't want employees, area residents, capital equipment, and manufacturing processes to be harmed. As a technical concept, risk is conventionally defined as something that can be given a numerical value by multiplying the probability of an outcome, typically one with negative consequences, with its severity. This expectancy value is used to estimate and compare risks that are perceived differently depending on the heuristics and biases each person uses to judge them.[13,14]

The EPA (1988) has characterized its safety, health, and community outreach initiatives under SARA in noble terms. The legislation, it suggests, "creates a new relationship among government at all levels, business and community leaders, environmental and other public-interest organizations, and individual citizens. For the first time, the law makes citizens full partners in preparing for emergencies and managing chemical risks."[15] This implied definition of risk management suggests that success comes when the people who fear the risks are informed about them, and feel confident that government and industry can control them. In other words, industry must responsibly exert controls in the public interest. The absence of such controls will fuel outcry from community activists, and damage the credibility of industry.

This state of affairs can be traced to the fact that SARA was driven by politics. It was aimed to force a standard of operating excellence on an industry thought by its critics to be indifferent to the interests of employees and people who live in the shadows of its industrial operations. These critics advocated for the interests of people who might meet with catastrophe through manufacturing explosions, derailed trains, exploding pipelines, and overturned trucks hauling explosive or hazardous materials. Reviewing the right-to-know provision for the Public Relations Society of America, Newman concludes, "The theory behind these toxic laws is that this information will not only help answer citizen questions about [chemical] releases, but will also assist them in pressuring government and industry to correct practices that threaten their health and environment."[16] Understanding the nature and impact of a source of risk is not the only factor involved in risk assessment, management, and communication. Another factor is power—a rhetorical struggle by parties engaged in negotiating levels of risk and standards of regulative or legislative control.

The fundamental elements of managing risk, including the risk of terrorism, in an industrial setting include the following: imagining potential risks, reducing their likelihood, mitigating the opportunities for attack, minimizing the consequences should one occur, and responding responsibly to citizens in harm's way. Terrorism in such settings can take many forms. Fundamental to each form is the risk of criminal behavior against property and human safety. One of the quintessential examples of risk management and industrial terrorism occurred when one or more persons, still unknown, tampered with Tylenol capsules in 1982. This person or persons terrorized residents in Chicago and around the nation by lacing extra strength Tylenol capsules with cyanide. People were afraid to use the drug for fear of drawing one of the poisoned capsules. Seven people had died by the end of the crisis.

Terrorism can have many faces, however. It can range from religious and culturally based hatreds to less intellectually or ideologically motivated criminal acts against a company, customers, and products. In one sense, the perpetrator of the Tylenol poisonings did not fit the operating definition of a terrorist, in that the motives for the acts remained unknown. The murders were committed for some reason. Perhaps the motives were more personal than philosophical. As is discussed elsewhere in this book, terrorists seem bent on advocating a cause as a vital and instrumental part of their actions. The person(s) who tampered with the Tylenol capsules may have been deranged or cleverly bent on committing a cleverly conceived murder. There seems to be no larger motive, but the sense of terror in the nation was nevertheless substantial. The Tylenol tragedy serves as an iconic case demonstrating how vulnerable a company can be, despite its vigilance and proactivity. However strategic the perpetrator of such crimes might be, from the company's perspective it is merely a matter of chance that such an event occurred when it did and with the consequences that followed.

In other words, such acts are like a game of cat and mouse. A crisis can be defined as a predictable event—but the timing of such events is unpredictable, and it is here that the element of risk comes into play. What can be done to compromise the security of products, services, and operations? Who will be harmed? What will be the magnitude of the harm? Such questions come to the forefront in security planning and communication planning. What is the responsible level of security, given that absolute security is impossible? What warning information should be shared with the community and employees? How can they be warned and know that response planning is in place without creating undue insecurity? How can we guard against complacency? Given the narrative of specific terrorists strategies and intents, how likely are we to need to be more alert, more secure? Terrorism of the kind that surfaced on 9/11 brought up new concerns and revitalized old ones. These concerns must be addressed in terms of the philosophy, principles, and operations of community right-to-know.

## IMPLEMENTING RIGHT-TO-KNOW POLICIES

The role of the terrorist changes the dynamics of risk. Many risks can be calculated by applying engineering principles to estimate the likelihood that a part or manufacturing process will fail. Calculations can be used to determine the likelihood of undesirable consequences, such as persons being harmed by taking routine medications or receiving inoculations from contagious diseases. In an industrial setting, maintenance schedules and other appropriate risk-assessment and risk-response procedures can reduce risks, but not eliminate them. Accidents and equipment failures happen. People make mistakes.

Such normal assessments lead to planning. Although the acts of terrorists are random in the scope of knowable events, there are some aspects that are predictable. The problem of predictability, however, is made more difficult by the human factor. Simply stated, it's difficult to guess when some individual or group might engage in a criminal action to make a rhetorical point and exert pressure.

In light of this uncertainty, risk professionals can look for signs of potential terrorist behavior and determine the likelihood that such acts will occur, albeit in a relatively subjective manner. Risk assessment entails the implementation of scenario assessment. This process consists of an analysis of the steady stream of events, (the narrative of life in general and industrial activities in particular), and imagines that at some point terrorism could occur. How can it be foreseen? How can it be managed, mitigated, even prevented? How does communication to employees, colleagues, and potentially affected communities factor into the risk assessment, mitigation, and response equation? Should people be warned of the potentiality of terrorism? If so, when and how?

Under community right-to-know legislation, people are supposed to be alerted to potential risks that could affect their health or safety. So, on one hand, responsible community relations and employee relations calls for effective, continual, and honest communication about risks and the best methods to prevent or mitigate the risk. Community right-to-know legislation assumes that people, indeed, have a right to know. On the other hand, what if information routinely available to people who work and live near industrial complexes could compromise their health or safety if it were to fall into the hands of terrorists? Questions such as this one frame the analysis provided in this chapter. It addresses the responsibility to predict, assess, and respond appropriately to potential terrorist events.

While an open stream of communication is the essence of community right-to-know, that information could, in fact, harm the community if it were made available in such ways that it easily could be obtained by terrorists and used maliciously. The risk is that terrorists can use information that citizens have a right-to-know. This information can be turned against citizens' interests by terrorists who want to make a statement through criminal violence that endangers livelihoods, health, and even lives.

Some argue that terrorists are less likely to engage in violent acts if their grievances are acknowledged as part of an ongoing dialogue that addresses their grievances. Unfortunately, persons who are responsible for the safe operation of facilities, such as the World Trade Center buildings or a chemical manufacturing facility, may not have much to do with determining the dynamics and content of such dialogues. They are merely the randomly selected targets of such violence. Nevertheless, they are responsible for the safety and protection of assets, employees, and residents who live near such facilities. For this reason they must assume they are a target. But they must take actions to prevent and minimize the threat to their facilities and to communicate with various members of the public in a responsible manner. They are often caught between a rock and a hard spot in their responsibility. Certain industrial complexes may be particularly vulnerable. For example, cities with a high concentration of chemical manufacturing, such as Houston, could serve as a target.

Scholarly journals in public relations, business, and communication, as well as textbooks and university courses, have explored crisis case studies on topics ranging from the 1992 Tylenol tampering incidents to the *Exxon Valdez* oil spill.[17] The latter occurred on March 24, 1989, when an oil tanker ran aground in Bligh Reef in Prince William Sound, Alaska, spilling more than 11 million gallons of crude oil. The spill was the largest in U.S. history and tested the abilities of local, national, and industrial organizations to prepare for, and respond to, a disaster of such magnitude. Likewise, the billion-dollar accounting scandals at Enron and WorldCom (now MCI), among other multinational corporate failures, represent a new age of organizational crises accompanied by communication challenges. For the oil and chemical industry—most notably refineries, chemical plants, storage terminals, and pipelines—the tragic events of 9/11 continue to generate strategic and tactical adjustments to methods of communicating about security.

## POST-9/11 SECURITY MEASURES

The Houston Ship Channel links Galveston Bay and the Gulf of Mexico with more than 100 industrial facilities. The Port of Houston Authority owns and operates the public facilities located along the Port of Houston, a 50-mile-long complex of public and private facilities that handle more than 175 million short tons of freight worth more than $60 billion annually. With about 6,000 ships passing through the channel annually, the port is one of the nation's largest in foreign cargo tonnage and serves most of the Gulf Coast refineries with their oil imports. The volume of marine cargoes of raw materials and finished products to and from the facilities make the channel one of the nation's busiest waterways. Often referred to as a "target of opportunity," along with airlines, airports, nuclear power plants, and other critical infrastructures, the Houston-area refining and petrochemical facilities have been at the front line of intensified security assessment and enhancement since 9/11. Upgrades in detection devices, lighting, fencing and other equipment; stepped-up training of security personnel; revised security procedures including more restricted site access; efforts to heighten workforce awareness; and closer coordination with local municipalities, law enforcement and the U.S. Coast Guard in some cases rapidly improved, while in others were rapidly developed among Houston Ship Channel facilities.

Security has always has been a high priority for the refining and chemical industry, but before 9/11, terrorism-related security was not. Plant security issues focused on vehicle break-ins, theft, perimeter access, trespassing, personnel problems, bomb threats and the like. Historically a second-tier industry issue when compared to health, safety, and the environment, security came into its own in a significant way after 9/11. Two forces that led to increased openness in security communications have been the ongoing, and at times relentless media interest, and a justifiably concerned public—primarily community residents near industrial facilities.

On September 11, 2001, industry communicators found themselves, hours after the attacks, pressured into talking about security, a subject that until that time was not typically discussed except within individual companies and the industry. Today, as it always has been, the interest level of local residents corresponds to their proximity to plants and refineries. The greater the distance between a community resident and a facility, the less likely it is that security is a top-of-mind concern.

Houston Ship Channel industry is good at preventing emergency incidents and, should they occur, responding to them in a timely and professional manner. Drills involving industry, municipalities and regulatory agencies test communication, coordination, and practical skills in scenarios such as fires, explosions, chemical releases, and product spills. Industry emergency-response plans and training also address hurricanes, flooding, freezing, electrical power failures, radioactive materials, medical calls, bomb threats, civil unrest, and other potential crisis situations. Revisions to many industrial emergency-response manuals were made after 9/11, with such headings as security, terrorism, site protection, and so on.

A key part of chemical industry operations is Responsible Care, a voluntary program implemented in 1988 by the American Chemistry Council (formerly the Chemical Manufacturing Association). This program works to achieve improvements in environmental, health, and safety performance. Its guiding principles include (1) to operate facilities and develop processes and products in a manner that protects health, safety, and environment; (2) to lead in the development of responsible laws, regulations, and standards; (3) to work with customers, carriers, suppliers, distributors, and contractors to foster the safe use, transport, and disposal of chemicals; and (4) to seek and incorporate public input regarding products and operations.[5]

A recent addition to Responsible Care is the Responsible Care Security Code, developed in response to 9/11, which safeguards against potential terrorist attacks, expands industry relationships with law enforcement, and a provides a model for chemical site protection. This security code, adopted June 2002, was developed in partnership with the EPA, the Office of Homeland Security, the FBI, the Department of Defense, the Coast Guard, and other agencies to protect citizens from possible threats.

According to the American Chemistry Council, the purpose of the security code is to help protect people, property, products, processes, information, and information systems by enhancing security, including security against potential terrorist attacks, throughout the chemical industry manufacturing chain.[5] The security code uses a risk-based approach to identify, assess, and address vulnerabilities; prevent or mitigate incidents; enhance training and response capabilities; and maintain and improve relationships with key stakeholders. Some specific examples include companies using tools to analyze the security of product sales, distribution, and cybersecurity; actions that protect facilities, such as the installation of new physical barriers, modified production processes, or materials substitution; measures to protect Internet commerce; additional screening of transportation providers; and improved lines of communication, a category that includes steps such as sharing effective security practices with others throughout industry and maintaining interaction with law-enforcement officials. The Responsible Care Security Code requires industry members to verify security enhancements through independent, third parties such as firefighters, law enforcement, and other state and federal officials.

Four other key information and communication programs related to the chemical industry are the Chemical Transportation Emergency Center (CHEMTREC), the Transportation Community Awareness and Emergency Response (TRANSCAER) program, the Chemical Sector Information Sharing and Analysis Center (ISAC), and the Emergency Response Mutual Aid Programs (ERMAP). When an emergency occurs, CHEMTREC provides first responders with technical assistance, information, and resources from product-safety specialists, toxicologists, and other industry experts. TRANSCAER provides information to communities through which hazardous materials are transported, offering community education, guidance in developing plans to respond to an incident, and training for local emergency responders. ISAC, established in June 2002, is a public-private partnership that shares vital security-related information between the multi-agency National Infrastructure Protection Center, which is based at the Department of Homeland Security, and companies that manufacture and use chemical products. ERMAP connects manufacturers of products that pose a very high risk if spilled or involved in an accident or catastrophe. These companies have developed a mutual aid agreement to provide immediate assistance in an emergency, agreeing that the closest capable response team will assist until the shipper or manufacturer of the products involved is able to take over at the scene.

A limited review of the chemical industry's steps to strengthen security at their facilities includes the following measures: (1) tightening access to facilities during deliveries of materials and at on-site parking facilities, and increasing perimeter protections, such as strengthening fences and exterior walls, creating setbacks and clear zones that eliminate hiding places, and installing additional lights; (2) recommending to federal law-enforcement officials that they should examine the licenses of all drivers transporting hazardous materials; (3) changing transportation standards, such as mandating that truck shipments cannot be left unattended and that no stops can be made between the plant and delivery, and communicating with local officials and briefing them on facility security efforts; (4) using the industry's existing risk-assessment tools for national security purposes; (5) permitting cleaning crews to work only during business hours; (6) improving information security measures, including the prohibition of radio and phone conversations about sensitive topics and use of voice encryption for some radio conversations; (7) increasing the number of properly trained security officers and developing a security center to better monitor and support security processes; (8) ensuring availability of backup systems for basic utilities such as electricity, water, sewer, and gas, as well as for communications, control centers, and computer servers; (9) improving marine and rail security by establishing protocols that correspond to standards set by the Homeland Security Administration and Marine Security levels; (10) improving security planning, training and drills; and (11) improving hiring and employment termination practices.[5]

One striking example of these new protocols in action occurred in Texas after the September 11 crisis. At an industrial complex in Deer Park, along the Houston Ship Channel, crews from two television stations and one radio station arrived less than one hour after the second plane crashed into the World Trade Center (WTC). Reporters were after the local angle: "Could a terrorist attack happen here, and if so, how bad would it be?" Live and taped interviews covered a range of questions that were predictable in light of the events in New York, Washington, DC, and Pennsylvania. For example, Are we in danger? What are you doing to protect this plant against an aerial attack? Are your security guards armed? Responses were carefully worded, couched in terms of not responding to speculation and emphasizing commitment to protecting employees and the community.

By noon on September 11, reporters quickly responded to a rumor that the Shell Deer Park facility, the sixth largest refinery operating in the United States, with a crude oil capacity of 340,000 barrels a day, had ordered employees to evacuate, setting off rumors that Houston Ship Channel industry was vacating its plants and refineries. What actually happened was that Shell Deer Park, like many businesses nationwide, was allowing "nonessential" employees to go home. These were mostly staff employees who were not deemed critical to the continued safe operation of the facility on a short-term basis. There is no turning off the lights and locking the door on your way out of a chemical plant or refinery. Eventually, the media clarified that the so-called mass evacuation really was the controlled release of employees, and that this practice was being followed all along the Houston Ship Channel area, achieving the result of assuring communities that industry was not deserting them.

By late morning, it had become evident that although the tragedy of September 11 was not a Houston Ship Channel crisis, the indirect impact it had by way of media attention and employee and community concern caused industry to behave as if there had been direct impact. Twenty-four-hour emergency operations centers were established at many facilities, security and off-duty police officers were added, statements were prepared for internal and external distribution, and industry and communities alike coped with the high level of personal anxiety that accompanies emergency status.

The Houston Ship Channel area is home to the East Harris County Manufacturers Association (EHCMA), one of the largest industrial associations of its type in the world. EHCMA is a nonprofit professional association of approximately 125 chemical manufacturers, refiners, and supporting distribution-terminal facility managers in east Harris County, Texas. By the afternoon of September 11, it was clear that if EHCMA members spoke with one voice about security, it would not only be more efficient than each facility speaking on its own, but it would have more impact because of the ability of industry to deliver consistent messages.

The Shell Deer Park security statement was revised to reflect an industry perspective and included "boilerplate" information about EHCMA and the industry. The EHCMA spokesperson then began handling industry media responses, while individual EHCMA-member facilities retained the responsibility of communicating beyond the industry effort as they saw fit.

Four key messages—all sound bite length—described industry's position: (1) safety and security are the top priorities; (2) industry is at the highest awareness and alert status; (3) industry is taking appropriate steps to protect its employees, facilities, and the community; and (4) industry is working closely with law enforcement, fire departments, regulatory agencies, the U.S. Coast Guard, and others.

The strategy involved aggressively communicating the statement via interviews, phone conversations, website postings, and group e-mails to media and other target audiences. It also required reaction, in the forms of responding to incoming telephone inquiries and on-site interviews. Media monitoring verified that the key messages were being widely distributed, and also identified concerns and questions about industry that required follow-up.

By September 13, when media and community interest in security of Houston Ship Channel industry had greatly decreased, it was clear that the strategy of industry speaking with one voice successfully conveyed prudent action and addressed public concern. It was acknowledged by industry communicators that any less open and forthright approach on

9/11, when questions greatly outnumbered answers and emotions ran high, would have been the wrong one.

## GETTING BACK TO BASICS

Although media relations is only one part of an overall strategy for effectively managing a crisis, it is at the top of the list because of its powerful function as a conduit with the public. Research has shown that in a large-scale emergency or crisis most people turn to the electronic media for information. By the nature of its business and the ever-present potential for incidents, the Houston Ship Channel industries understand the value of effective communication in a crisis—even when the crisis is half a continent away, as it was on 9/11.

One ongoing challenge for industry since September 11 relates to communicating security in the context of scenarios proposed by media, employees, and residents regarding vulnerability to terrorist acts. Basic media-relations practice dictates not going down the road of speculation; yet the intensity of 9/11 introduced a harsh new reality into what had been a more or less a "no comment" approach.

The so-called CAP rule of expressing "concern," "action," and "perspective" was tailor-made for September 11 communications. All three rules came into play in the Houston Ship Channel incidents. Residents of nearby communities wanted assurances that industry was concerned for their welfare. Residents are sensitive to how this concern is demonstrated by what industry says, how industry says it, and how industry appears. Action has to do with describing what is being done or will be done to improve security—real steps, not just intent or policy. Perspective requires industry spokespersons to put themselves in the same emotional frames of mind as facility neighbors, as well as media consumers, and to articulate in a manner that is genuine, empathetic, and informative.

Communications often is a combination of both reactive and proactive strategies, as was experienced by industry on 9/11, and the tough questions continue to be: What is different today at your facility as a result of the September 11 events? How vulnerable is your facility? What are you doing to protect your employees and the public? How safe is your facility? How should people near your facility feel? By the same token, industry asks itself: Do we know all of our stakeholders? Are we reaching them with our key messages about security? What steps should we take to provide the ongoing assurance they seek, stopping short of guarantees? What do we say, and how do we best communicate with an alarmed, anxious community on a continuous basis? How do we know if we are communicating effectively? Responses to these questions have been edited over time to reflect industry's changing security profile and the public's desire for information.

## STRATEGY AND WALK-AWAY POINTS

Communicating after a crisis, assuming it is evident that a state of crisis has diminished to the point where an "all hands on deck" approach is not required, is a call often triggered by less negative media attention, stabilizing of public response or outcry, and a general return to status quo. There is a school of thought in industry that the "crisis" ceases when the fire is out, the chemical release is over, the highway reopens, the evacuation ends, or any number of other major situations conclude. Savvy communicators, however, recognize the potential for a nonoperational crisis to emerge from an operational crisis that is poorly handled. Commonly, this manifests itself as legal or regulatory action, consumer boycotts, sustained negative media coverage, poor employee morale, and hits to public reputation or image. The communication groundwork laid at the outset of a crisis can do much to offset lingering problems when the immediate and more apparent crisis is under control. Taking victory laps when the "all-clear" siren sounds or the last television crew departs can be naïve.

Industry communicators were as stunned by the events of 9/11 as anyone else. Before the attacks, industry was unprepared to quickly communicate about terrorism and the potential for terrorist acts at an industrial facility. What has worked well in the past has been communicating messages of protecting people and assets, minimizing impact on the community and the environment, and reestablishing normal operation—backed by action to support those messages. The media and public were forgiving on September 11 because they recognized that having crisp, solid responses to questions about terrorism vulnerability at refineries and plants were difficult to come by, as it was with other businesses and industries interviewed that day across the nation.

Looking back, the basics of communication carried the day for Houston Ship Channel industry. Factual information about security, a very sensitive topic, was developed and communicated under stressful conditions in a consensus manner—industry, as an entity, crafted and delivered messages. Key walk-away points included the importance of being accessible to the community and media, acknowledging early on that security is a high priority and has industry's full attention, emphasizing commitment to security, demonstrating action, meeting employees' communication needs, being creative in getting security-related information to various stakeholders (using Internet postings, group e-mails, telephone recordings, media statements and interviews), and knowing what to say to distraught residents who called wanting to know what is being done to protect families one-quarter mile from the facility property line.

Validating the effectiveness of crisis communications during and following 9/11 comes through media analysis, personal discussions with stakeholders, and formal community surveys coordinated by industry. It's also important to recognize that the security world we knew before 9/11 no longer exists. The public's security concerns may decrease during sustained periods without terrorist activity, and likewise escalate when national alert-levels rise, yet security as a major issue with crisis potential will never go away. Communicators must always expect the unexpected, and should never underestimate the value of their role in connecting the information dots regarding security or other sensitive topics.

## NARRATIVE THEORY FOR RISK AND CRISIS PREPARATION

This section explains narrative theory and how it can help explain how persons responsible for predicting and responding to threats can approach such situations as though they were narratives. Knowing the common narratives of a group, organization, or society provides a framework for scanning, analyzing, identifying, and monitoring for nonnormative narratives that might alert critics. Such critics can be activists who seek to change corporate policies, procedures, and actions through public policy pressure. At the extreme, such activist critics may engage in the sort of criminal behavior that is characterized as terrorism.

### Narrative Theory and Culture

Narrative theory, created by Fisher, adds depth to the view that people enact their lives as actors in an undirected play.[18-23] As is true of a theatrical production, members of companies and their communities, as well as their customers, must create and enact shared perspectives, characters, scripts, plots, and themes. Narratives and metaphors, the stuff of theater, serve this purpose, as people create and share views of life and living that allow for coordinated activities, and even the creation and management of conflict. Enactment of various narratives involves creation, perception, attention, and retention. People focus on some elements of their environment as they interact with one another, and they ignore other aspects. Recurring selections of views of life and living are known as schema—patterned and predictable ways of perceiving and thinking. Information derived from this process becomes retained in individual and collective memories. It is translated into customs, mores, and public policies.

What is a narrative? "A narrative generally is recognized to be a way of ordering and presenting a view of the world through a description of a situation involving characters, actions, and settings."[24] At first glance, we may think of a narrative, or story, as nothing more than a descriptive recounting of events. It is more. "A narrative, as a frame upon experience, functions as an argument to view and understand the world in a particular way, and by analyzing that narrative, the critic can understand the argument being made and the likelihood that it will be successful in gaining adherents for the perspective it presents."[24]

In other words, narratives are a way of thinking, a way of ordering events that would otherwise seem unpredictable or incoherent. As people construct narratives in meaningful patterns, those patterns—scripts and themes—express their values and guide their actions. Of course, not everyone thinks and acts in the same way. Narrative analysis assumes that people choose among competing stories that account for a given event. Thus, the question often is not whether, but which narrative best explains events.

Through narratives, people structure their experiences and actions. Narratives give meaning to the world. Through stories, the world and people's actions reflect a logic that explains what happens, why it happens, who makes it happen, when it happens, and how to respond. Each narrative expresses a set of preferences that correspond to the values of those who opt for it. The world of human events is understood in terms of a thematic logic that begins with "once upon a time," progresses through "and then she said to him," and resolves into "and all ended well for both." For businesses, a narrative might be, "and after that, the company had to file for bankruptcy." The desired resolution of a story would be, "and all ended well."

Scripted logics allow people to create and share a variety of social realities. Stressing this point, Gergen and Gergen conclude that "narratives are, in effect, social constructions, undergoing continuous alteration as interaction progresses. The individual in this case does not consult an internal narrative for information. Rather, the self-narrative is a linguistic implement constructed by people in relationships and employed in relationships to sustain, enhance or impede various actions. It may be used to indicate future actions but it is not in itself the basis for such action. In this sense, self-narratives function much as histories within society do more generally. They are symbolic systems used for such social purposes as justification, criticism, and social solidification."[25]

Narratives have substantial rhetorical potency because they are a conventional and convenient means for understanding the theme that runs throughout a series of events—including a crisis such as a terrorist act, or a set of similar crises such as airline crashes. Narratives simplify; even when they are profoundly incorrect, they can facilitate the attribution of motivation. Narrative is fraught with motive because even—or especially—as children, people learn that the characters in stories respond to and enact motives. The motives of a society are embedded in and expressed by its culture.

Culture, a driving force of narratives, shapes people's thoughts and actions. It accounts for how groups view and evaluate their physical and social worlds, as Sapir writes.[26] Culture, as Morgan defines it, is "a process of reality construction that allows people to see and understand particular events, actions, objects, utterances, or situations in distinctive ways."[27] It helps people to hold views that they knowingly share with other members of their organization. Within the chemical manufacturing business, culture consists of jargon unique to each company, and to each of its subunits and industries. It includes knowledge of the company (expressed as beliefs and attitudes), as well as company values, roles, and rules—those relating to communication activities, work, and messages.

As such, culture can be seen as a set of unique opinions and a way that groups think about their own identity and actions, and also about the world around them. Through culture, groups of people create a shared social reality that expresses values, defines roles, and establishes relationships to socioeconomic and sociopolitical systems. As such, culture helps people evaluate the rewards and costs that they encounter.[28] For example, a culture that rewards certain economic realities or personal liberties, such as privacy, might find the costs of absolute homeland security too high.

In other words, culture is connected to narratives and ultimately to risk perception. Douglas underscores the point when she defines cultural theory as "a way of thinking about culture that draws the social environment systematically into the picture of individual choices. It provides a method of analyzing public debates as positions taken in a conflict between cultures."[1] The culture of each entity (business, government, and citizen) influences its decision-making processes and expectations relevant to the formation of social mores, and corporate or governmental policy. For example, the culture of one organized group is likely to spawn others, including supporters, detractors, nonactivist community members, and groups whose culture is latent. Thus, for public relations and risk communication, culture may partially account for why groups collide with one another. Through culture, people express standards they expect others to meet. For instance, while one group or society may define terrorism as amoral and an unreasonable political and military tool, other groups or societies may support terrorism as culturally acceptable to accomplish societal goals.

Narratives give people the scripts and perceptual structures they need to identify with and understand the events, actions, and expectations of one another. Narratives embed beliefs, attitudes, and values as ideologies that reflect and guide people's judgments and evaluations. Narrative content and theme allow people the means for predicting the actions of others, and coordinating their own actions with them. For this reason, savvy public-relations professionals need to be aware of, consider, and use the several available narratives to predict how key groups may react to the events of a crisis, and to media reporters' accounts of them. Public-relations practitioners come to realize that some stories work as the basis for explaining and justifying a set of circumstances related to a crisis, and others do not.

## Narrative and Terrorism

As shared organizational meaning changes for the people who make each organization function, so does organizational structure because they enact the scenes they know and expect to be rewarding. Therefore, to change organizational structure requires a redefinition of the meaning they use to interpret scenes or of the actions that are appropriate to each scene. Creating and sharing meaning allows people to identify with other members of the organization and with the organization itself. People's understanding of physical and social reality is never free from the words they use to talk and think about it. Therefore, their experiences may not be as important as the terms they use to discuss them. The terminology people use to enact that reality is crucial to the enactment, whether they have engaged in actions or merely have terms that refer to those actions. Thus, "language is a way of acting together by living the substance of the perspectives captured in each idiom."[29]

This view of enactment is based on the principle, as Burke reasons, that "a motive is not some fixed thing like a table, which one can go and look at. It is a term of interpretation, and being such it will naturally take its place within the framework of our *Weltanschauung* as a whole."[30] How people enact roles on behalf of and in response to each other and their work depends on the perspectives they hold and share in common. They enact their roles as though they were "dancing an attitude," the essence of symbolic action.[31]

Ultimately, narrative is central to the human experience. Kenneth Burke elaborates on these themes:

> Surrounding us wordy animals there is the infinite wordless universe out of which we have been gradually carving our universes of discourse since the time when our primordial ancestors added to their sensations <u>words</u> for sensations. When they could duplicate the taste of an orange by <u>saying</u> "the taste of an orange," that's when STORY was born, since words <u>tell about</u> sensations. Whereas Nature can do no wrong (whatever it does is Nature) when STORY comes into the world there enters the realm of the true, false, honest, mistaken, the downright lie, the imaginative, the visionary, the sublime, the ridiculous, the eschatological (as with Hell, Purgatory, Heaven, the Transmigration of Souls, Foretellings of an Inevitable wind-up in a classless society), the satirical, every single detail of every single science or speculation, even every bit of gossip—for although all animals in their way communicate, only our kind of animal can gossip. There was no story before we came, and when we're gone the universe will go on sans story.[32]

If, as Burke reasons, story is basic to human existence, we are challenged to explain the role of story in terrorism, and in crisis response to terrorism.

Terrorism can be viewed as a narrative that competes and collides with the normal narrative that guides policies and actions at any particular time in a society. In a business, this normal narrative is "ordinary" business procedures. Companies create and enact strategic business plans. These plans lead to employment, production of products, creation and delivery of services, and the generation of income of various types. Such plans reflect and conform to the larger narratives of a free enterprise, free market society. Strategic plans also feature narratives that are brought to life by specific characters enacting roles of various kinds. These characters play roles that are guided by plots and themes that, in turn, are expressed, or lived, scripts. Managers and employees define the routine or ordinary activities that are used to meet the expectations of other members of society. In this way, their shared perspectives result in orderly actions with predictable events and interactions.

Against this "ordinary" narrative society, corporate organizations encounter a variety of counternarratives. These are enacted by characters who play roles that advocate different policies and procedures. One set of counternarratives comes from critics of corporate performance. Some critics are environmental activists who call for policies that result in cleaner air and water. Others are activists who call for increased standards of public health and safety. Still others are union members. All of these counternarratives, together with the ordinary business narrative, help frame the lives of people who live in communities near manufacturing.

Into this drama of compatible and incompatible narratives enters another possibility, the terrorist narrative, which is willing to counter the prevailing corporate narrative with violent criminal activities. The goal of terrorists is to replace or dramatically modify the narratives they criticize. Terrorist attacks have two dimensions, one symbolic and one strategic. The terrorist narrative seeks to destroy hated symbols that violate the terrorist's values. In this sense, terrorists want to attack the symbolic rationale for society, or a key segment of society, to discredit it and therefore justify its replacement.

Strategic attacks are even more threatening. During the post-9/11 era, for instance people worried that sources of drinking water and electricity were vulnerable. If the water supply of a major city could be compromised, the terrorists would truly bring terror to the hearts and minds of society. But a strategic attack on the water supply is still symbolic, in that the inability to protect against the attack demonstrates lack of authority. For days after 9/11, the airline industry was crippled by the strategic attack on this vital part of the transportation industry in the United States. Similar attacks would be predicted against the refining and chemical manufacturing industries, which have strategic value to the economy and lifestyle of the United States. These industries are vital to the commercial viability of their communities, and to the nation.

Narrative theory has proved valuable to scholars and practitioners in preparing for crisis and for analyzing the conditions that can lead up to and result from a crisis. This theory is particularly rich in implications for the monitoring, operational preparation, communication preparation, and response to crises, including terrorism. In the sense of terrorism, the logic is that criminal acts of violence against people and property can pose a crisis as interpreted according to the narratives of risk management that exist for each industry and the people whose lives they affect. Such is the case, for instance, with the iconic criminal acts against people of Chicago using Tylenol capsules as murder weapons. People are constantly at varying degrees of risk. When the risk potential manifests itself, organizations responsible for people's welfare must respond.

The essence of this response is the telling of a lived story. This view of planning and response fits nicely with journalistic reporting that focuses on the narrative elements of life: Who, when, where, why, what, and how. Responses to these traditional news reporting story lines must in some way conform to the narrative expectations of people in a community.[28,33,34]

Researchers and public-relations practitioners study and engage in (or counsel) communication response during crises. They examine how persons caught up in a crisis can and should design messages and respond to media and other investigative inquiries in ways that are ethically and rhetorically sound. One method of meeting this challenge grows out of analysis that reasons that life is narrative and humans can best be characterized as storytellers who think and live in terms of the stories they tell.

The narrative paradigm suggests that structure and content (or form and substance) are connected in "undirected plays." This concept emphasizes that interaction occurs during communication episodes, in which members of an organization enact their various narrative views about the company. These interactions result in the development of relationships. Given time and a number of such communication episodes, the relationships become organized around shared themes. The content and form of these narratives help explain how members of an organization comprehend thoughts and, over time, translate them into action. People, who are familiar with the principles central to their narrative plots, enact roles in response to enactments by others who also know those themes and plots. A narrative framework explains how company members attribute motives to one another, episode by episode and scene by scene.

Because narratives privilege certain interests and practices, we must be able to unlock the way this hegemony occurs. People throughout an organization tell stories, often quite unintentionally, and perhaps for no other motive than ventilation ("You won't believe what happened") and amusement ("John/Joan did X again"). Several stories may exist that provide different versions of the same event. To advance the scope of narrative analysis, we need to explain how these competing stories interlock in a coherent narrative fabric so that the order of the company is made apparent and enactable, even though individuals may disagree and experience conflict.

Narratives provide perspectives through which people coordinate behavior. Their content informs "tellers" and "hearers" about the cost/reward ratios that exist for each effort they consider undertaking or avoiding. Given a choice between complying or defying norms, or expectations, within the company, stories help people predict the probable rewards or punishments for their behavior. Tellers, as well as hearers, use each story as a mirror that reflects themselves in contrast to others. The grammar of such narrative form is reflective, transitive, or intransitive. Stories are a means for thinking aloud. Some stories moralize, while others are told to imagine and examine certain conditions of the organization. In this way, the meaning contained in stories is a fabric of thought, a constellation of symbols by which each organization exerts its uniqueness. This meaning expresses performance expectations.

Interpretations of the relationship between symbols, thoughts, and actions begin by approaching narratives as perspectives, or terministic screens.[35] The assumption is that people see the physical and social world the same way if they view it through the same set of terms, which serve as terministic screens that feature certain interpretations. As people share perspectives embedded in symbols made meaningful by their shared narrative content and form, they will think and act in predictable, interlocking ways. Such is the case even if their actions result in conflict and uncooperativeness. Competition requires cooperation, as does war. The dialectical tensions of war require persons who know how to engage in combat. Democracy is "a political structure that gives full opportunity for the use of competition to a cooperative end."[31]

What Fisher calls the narrative paradigm allows us to look beyond individual stories to think of many cooperative and competing narratives as bringing people together and putting them at odds with one another.[19-21] Narrative has this capacity regardless of whether the content is scientific or mythical. It assumes that "there is no genre, including technical communication, that is not an episode in the story of life (a part of the 'conversation') and is not itself constituted by logos and mythos."[19] Even technical discourse contains myth and metaphor, and aesthetic communication has "cognitive capacity and import."[19] People are valuing and reasoning animals who examine and express thoughts in the context of large, dominant narratives, against which each specific narrative is compared and interpreted. In making this point, Fisher concludes that knowledge "is ultimately configured narratively, as a component in a larger story implying the being of a certain kind of person, a person with a particular worldview, with a specific self-concept, and with characteristic ways of relating to others."[20]

This analysis suggests that discourse in organizations ranging from private companies to terrorist organizations can be interpreted as narrative, even though it does not "tell a story" in the literal sense. Exchange of correspondence (such as memos and letters, as well as conversations and telephone calls) occurs as episodes in a drama; if someone were to describe these events, chances are they would be presented narratively: "I said." "He said." "She said." Some documents, such as policies and procedures constitute scripts: "Do this and say this." Procedures are often narratively based on temporal progression of steps: "Do this." "Next do this." Meetings transpire temporally as episodes with engaged actors. Not only is each meeting an episode, but also the discussion of each meeting is episodic. Meetings, as is true of other kinds of discourse, progress as players enact what they think to be an appropriate role, or persona, as they contribute to the discussion. A sense of theme—shared social reality and shared development of a reality— guides the discussion, as each person's comments help shape the progression of some theme, a guiding principle in the narrative enactment. Narrative development of themes gives the continuity to the enactment of these episodes.

## RISKS AND CRISIS RESPONSE: THE DYNAMICS OF COMMUNITY

On any day, people can suffer terrorism in any aspect of their life. At certain times that risk might be higher or lower, but the possibility always exists. Where and when such attacks occur reflects a random model with modest amounts of predictability. In fact, the essence of terrorism is to be unpredictable. Terrorists want their threat to be present, but they want to control when and where the attack might occur and whom it might harm.

Thus, one of the underpinnings of terrorism is an attack on the efforts by others in society to create and implement the orderliness of control. The strategic challenge of terrorism is an attack on that orderliness that damages and alters the ordered control of society. The symbolic challenge of terrorism aims at delegitimizing the people and organizations that are expected to exert control in the name of the "people." In the days after the fall of Iraq to the British and American forces, the efforts of terrorists, insurgents, or freedom fighters (whatever rhetorical view of these people one might have) was launched against symbolic targets including symbols of America—including government officials—and even organizations providing humanitarian aid. More importantly, such attacks sought to destroy strategic efforts to restore civil society and commerce. Thus, the targets included pipelines and Iraqi police stations, for instance.

## Crisis Response

In his analysis of the narrative response to crisis, Heath asks: "Does the narrative enacted by the organization responsible for the crisis demonstrate that the organization has not lost control or that its efforts will restore or achieve control; is the resolution of the story satisfactory to the key publics?"[34]

History is a drama of people assessing, communicating about, and creatively preventing or adapting to risks.[2] A crisis results when groups within the public are confronted with events that lead them to feel uncertainty, concern, and even outrage regarding some condition that both threatens their well being, and violates their expectations of responsible organizational performance. Paramount in the thinking of persons in this century are the hazards they encounter as they seek the benefits of technology. Science has dramatically improved the quality of life, but some members of the public are convinced that innovation is not without dire consequences. Such worry is not new, but has become heightened in this age of national and international terrorism.

The fact that people and organizations face an enormous variety of crises on a daily basis is not new. Life hazards are a part of everyday existence in a modern, industrialized, and politicized society. Recent potential or actual crisis issues, from foot-and-mouth disease in the United States to the fluctuations of the Homeland Security terrorist-threat levels, remind people of the perceived, potential, probable, or likely dangers and risks. Typical modern crises reflect the increasing influence and complexity of science, technology, and industry, and crisis managers must address these areas.[36] These increasingly complex risks are even more heightened following 9/11 and the ever-present media coverage of terrorism. Moreover, the political, social, and cultural aspects of terrorism pose an even more difficult challenge for communicators.

A crisis is typically defined as an untimely but predictable event that has actual or potential consequences for stakeholders' interests, as well as the reputation of the organization suffering the crisis, thus causing harm to stakeholders and damage to the organization's relationship with them.[37]

In dealing with these modern crises, public relations and risk communication can guide organizations to better understand, evaluate, and manage relationships as well as understand and respond to individuals' and groups' construction of crisis narratives.[28] In a similar vein, crisis management and risk management can be viewed as the understanding of and the relationship management of the numerous narratives of multiple cultures before, during, and after a crisis. This view of public relations and crisis management presumes that each society and group of stakeholders (and the subcultures that comprise these groups) develops a unique culture that reflects its view of what is and ought to be.[38] The culture of each group influences how it evaluates commercial and nonprofit activities and governmental policies. Other members of society also use their narratives to evaluate commercial and nonprofit activities and governmental policies. How each organization forms and implements strategic crisis-management policy reflects its unique culture. How each organization communicates during a crisis with various public groups, whether they are internal or external, reflects the organization's culture and furthermore, should be sensitive to the culture of each group.[39] These concepts are an internal component of crisis management and risk communication.

Sophisticated crisis-management practitioners and scholars focus their agenda on the proactive management of key stakeholders' cultures. Part of that proactive management, according to public-relations best practices, includes utilizing organizational narratives to guide the thoughts, actions, and responses—culture expressed in communication—during a crisis.

Ideally, crisis management specialists can help foster the understanding and agreement needed to build harmony between an organization's narrative and those of key members of the public prior to the onset of a crisis. If so, this harmony benefits all parties during an actual crisis. However, when a crisis does occur, crisis communication comes to the forefront of organizational response. As such, it is critical that savvy practitioners gain additional insights into the content of crisis discourse. One element of crisis discourse is the role that narratives play in crisis management. Appropriate and cocreated narrative elements embedded in crisis and risk communication should be a part of the organizational culture, continuous risk communication materials, and an integral part of crisis spokespersons' comments.

Fearn-Banks defines crisis communication as "the communication between the organization and its public prior to, during and after the negative occurrence.[40] The communications are designed to minimize damage to the image of the corporation. Effective crisis management includes crisis communications that not only can alleviate or eliminate the crisis, but can sometimes bring the organization a more positive reputation than before the crisis."[40] The purpose of narrative analysis is to see how respondents impose order on the important experiences of their lives and to make sense of those events—particularly during crises, such as traumatic events and transitions in life.

Individuals and groups define social reality by following rhetorical prescriptions. These prescriptions, in turn, affect the understanding and interpretation of particular experiences. Thus, "crisis" is in fact an interpretation of an actual event. Some crisis-management studies and prescriptions take an information-based approach that features a source, with scientific or managerial credentials, which offers a variety of approaches to dealing with crises. Such prescriptions, however, do not incorporate issues of conflict and negotiation. Nor do they address the perspective of concerned members of the community who believe they have reason not to trust any statement regarding the crisis situation.

Heath and Millar suggest a variation of this view is to treat crisis as an interruption of a narrative.[37] Individuals, organizations, and other actors play a role in this crisis narrative. Some elements in the event have narrative implications.

A crisis not only is an interruption of one narrative—the normal activities of an organization—but it also begins its own narrative, one that may or may not end happily ever after. During a crisis narrative, the exigency is to manage actions and rhetorical statements that demonstrate that the organization understands the crisis and has the resources—intellectual, managerial, financial, rhetorical, and ethical—to restore an acceptable narrative.[37]

Much of the traditional crisis-management literature descriptively highlights the value of developing, implementing, and maintaining a crisis-management plan.[41] Crisis management plans are advocated because they guide organizations during times of crisis. The crisis-management plan (CMP) or crisis-communication plan (CCP) are both considered primary tools that prepare for a crisis, and guide members of an organization through one. Fearn-Banks describes a CCP as "providing a functionally collective brain for all persons involved in a crisis, persons who may not operate at normal capacity due to the shock or emotions or the crisis event."[40]

An unlimited number and variety of crisis situations make a specific or paradigmatic guiding principle of crisis management nearly impossible.[42] However, developing a broad base of narratives that guide an organization through its response to terrorism and other crisis events can be a strong start to developing an effective and immediate response.

A spokesperson or persons is a critical element of any CMP. The spokesperson is often the most visible representation of the organization during a crisis and acts as the voice of the organization.[43] The spokesperson's main responsibility is an accurate and consistent organizational message.[44] Researchers and practitioners thoroughly address tasks, functions, roles, and technical communication delivery skills. For example, Coombs provides a thorough list of tasks, knowledge, and skills, but does not address the role of organizational culture among the numerous requisite attributes for crisis communication.[43] The narratives developed for use by organizations following a terrorist attack can have a dramatic effect on the industry's sense of trust and control in response to terrorism.

Marra correctly argues that more is required than a checklist of prescriptive advice for managing crisis situations, though these lists are critical for the development of best practices and descriptive research within crisis management.[45] Marra found that the underlying culture of organizations is also a critical component of effective best practices in preparing for and managing a crisis situation. Overall, crisis management is an organizational state of mind that should guide institutional thinking. In best cases, organizations facing crisis situations are guided by values that are deeply ingrained in their cultures.[46] These values must be shared with affected members of the public through narrative discourse, and the values of terrorist groups must be identified through narrative theory.

As such, a rhetorical approach to crisis acknowledges that the responsibility for the crisis, its magnitude, and its duration are all contestable. As Heath and Millar note, this approach stresses the aspects of crisis response that include the development and presentation of a message.[37] "It underscores the role that information, framing, and interpretation play in the organization's preparation for a crisis, response to it, and post-crisis comments and actions."[37] As such, it features discourse, one or more comments made over time, which work to carry the narrative of trust and control following acts of terrorism.

Overall, an organizational crisis related to terrorism can harm stakeholders, as well as the organization's relationship with them and other key constituencies. Regardless of who is to blame for this harm, it can have a long-term impact. The organization must ease the minds of its stakeholders about its responsibility for creating or allowing a terrorist-caused crisis, and reassure them that future attacks can be prevented. Ultimately, the manner in which the organization addresses these responsibilities can serve as the turning point to reestablishing a positive relationship with key stakeholders.

## Risk-Communication Response

As a technical concept, risk is conventionally defined as something that can be given a numerical value by multiplying the probability of a typically negative outcome by its severity. This expectancy value is used to estimate and compare risks that are perceived differently, depending on the heuristics and biases each person uses to judge them.[13,14] People look to government and other sources of sociopolitical power to help discover risks, assess their severity, and solve them by reducing their chance of occurring or mitigating their negative consequences. Evidence abounds that risk perceptions and estimates are affected by decision heuristics that reflect the cultures of key groups, based largely on their roles in society. For instance, policymakers' attitudes tend to be more favorable toward risk conditions than are the opinions of the lay public.[47]

Risk communication, as an integral part of risk assessment and risk abatement, serves several purposes. It provides the opportunity to understand and appreciate stakeholders' concerns related to risks generated by organizations. It also encourages dialogue to address differences and concerns, carry out appropriate actions that can reduce perceived risks, and create a climate of participatory and effective discourse that reduces friction and increases harmony and mutuality.

Such a perspective, rooted in community infrastructure, leads risk assessors and communicators to the realization that each key group within the public makes an idiosyncratic response to each risk based on its unique decision heuristic. Each of these groups has an inclination to engage in, or at least support, activism to effect public-policy solutions that correct what they see as intolerable risk.

Risk communication is grounded in various academic and applied disciplines. These include an actuarial approach utilizing statistical predictions; a toxicological and epidemiological approach that includes ecotoxicology; an engineering approach that includes probabilistic risk assessments; an economic approach that includes risk-benefit comparisons; a psychological approach that includes psychometric analysis; and cultural and social theories of risk.[48]

Risk-communication campaigns typically involve large organizations, such as manufacturing facilities or transportation companies, whose activities pose a risk to communities. Strategic risk communication contends that people in key communities need to understand the levels of risks that they face as a result of working or living in proximity to risk sources. Moreover, it posits that they can reduce their risks when they understand the prevailing risk and collectively take action. Risk communication based on this shared, social-relations or community-infrastructure approach works to achieve a level of discourse at which the technical assessments of risk can be shared. Reaching this level, however, requires attention to the quality of relationships, as well as the political dynamics of the participants.

Views of risk communication have evolved from at least three separate streams of thought to guide the way risks are calculated, evaluated, and controlled: (1) scientific positivism, whereby community efforts to ascertain the degree of risk faced, as well as communications from the organization, are based upon data and scientific methodologies; (2) constructivism/relativism, which assumes that everyone's opinion has equal value, so that no opinion is better or worse than anyone else's; and (3) dialogue, or collaborative decision-making, whereby scientific opinion becomes integrated into policies which are vetted by values.

A fourth foundation for risk communication features complex social relations operating within community infrastructures. "Risk communication requirements are a political response to popular demands. . . . The main product of risk communication is not information, but the quality of the social relationship it supports. Risk communication is not an end in itself; it is an enabling agent to facilitate the continual evolution of relationships."[49] People often decide what levels of risk are acceptable based not on technical data analysis, but on a question of value, such as fairness.[2] Though people may debate their perceptions of risk in terms of values, experts remain examiners of the actual risk, though not entirely removed from value judgments. In short, perceived risk has a structure that differs from that of expert judgments about risk.[50]

As Fischhoff models, the risk communication process can be viewed as consisting of developmental stages: getting the numbers regarding risks correct, putting those numbers out to a community at risk, explaining what they mean, showing that members of the community have accepted similar risks, showing the benefits of risks, treating the public with respect, and creating partnerships to understand and properly control risks.[51] The strongest component of this progression is the creation of meaningful partnerships that respond to the concerns and needs of community members for information and to bring collective wisdom and judgment to bear on problems. This stress on "we" gives a community grounding for two-way communication and partnership development.[52]

One way to foster that "we" is to develop narratives that address infrastructural risk-communication process variables. Numerous researchers from a variety of academic and professional fields, including public relations, risk communication, risk management, psychology, rhetoric, political science, engineering, sociology, and anthropology, have developed this broad typology. For example, Heath and Abel introduce a model that includes variables such as uncertainty, trust, information seeking, and cognitive involvement.[10] Palenchar and Heath develop a model that focuses on uncertainty, control, internal and external involvement, and support/opposition.[53] Other key variables include credibility, firsthand experience, knowledge, and perceived economic benefit, to name a few.[54-56]

Within the discussion of terrorist threats and acts, three key risk-communication process variables have been identified: uncertainty, control, and trust. Uncertainty, for example, is a central variable in risk perception and the risk-communication process. Risks, by definition, are matters of uncertainty. In light of this, Albrecht defines uncertainty as the lack of confidence about cause-effect patterns.[57] Different groups within the public want to reduce uncertainties about the subjects under consideration and about the people who are creating those uncertainties. Thus, uncertainty is a measure of confidence regarding the ability to estimate risk and its consequences, and the ability to communicate knowledgeably on the facts and issues surrounding any specific risk.

Concerning communication related to terrorist acts, it is understandable that for lay persons risk messages can be confusing: They come from a variety of sources that involve multiple parties and often reflect competing scientific conclusions. Experts and regulatory agencies often operate on the assumption that they and their audiences share a common framework for evaluating and interpreting risk information. This confusion also stems from the fact that prominent government officials take different and often opposing viewpoints about environmental, health, and safety risks and participate in highly public debates about risk estimations.[3,58]

Uncertainty is a motivator because it is uncomfortable. Uncertainty reduction theory uses this principle to explain the human incentive to seek information.[59] Driskill and Goldstein define uncertainty "as the perceived lack of information, knowledge, beliefs, and feelings necessary for accomplishing organizational tasks."[60] When facing uncertainty about the future, people use the best information available to reduce their fears, to achieve a sense of control over the future, and to feel better about what they have to do—face uncertainty with incomplete information. Adopting this line of reasoning, Albrecht defines uncertainty as "the lack of attributional confidence about cause-effect patterns."[57]

Risk assessment, specifically terrorist risk assessment, and uncertainty are interrelated.[61] Risk is a product of uncertainty about whether an event will occur and the possibility its consequence will be good or bad. To complicate matters, uncertainty thrives in risk communication issues. Otway suggests that scientific knowledge is often most uncertain in precisely those policy decisions regarding technological risks.[49] During crises or other troubling times, uncertainty is likely to increase. The same is true regarding terrorism. This concept is evident in the ever-changing color-alert status for terrorist threats used by the U.S. Department of Homeland Security. "In turbulent times, uncertainty and distrust soar. Highly involved people struggle to control sources of risk that affect their self-interests. Information and knowledge become less relevant to the need to exert control because they are only loosely related to risk tolerance."[62]

Numerous views of communication, however, continue to identify understanding as the final dependent variable. People may understand, for example, the meaning of each color of the Department of Homeland Security's terrorist alert system. Yet they may not agree that the risk assessments corresponding to those colors are founded on the proper levels of risk. This line of reasoning makes explicit the fact that risk communication is not merely a scientific- or knowledge-based activity.

The requisite processes for anticipating, preventing, mitigating, and responding to terrorism pose substantial challenges for corporations. Standard approaches to risk perception find that key groups within the public believe that responsible organizations must exert efforts to control the likelihood that terrorism will affect their interests. Controllability refers to the ability of knowledgeable and responsible people to prevent the occurrence of the risk or its consequences. Risks are uncertainties that experts attempt to reduce to probabilities that some persons out of a population will suffer. Who will the victims be? Dread refers to the seriousness or magnitude of the outcome: the number of people harmed or the agony of the effects of encountering that risk. Uncertainty is a concept that is routinely used to define risk. Risk is the probability that an event will occur and whether its effects will be tolerable or severe.

Many studies have demonstrated that control is a key variable in risk communication. Community-based control means that members of a community seek to enforce standards for corporate responsibility on organizations that generate risks, as well as upon their watchdog counterparts (including government and nonprofit organizations). Thompson defined control as the belief that an individual or organization can influence an event, or at least has the ability to do so.[63] Control can be exerted to reduce the likelihood of a risk event or to minimize its impact.

Johnson, as well as Hance, Chess, and Sandman, determines that risk communication is likely to fail if it does not increase residents' control in the decision-making process.[64,65] A risk is more acceptable to persons if they have some degree of control over the situation, so reasons Covello.[66] Thus, at-risk groups are more willing to accept risks if they have some control over them.[67,68] Kasperson discovered a relationship between people's belief that they can control the gathering of information and the support for risk-communication programs.[69]

These theories rest upon an understanding of control as a personal trait, which can be internal when control rests with the individual, or external when control belongs to someone else. Internal control occurs when persons feel some control over their destinies. External control results when outside forces are perceived to have control over a risk source. In this regard, Sims and Baumann find that the more a person feels in control (internally or externally) the less s/he should feel that local chemical plant activities will affect their life.[9] Personal control extends to perceptions of speed of onset, scope (area), and duration of impact of the risk, as well as the quality of emergency preparedness.

Control is a key factor in risk assessment because risk is associated with uncertainty. Risks are by nature matters of uncertainty. Uncertainties of risks come in three kinds: the likelihood that some risk event will occur (positive or negative), the likelihood that the outcome of the event will harm specific individuals, and the likelihood that the outcome will be serious (such as death) as opposed to slight. As people think about risks, they ask many questions: Will something happen? Will it be bad? Will I suffer from the damage? To compensate for feelings of uncertainty, people want to exert control. In an academic setting for instance, students try to exert control over the outcome of an examination by trying to reduce uncertainty by knowing which questions will be asked and which answers are correct. Thus, uncertainty is a motivator and control is a means for reducing uncertainty.

As control declines and a sense of risk increases, people's cognitive involvement also increases, especially if the risk is seen to affect their self-interests or the interests of persons and entities for which they have concern. In this regard, uncertainty (doubt as to facts and conclusions) and cognitive involvement (belief that self-interests are at stake) lead to increased communication activity. Trust predicts what affected people believe and the sources on which they rely. The infrastructure exhibits social amplification as various players receive, comment on, and pass along information and opinions.

Trust is a vital part of this narrative. People in each community where risks occur must be able to trust the efforts to achieve reasonable levels of security. Such levels need to withstand the "smell" test of the area residents; that means the announced levels of security have to seem correct, the right and logical thing for companies to do. Specifically, community members must feel they can and should trust industry to achieve a reasonable level of security, and to communicate in ways that increase rather than decrease citizens' security.

Trust is a counterpart of control. It assumes that when people are vulnerable in to one another, the matter of trust becomes relevant. Industry would like to say, "trust us because we have planned and launched policies that will reasonably protect your interests, your security, and safety." People are vulnerable to the quality of planning by industry. Industry is vulnerable to the cleverness and treachery of terrorism. Employees, investors, customers, and community members are vulnerable to terrorism to the extent that the relevant industry is vulnerable.

Trust is a central factor in predicting whether members of a community accept and rely on the conclusions and recommendations of people who are trained in science, national security, business operations, engineering, emergency management, and public policy. Risk assessments require scientific and decision-making techniques that are often foreign to lay persons. If these expert risk estimates conflict, decisions become even more complex and require even greater amounts of trust. For effective risk communication, groups within the public must trust the source of information and advice.[54]

Trust is demonstrated in word and deed. It is groomed and maintained. It can be lost or destroyed. Thus, it is a precious ingredient in community relations. If citizens cannot trust individuals to be responsible, they will turn to other entities—government bodies and activists—to force appropriate operating standards. Thus, industry has a moral and strategic business-planning obligation to motivate and guide its planning and operations.

These factors influence how, what, when, and to whom the industry will communicate. In essence, when it comes to terrorist-related risk and crisis communication, issues such as uncertainty, control, and trust remain key elements of the stakeholders' narratives that provide insight into both risk-management and risk-communication protocols.

## CONCLUSION

Terrorism and risk communication are narrative enactments of culture. Risk management and risk communication help organizations enact and comanage cultures with key groups within the public. To support this view, we draw on Fisher, who sees narrative as the paradigm of all communication.[19,20] People think and act in terms of narratives. Narrative form and content connect and give meaning to events. In the narrative of ocean travel, the sinking of the *Titanic* is an iconic narrative, as is the *Exxon Valdez* in the transport of crude oil. Not only do such events happen over time, as narrative, but they also are part of larger narratives of transportation and industrial activities. Each news story frames events, characters, and meaning in terms of who, when, where, why, what, and how. These narrative elements correspond to how people think. For this reason, risk- and crisis-communication statements made by organizations are more likely to be meaningful and effective when they address the narratives that key groups use, as reflected in their particular cultures. At the same time, communicators must monitor the narratives of conflicting groups, as a means to prevent and respond to terrorist-related crises.

The best risk prevention and crisis-response preparation is that which is never used. Research shows that many plans are developed, but never drilled. Communication strategies are developed, but not employed. Management is lulled into complacency. Managers look in the wrong direction, or not at all.

The tragedies of Bhopal, Tylenol, and the World Trade Center remind professionals of what they "should have done." Management often scolds professions in risk and crisis—why didn't you do more to warn us of what could happen. Analysis that follows each incident is best when it reviews the success of planning, not the need for planning. Such is the burden shouldered by managements to earn and maintain the trust to stakeholders and stakeseekers.

## NOTES

1. Douglas M. Risk and blame: essays in cultural theories. London: Routledge; 1992.

2. Plough A, Krimsky S. The emergence of risk communication studies: social and political context. Sci Technol Hum Values 1987;12(3/4):4–10.

3. Krimsky S, Plough A. Plant closure: the ASARCO/Tacoma copper smelter. Environmental hazards: communicating risks as a social process. Dover, MA: Auburn House; 1988.

4. Fischhoff B. Managing risk perceptions. Issues Sci Technol 1985;2:83–96.

5. American Chemistry Council. ACC media kit on security. 2004. Available from: www.americanchemistry.com. Accessed January 29, 2004.

6. Hunter D, Mullin R. Responsible care: the challenge of communication. Chem Week 1992 Dec 9:22–33.

7. Walsh EJ. Challenging official risk assessments via protest mobilization: the TMI case. In: Johnson BB, Covello VT, editors. The social and cultural construction of risk: essays on risk selection and perception. Dordrecht, Netherlands: Reidel; 1987. p. 85–101.

8. Rosenblatt R. All the world gasped. Time 1984 Dec 17:20.

9. Sims JH, Baumann DD. Educational programs and human response to natural hazards. Environ Behav 1983;15(2):165–89.

10. Heath RL, Abel DD. Proactive response to citizen risk concerns: increasing citizen's knowledge of emergency response practices. J Public Relations Res 1996;8:151–71; See also Heath RL, Palenchar M. Community relations and risk communication: a longitudinal study of the impact of emergency response messages. J Public Relations Res 2000;12(2):131–61.

11. Heath RL, Bradshaw J, Lee J. Community relationship building: local leadership in the risk communication infrastructure. J Public Relations Res 2002;14(4):317–53.

12. Freudenberg N. Not in our backyards! Community action for health and the environment. New York: Monthly Review Press; 1984.

13. Hansson SO. Dimensions of risk. Risk Anal 1989;9(1):107–12.

14. Tversky A, Kahneman D. Judgment under uncertainty: heuristics and biases. In: Arkes HR, Hammond KR, editors. Judgment and decision making. Cambridge: Cambridge University Press; 1986. p. 38–55.

15. Environmental Protection Agency. Seven cardinal rules of risk communication. Washington, DC: Environmental Protection Agency; 1988.

16. Newman KM. Toxic chemical disclosures: An overview of new problems. New opportunities for the professional communicator. New York: Public Relations Society of America; 1988.

17. Heath RL. Strategic issues management: organizations and public policy challenges. Thousand Oaks, CA: Sage; 1997; Toth, EL, Heath, RL, (editors). Rhetorical and critical approaches to public relations. Mahwah, NJ: Lawrence Erlbaum Associates, 1992.

18. Fisher WR. Narration as a human communication paradigm: the case of public moral argument. Commun Monogr 1984;51:1–22.

19. Fisher, WR. The narrative paradigm: an elaboration. Commun Monogr 1985;52:347–67.

20. Fisher WR. Human communication as narration: toward a philosophy of reason, value and action. Columbia: University of South Carolina Press; 1987.

21. Fisher WR. Clarifying the narrative paradigm. Commun Monogr 1989; 56:55–8.

22. Pearce WB, Cronen VE. Communication, action, and meaning. New York: Praeger; 1980.

23. Cronen VE, Pearce WB, Harris LM. The coordinated management of meaning: a theory of communication. In: Dance FEX, editor. Human communi cation theory: comparative essays. New York: Harper & Row; 1982. p. 61–89.

24. Foss SK. Rhetorical criticism: exploration & practice. 2nd ed. Prospect Heights, IL: Waveland Press; 1996. p. 400.

25. Gergen KJ, Gergen MM. Narrative and the self as relationship. In: Berkowitz L, editor. Advances in experimental social psychology. New York: Academic Press; 1988. p. 17–56. (vol 21).

26. Whorf BL. Language, thought, and reality. Cambridge, MA: MIT Press; 1956.

27. Morgan G. Images of organization. Newbury Park, CA: Sage; 1986. p. 128.

28. Heath RL. Management of corporate communication: from interpersonal contacts to external affairs. Hillsdale, NJ: Lawrence Erlbaum; 1994.

29. Heath RL. Realism and relativism: a perspective on Kenneth Burke. Macon, GA: Mercer University Press; 1986. p. 121.

30. Burke K. Permanence and change. 2nd ed. Indianapolis: Bobbs-Merrill; 1965. p. 25.

31. Burke K. The philosophy of literary form. 3rd ed. Berkeley, CA: University of California Press; 1973. p. 9.

32. Burke K. Dramatism and logology. Times Literary Suppl 1983 Aug 12;859.

33. Heath RL. Strategic issues management: organizations and public policy challenges. Thousand Oaks, CA: Sage; 1997.

34. Heath RL. Telling a story: a narrative approach to communication during a crisis. In: Millar DP, Heath RL, editors. Responding to crisis: a rhetorical approach to crisis communication. Mahwah, NJ: Lawrence Erlbaum; 2004. p. 167–87.

35. Burke K. Language as symbolic action. Berkeley, CA: University of California Press; 1966.

36. Lerbinger O. The crisis manager: facing risk and responsibility. Mahwah, NJ: Lawrence Erlbaum; 1997.

37. Heath RL, Millar DP. A rhetorical approach to crisis communication: management, communication, processes, and strategic responses. In: Millar DP, Heath RL, editors. Responding to crisis: a rhetorical approach to crisis. Mahwah, NJ: Lawrence Erlbaum; 2004. p. 1–17.

38. Barnes B. The nature of power. Urbana, IL: University of Illinois Press; 1988.

39. Sriramesh K, Grunig JE, Buffington J. Corporate culture and public relations. In: Grunig JE, editor. Excellence in public relations and communication management. Hillsdale, NJ: Lawrence Erlbaum; 1992. p. 577–95.

40. Fearn-Banks K. Crisis communications: a casebook approach. Mahwah, NJ: Lawrence Erlbaum; 1996.

41. Penrose JM. The role of perception in crisis planning. Public Relations Rev 2000;26(2):155–74.

42. Burnett JJ. A strategic approach to managing crises. Public Relations Rev 1998;24(4):475–88.

43. Coombs WT. Ongoing crisis communication: planning, managing, and responding. Thousand Oaks, CA: Sage; 1999.

44. Carney A, Jordan A. Prepare for business-related crises. Public Relations J 1993;49:34–45.

45. Marra FJ. Crisis communications plans: poor predictors of excellent crisis public relations. Public Relations Rev 1998;24(4):461–74.

46. Pearson CM, Clair JA. Reframing crisis management. Acad Manag Rev 1998;23(1):59–76.

47. Thomas K, Swaton E, Fishbein M, Otway HJ. Nuclear energy: the accuracy of policy makers' perceptions of public beliefs. Behav Sci 1980;25:332–344.

48. Renn O. Concepts of risk: a classification. In: Krimsky S, Golding D, editors. Social theories of risk. Westport, CT: Praeger; 1992. p. 53–79.

49. Otway H. Public wisdom, expert fallibility: toward a contextual theory of risk. In Krimsky S, Golding D, editors. Social theories of risk. Westport, CT: Praeger; 1992. p. 227.

50. Brehmer B. The psychology of risk. In: Singleton WT, Hovden J, editors. Risk and decisions. New York: Wiley; 1987. p. 25–39.

51. Fischhoff B. Risk perception and communication unplugged: twenty years of process. Risk Anal 1995;15:137–45.

52. Chess C, Salomone KL, Hance BJ, Saville A. Results of a national symposium on risk communication: next steps for government agencies. Risk Anal 1995;15:115–25.

53. Palenchar MJ, Heath RL. Another part of the risk communication model: analysis of communication processes and message content. J Public Relations Res 2002;14(2):127–58.

54. Renn O, Levine D. Credibility and trust in risk communication. In: Kasperson RE, Stallen PJ, editors. Communicating risks to the public. Dordrecht, Netherlands: Kluwer; 1991. p. 175–218.

55. Baird B. Tolerance for environmental health risks: the influence of knowledge, benefits, voluntarism and environmental attitudes. Risk Anal 1986;6(4):425–35.

56. Covello VT, von Winterfeldt D, Slovic P. Communicating scientific information about health and environmental risks: problems and opportunities from a social and behavioral perspective. In: Covello VT, Lave LB, Moghissi A, Uppuluri VR, editors. Uncertainty in risk assessment, risk management, and decision making. New York: Plenum; 1987. p. 221–39.

57. Albrecht TL. Communication and personal control in empowering organizations. In: Anderson JA, editor. Communication yearbook. Newbury Park, CA: Sage; 1988. p. 380–404. (vol 11).

58. Covello VT. Risk communication: an emerging area of health communication research. In: Deetz SA, editor. Communication yearbook Newbury Park, CA: Sage; 1992. p. 359–73. (vol 15)

59. Berger CR, Calabrase RJ. Some explorations in initial interaction and beyond: toward a developmental theory of interpersonal communication. Hum Commun Res 1975;1:99–112.

60. Driskill LP, Goldstein JR. Uncertainty: theory and practice in organizational communication. J Bus Commun 1986;23(3):41–56.

61. Weterings R, Van Eijndhoven J. Informing the public about uncertain risks. Risk Anal 1989;9(4):473–82.

62. Heath RL. Corporate environment risk communication: cases and practices along the Texas gulf coast. In: Burleson BR, editor. Communication yearbook. Thousand Oaks, CA: Sage; 1995. p. 273. (vol 18).

63. Thompson SC. Will it hurt less if I can control it? A complex answer to a simple question. Psychol Bull 1981;90(1):89–101.

64. Johnson BL. Health risk communication and the agency for toxic substances and disease registry. Risk Anal 1987;7(4):409–12.

65. Hance BJ, Chess C, Sandman PM. Setting a context for explaining risk. Risk Anal 1989;9(1):113–7.

66. Fischhoff B, Slovic P, Lichtenstein S, Read S, Combs B. How safe is safe enough? A psychometric study of attitudes toward technological risks and benefits. Policy Sci 1978;9:127–52.

67. Covello VT, Sandman P, Slovic P. Risk communication, risk statistics, and risk comparisons: a manual for plant managers. Washington, DC: Chemical Manufacturers Association; 1988.

68. Lindell MK, Earle TC. How close is close enough: public perceptions of the risks of industrial facilities. Risk Anal 1983;3(4):245–53.

69. Kasperson RE. Six propositions on public participation and their relevance for risk. Risk Anal 1986;6(3):275–81.

# 8 Constructing the "New Normal" through Post-Crisis Discourse

*Timothy L. Sellnow, Matthew W. Seeger, and Robert R. Ulmer*

Crises, particularly in the early stages, create a need to understand causes, consequences, and levels of harm.[1-3] In acts of terrorism, uncertainty is at once the most alarming and pervasive consequence of the attack-induced crisis. This uncertainty is further intensified by the terrorist's intentional effort to cause maximum harm and fear. Lerbinger explains that, "in particular, it is the psychological element of malice that makes each terrorist act, no matter how small, deeply repugnant" (p. 145).[4] Terrorism-inspired fear is based largely on its seemingly random assault on innocent victims. Thus, the nature of terrorism creates a level of uncertainty that is both a natural consequence of the event and the ultimate objective of the terrorists.

The uncertainty produced by terrorism also creates an urgent need for information.[5] Because terrorist acts typically have a political objective, government agencies are an essential means for gathering and disseminating information. Moreover, governmental organizations have a primary responsibility for managing those crises that produce widespread public harm. A dramatic example of this responsibility was the Centers for Disease Control and Prevention's (CDC) primary role in addressing the anthrax crisis. This crisis began within days after the September 11, 2001, terrorist attacks on the World Trade Center (WTC) and Pentagon. Letters laced with anthrax spores were mailed to the offices of the tabloid the *Sun*, in Boca Raton, Florida; to NBC news anchor Tom Brokaw in New York City; to the offices of the *New York Post*; and to Senate Majority Leader Tom Daschle in Washington, DC. The conflation of the 9/11 attacks and the anthrax poisonings created a unique level of alarm and fear that a widespread bioterrorism attack was possible.[6] When individuals who handled the mail became infected through skin contact with cutaneous anthrax, and in some cases, the more dangerous inhalation anthrax, a fearful nation turned to the CDC for information regarding vulnerability and appropriate medical responses to the assault.

The CDC's public response to the crisis became extremely controversial. Responding in a somewhat routine manner to what many experts initially assumed was a familiar form of anthrax, CDC spokespersons attempted to calm those who assumed they had been exposed. Moreover, CDC officials sought to assure the public that there was little threat of widespread harm from cutaneous anthrax, and that inhalation anthrax was rare. These early characterizations proved regrettable, as the number of victims and the severity of their infections steadily increased. Throughout the crisis, the CDC was resoundingly criticized by a wide variety of sources. Critics claimed that the CDC failed to account for the complexity of the infectious agent, failed to protect postal workers, and provided conflicting information. This criticism, and the CDC's own internal assessment, have since led to notable changes in how the agency communicates in crisis situations. Simply put, the terrorist attack produced a level of uncertainty and complexity that forced the CDC to reorganize its crisis-communication functions. The lessons learned from the anthrax crisis relate to all aspects of the CDC's risk communication and crisis planning. As Covello explains, the anthrax crisis "presents a unique opportunity for public health agencies to assess and elevate their level of communication preparedness for all risk and crisis scenarios" (p. 5).[7]

In this chapter, we examine the CDC anthrax crisis as a case study to explore two issues: (1) the means by which organizational learning is inspired by a crisis event, and (2) the way such learning leads to necessary changes in the structure and planning functions of an organization. Specifically, we explore the complex process of coming to terms with a crisis event, or "sense making," and the role this process plays in organizational learning about crisis. We examine a number of ways in which the CDC learned from the anthrax event and describe implications for other organizations facing crisis. We describe the process through which, in crisis circumstances, learning can generate the emergence of a "new normal," as the public and response agencies construct a new understanding of risk and threat.[8] Finally, we outline conclusions and implications for organizations as they seek to learn and adapt in response to crisis events.

## THE "NEW NORMAL"

The new normal was a term that emerged in public discourse following the 9/11 terrorist attacks. It came to signify both a broader public understanding of new risks, and specific organizational responses to that risk, such as risk-avoidance processes and procedures. The new normal, for example, was often used to describe heightened airline safety, including more rigorous inspections of passengers. It is applied to new antiterrorism laws by civil liberty advocates and to the artistic, literary, and musical tributes to the 9/11 victims. Observers have noted that new normal involves the public stockpiling of antibiotics and gas masks, heightened anxiety and stress-related illness, and the acts of civility and selflessness that emerged following the 9/11 attacks. New normal, then, represents a broadly reconstituted order that incorporates new understandings and interpretations of a crisis into a revised status quo.

Researchers using chaos theory to examine crises have described this revised status quo as emerging after a dramatic disruption of a system's order.[9,10] Through natural self-organizing processes, new forms, structures, procedures, hierarchies, and understandings emerge, while outdated procedures, technologies, and assumptions are discarded. The result is a fundamentally new form or shape to the system. In part, this process takes place because the disruption of crisis dramatically reveals the inadequacy of the status quo. Thus, crisis severely weakens resistance to change within an organization. Previous procedures and assumptions may be refined or replaced when appropriate, or they may simply be discarded. Self-organization and the emergence of a new normal is one the most optimistic outcomes of a crisis. In some cases the new normal may even involve a dramatic renewal or rebirth of the organization.[11]

## CRISIS AND SENSE MAKING

By their very nature, crises are shocking events. Victims of crises must make sense of an event they did not anticipate and cannot hope to fully understand.[2] Karl Weick refers to this process as retrospective sense making.[12] Crisis situations disrupt normal patterns and routines and demonstrate the inadequacy of existing assumptions. As a consequence, they create high levels of uncertainty as victims, government agencies, and members of the public struggle to make sense of what happened. Communication is central to this process, as members share interpretations of the event and construct a collective understanding of the crisis.

The principal problem for organizations, particularly during crisis, is that of resolving or reducing this high environmental uncertainty or ambiguity.[3,13] Ambiguity in this case refers to the various possible meanings the crisis event could have. One way organizations reduce ambiguity and reach consensus about meaning is through enactment, that is by taking some action to understand a crisis and then evaluating those actions. Acting toward a crisis situation in essence allows members to begin the process of reconstituting some new understanding that includes the crisis experience.

Organizations often mistakenly believe, however, that the future will look much like the past. This may be a serious mistake, particularly when dealing with nonroutine, complex crises. Crises are inherently dynamic events that more often than not evolve in unexpected and surprising ways. If organizations fail to recognize the multivariate and dynamic components of a crisis situation, they are likely to respond in a routine manner, thereby unwittingly increasing the potential severity and impact of the crisis. The result is what Weick terms stunted enactment.[12]

The enactment and sense-making process is often severely constrained during a crisis. Crisis creates entirely new and threatening situations. Often, irrevocable decisions must be initiated without time to fully consider their implications. The result may be a collapse or severe reduction in sense making. These collapses are associated with the onset of a threatening situation, followed by maladaptive responses that accentuate harm. Organizations may find themselves in a downward spiral as they struggle to manage a novel crisis situation in ways that make sense. Weick describes these basic losses of meaning as occurring "when people suddenly and deeply feel that the universe is no longer a rational, orderly system. What makes such an event so shattering is that both the sense of what is occurring and the means to rebuild that sense collapse together" (p. 633).[14]

These episodes involve a basic loss of understanding of what is happening and what can be done about it. In some rare cases, decision-makers and those affected by the crisis may become so completely disoriented that they simply lose the capacity to respond. Such losses in sense making are not uncommon during the periods of high uncertainty, high stress, and short response time typical of many crisis situations.

One of the implications of Weick's analysis is that previous experience with a crisis may enhance the ability of members to make sense of a similar event. In other words, experiencing a crisis may be a learning experience that teaches participants how to respond. Conversely, individuals may also interpret or enact a serious event using their previous experience with a routine event. Rising water, for example, may be interpreted as a routine minor spring flood and when in fact it is a much more serious flood.[15] In this way, minor crises may actually create additional blind spots, particularly with organizations like the CDC that routinely experience moderate threats and disruptions. If an organization initially responds to a crisis with a routine response that fails, its ability to make sense of the event and respond effectively may be reduced.

## ORGANIZATIONAL LEARNING

Organizational learning concerns the processes of adaptation. Learning emphasizes a system's openness and flexibility as essential for accommodating changing conditions and new understandings.[16] Through learning, organizations add new know-how, competencies, skills, and capacity, often replacing those previously learned. Events that provide an opening for learning may range from comparatively minor modifications of routine, such as a change in work schedules, to full-blown crises. As discussed earlier, crises often demonstrate the inadequacies of established structure, procedures, and beliefs. Thus, as organizations respond to crises, they must abandon the status quo and adapt to what becomes a new normal.[8]

Barry Turner offers a detailed six-stage model that describes how crises develop and how organizations accommodate to lessons learned from these events.[17] Among these adaptations is the development of a new sense of what is "normal," including new beliefs, norms, structures and procedures. Using Turner's model, we illustrate the process by which organizations learn from crises.

### Six Stages in Failure of Foresight

Turner's developmental model is based on his analysis of public inquiries into disasters. He argues that crises can be understood as "large scale intelligence failures" or "failures in foresight." "A disaster occurs because of some inaccuracy or inadequacy in the accepted norms and beliefs" that "rarely develops instantaneously" (p. 381).[17] Most organizations successfully manage many day-to-day problems by relying on well-established beliefs about the world, its hazards, and what constitutes reasonable precaution. At any particular point, Turner argues, these established beliefs help constitute a sense of what is normal operation. In fact, most problems are effectively resolved through these routine, normal structures, and require little or no attention. One fundamental difficulty organizations face, then, is to determine which problems can be trusted to routine procedures and which should be attended to with novel actions. When an organization misses some critical cue regarding an emerging threat, it experiences what Turner calls a "failure in foresight," or a "collapse of precautions which have hitherto been regarded culturally as adequate" (p. 380).[17] Crisis events often erupt when problems that are seen as insignificant interact with precautions that were considered adequate. Crisis, then, is the result of a widespread and dramatic failure in the organizational status quo. As an organization emerges from a crisis, it consequently must reconstitute a new status quo.

Turner's first stage (see table 8.1) is a time of normal operations and routine procedures. Members have a set of culturally accepted beliefs about the world and its hazards. Associated precautionary norms, which may be set out in laws, codes, and practices, as well as mores and folkways, are generally considered adequate (p. 381).[17] Accepted beliefs, policies, and procedures, for example, may govern handling of dangerous chemicals, dealings with agitated employees, inspection of airline baggage, or methods for reporting profits and losses. These beliefs, norms, and associated procedures are highly interdependent, so that a change in one would require changes in others.

The second stage, the crisis-incubation period, features an accumulation of events that don't conform to accepted beliefs about hazards, or norms for avoiding crisis. Turner argues that these events are either unknown, or known but not fully understood. Often a collective blindness develops that resembles Weick's concept of stunted enactment.[3] This blindness allows minor problems to incubate, fester, grow, and

Table 8.1
Turner's Five Stages of Failures of Foresight

| Stage | Features |
|---|---|
| I: Normal operations | Risk-management norms (beliefs, procedures) are codified |
| II: Incubation | Unnoticed events challenge norms |
| III: Preciptation | Noticed event brings norms into question |
| IV: Onset | Norms collapse; crisis becomes evident |
| V: Rescue and salvage | Ad hoc adjustments made to norm |
| VI: Cultural adjustment | Assessment results in changes to the norms |

Source: Turner B. The organizational and interorganizational development of disasters. Admin Sci Q 1976;21:381

perhaps interact with other unnoticed problems, resulting, finally, in a severe threat. Turner suggests that incubation often occurs because a problem or issue is poorly structured or defined, and, consequently, cannot be attended to easily.[17] Such problems are more difficult to perceive and make sense of.

In the third stage, the crisis is first sensed through a "trigger event." This dramatic event signals a fundamental inadequacy of dominant beliefs about hazards and the associated norm for avoidance. A trigger event may be a consumer harmed by product failure, a lawsuit, some extensive disruption of operations, an explosion, a violent act, or a media report that signals the eruption of a threat into a crisis.[18] In short, the event's disruptive power is so great that the distinction between it and normal, routine operations is so clear that it cannot be ignored. The crisis, however, is still very difficult to define or understand. It is clear that something is dramatically wrong, but the significance of the event is not clear, nor are the consequences.

Turner's fourth stage is the onset of the crisis. During this stage, immediate, direct, and unanticipated consequences become manifest. This damage varies widely in intensity and scope from one crisis to another. Stage four is the period in which the crisis is in operation—when direct impact and harm occurs. In many instances, such as the attacks on the WTC and Pentagon, this stage may last only a matter of minutes or hours, but in that time, a significant proportion of the harm accumulates. Reducing the duration of stage four is a primary goal of crisis management. Crisis containment means that some level of control has been reasserted, and the major risks are past, although secondary risks and outbreaks are possible. The conclusion of this stage, however, often either goes unrecognized or is prematurely declared. Because crisis events represent novel circumstances, it is often impossible to know when containment has been successful or if risk is still high.

Stage five is rescue and salvage, when members of the organization recognize the collapse of their past avoidance norms and beliefs about the world and its hazards. This recognition allows for initial and rapid ad hoc adjustments and responses, and the initiation of rescue and salvage efforts. At this point, the organization may activate its crisis plans and make strategic adjustments in its crisis response in ways that reduce, mitigate, and contain harm. Efforts are undertaken to mitigate harm, protect property, provide treatment to victims, recover bodies, quarantine dangerous areas, and assess the level of damage. These responses often require high levels of coordination between the organization, outside agencies, and the public. This coordination, in turn, requires some consensus about the nature of the crisis and appropriate mitigation strategies. Stage-five coordination also requires restoration of communication channels often disrupted during a crisis.

Finally, Turner's sixth stage involves what he has described as a full cultural adjustment of beliefs about the world, its hazards, and its avoidance norms so that they are once again compatible with new insights and understandings gained during the crisis. New norms, structures, policies, and procedures are instituted so that similar events do not reoccur. This final stage requires some general consensus about cause, blame, and responsibility. Often, as with the National Transportation Safety Board (NTSB), a formal inquiry or investigation of the crisis is undertaken by outside agencies to identify probable cause and responsibility. Strategies for rebuilding public trust during stage six may include excuses, justification, ingratiation, denouncement, and distortion.[19] In terms of learning, stage six is also the point at which a critical event becomes a narrative history about risk, its potential for crisis, and its avoidance. In some instances, the process of learning from crisis is highly structured, such as the NTSB's issuing of probable-cause findings and recommendations. In other instances, stage-six adaptations are more informal, as participants reach a new consensus regarding risk and choose to behave differently. In either case, Turner argues, a new understanding regarding what constitutes normal arises. This new understanding is reflected in post-crisis adaptive responses that become standardized parts of the organization's operations—a new normal.

Turner also suggests that the sixth stage leads back to the first, a point of normal operation and procedures.[17] At this point, the crisis resolves into the full acceptance of a new normal, including new beliefs, norms, structures, and procedures. From an organizational learning perspective, then, crises are long term and broadly cyclical processes with stage six (full cultural readjustment) leading back to stage one (initial accepted beliefs about the world and its hazards and its avoidance).

The stages of Turner's model are particularly useful for assessing the CDC's response to the anthrax crisis. The agency's initial failure to grasp the severity of the crisis, the lingering intensity of the attack, the continued sense making and adjustments throughout the crisis, and the establishment of a new normal in response to the crisis are all evident in the CDC's protracted response. In the following section, we describe the criticism and organizational learning the CDC experienced during, and in response to, the anthrax crisis.

## CRITICISM OF CDC'S RESPONSE TO THE ANTHRAX CRISIS

After the September 11, 2001, attacks on the WTC and the Pentagon, the CDC adopted a heightened state of observation for the occurrence of biological terrorism. Although anthrax had been mentioned as a likely tool of biological terrorism, the CDC consistently indicated that, because anthrax is not communicable, its viability as a terrorist weapon in the United States was limited. Moreover, anthrax was believed to be well understood, relatively easily controlled, and difficult to disseminate to the larger population. Thus, the CDC remained in Turner's stage two, relatively comfortable with its routine knowledge for coping with an anthrax episode. When the first cases of anthrax appeared in Florida and New York (see table 8.2), the CDC did not appear overly alarmed and undertook what could be described as a largely routine response. The agency addressed the precipitating event, Turner's stage three, with established procedures and structures. As the number of anthrax cases climbed in the following months, however, and the crisis moved into stage four, the CDC was severely criticized for what was perceived to be an inadequate response. For example, Congress, state health officials, postal workers, and the general public disparaged the CDC for its ineffectiveness at the onset of the crisis, including its perceived failure to issue effective, timely warnings and recommendations.

The CDC's response to the anthrax crisis was based on routine knowledge of the biological agent. In its cutaneous form, the disease is not uncommon in the cattle industry and is easily treated. The much more serious inhalation anthrax had always been rare but was associated with the leather and hide processing industry, and had essentially been eradicated in this country. At the onset of the crisis, however, CDC administrators did not recognize the virulence of the anthrax spores disseminated through contaminated letters. More importantly, the agency was initially unprepared to accurately project the infection rate caused by the mailed anthrax spores, which had been processed into a sophisticated aerosol form. These complicating factors led the CDC to respond routinely in a manner perceived by its stakeholders as inadequate. In its defense, the agency was dealing with a form of anthrax it had never before encountered and thus could not accurately project how the spores would spread. Moreover, no one could have predicted how anthrax spores might be spread through a complex mail system involving delivery routes, mail carriers, and automated sorting technology.

## Table 8.2
## A Timeline of Events Related to the Anthrax Crisis of 2001

| Date | Event |
| --- | --- |
| September 18 | Letters postmarked in Trenton, NJ, sent to *New York Post* and NBC anchor Tom Brokaw. The letters test positive for anthrax. |
| September 22 | *New York Post* editorial assistant Johanna Huden, who opens letters to the editor, notices blister on her finger. |
| September 27 | Teresa Heller, letter carrier at the West Trenton post office, develops lesion on her arm. |
| September 28 | Erin O'Connor, assistant to Brokaw, notices a lesion. |
| October 1 | Ernesto Blanco, mailroom employee at American Media, Inc., publisher of the *Sun* is admitted to the hospital. O'Connor begins taking ciprofloxacin. |
| October 4 | Authorities confirm first case of anthrax. Bob Stevens, photo editor at the *Sun*, is diagnosed with inhaled form of anthrax. |
| October 5 | Stevens dies. First U.S. death from inhaled anthrax since 1976. |
| October 9 | Letter postmarked in Trenton, NJ, sent to Senate Majority Leader Tom Daschle. The letter tests positive for anthrax. |
| October 12 | Officials announce that O'Connor at NBC developed skin anthrax after opening the letter. |
| October 15 | Letter containing anthrax opened in Daschle's office, which is quarantined. Officials say infant son of an ABC producer in New York developed skin anthrax. |
| October 17 | Thirty-one people at U.S. Capitol test positive for exposure to anthrax. Later tests showed 28 were actually exposed. |
| October 18 | Claire Fletcher, assistant to CBS News anchor Dan Rather, tests positive for skin anthrax. |
| October 19 | *New York Post* announces Huden is diagnosed with skin anthrax. Another New Jersey postal worker tests positive for skin anthrax. |
| October 21 | Washington postal worker Thomas L. Morris Jr dies of inhalation anthrax. Officials begin testing thousands of postal employees. |
| October 22 | Another postal worker, Joseph P. Curseen, dies of inhalation anthrax. |
| October 23 | Anthrax is found on machine at military base that sorts mail for White House. Unidentified New Jersey postal worker at Hamilton office is hospitalized with suspected case of inhalation anthrax. |
| October 25 | State Department mail facility employee is hospitalized with anthrax. |
| October 28 | CDC confirms a female New Jersey postal worker has inhalation anthrax. |
| October 29 | A 51-year-old Hamilton Township, NJ, woman with no connection to the postal service or media is diagnosed with skin anthrax. Anthrax is confirmed in a Hamilton Township mailroom. |
| October 30 | Officials confirm New Jersey's second case of inhaled anthrax—a postal worker. |
| October 31 | New York woman, Kathy T. Nguyen, dies of inhalation anthrax. |
| November 8 | President Bush visits CDC. |
| November 21 | Ottilie W. Lundgren, a 94-year-old retiree, dies of inhalation anthrax in Connecticut. |
| February 22 | Koplan announces his resignation as director of CDC. |

*Source*: Barrett SM, et al. CDC and anthrax: a communication study. North Dakota State University, Department of Communication; 2002

Turner's stage five of the crisis, rescue and salvage, emerged as the media descended on the CDC during the crisis. The media portrayed the agency as the primary means for combating and resolving the anthrax crisis. Reporters, however, also suggested that the CDC was unprepared for a crisis of this magnitude. They described its laboratories and ventilation systems as outdated. Moreover, they suggested that the agency's authority to regulate U.S. laboratories possessing anthrax, to say nothing of its existing anthrax knowledge base, were inadequate. Furthermore, the CDC was criticized for the amount of time it needed to confirm cases of anthrax and to locate dormant anthrax spores. Thus, in addition to criticism regarding its communication, the CDC was portrayed as functionally unprepared to fulfill its role in managing the crisis.

As the number of cases intensified (see table 8.2), the CDC was further accused of inconsistency by state agencies, and groups of individuals who were thought to have been exposed, or were considered at high risk of infection. Specifically, the agency was criticized for sending inconsistent messages regarding the use of antibiotics among postal workers. The issue was complex because, in addition to the general risks of using antibiotics, the approved anthrax medication, ciprofloxacin, often causes severe gastrointestinal distress. Initially, the agency did not believe postal workers had been exposed, because Anthrax in its natural form, the form with which the CDC was most familiar, could not easily be dispersed from a sealed envelope. Later, the fallacy of this assumption would become dramatically evident when individuals with no known shared connection became ill and died from inhalation anthrax. This group included both postal workers and individuals who were later discovered to have been exposed by cross contamination of letters. When a vaccination was made available, the CDC was accused of being equivocal in the recommendations. Vaccinations carry their own risk, albeit small, and the agency could not predict adverse side effects if large numbers of the general public began receiving vaccinations. Public-health officials in states other than those where cases of anthrax had already been confirmed claimed that the CDC did not allow them access to information they needed to ready themselves for a possible outbreak in their states.

When the intensity of the crisis waned in December 2001, the CDC devoted considerable energy toward moving to Turner's level six: full cultural adjustment. Despite receiving praise from his peers in the medical community, CDC Director Dr. Jeffrey Koplan resigned on February 22, 2002. As Koplan prepared for his departure, CDC employees at every level engaged in a series of debriefings and planning sessions designed to improve the agency's capacity to respond to bioterrorist attacks. A primary component in this planning focused on effective communication with stakeholders, including the public. The innovations proposed and adopted by the CDC framed what is now a return to Turner's level one, a new normal for the agency.

## THE NEW NORMAL FOR THE CDC

Reflecting on the CDC's experiences during the anthrax crisis, Vicki Freimuth, the CDC's director of communication at the time, wrote frankly: "[On] 9/11/01 the world changed [and on] 10/04/01 the world changed again" (p. 1).[20] The anthrax crisis, in effect, created an organizational learning opportunity that ultimately produced a fundamentally new understanding of normalcy for the CDC. Freimuth explains that as a result of the failure and subsequent criticism related to the anthrax attacks, the CDC permanently altered its strategy for communicating publicly during crises.

In this section, we describe the changes the CDC made in its sensemaking process and public communication during crises, first by discussing the failures the CDC identified in its response to the anthrax crisis, and then by identifying how the agency learned, and how the lessons of failure have created a new normal in its operations.

### Perceived Failures

In retrospect, Freimuth explains that the sense-making process communicated by the CDC during the anthrax crisis was problematic.[20] She identifies five challenges her employer faced while attempting to publicly address the uncertainty created by the anthrax crisis. Two of these challenges were related to available information, and three concerned assumptions regarding public communication.

#### Uncertainty

Simply stated, during the initial stages, the CDC did not have the information it needed to respond accurately to the anthrax crisis. First, as Freimuth explains, "[T]he attacks were unprecedented" (p. 3).[20] The centers had not previously responded to an act of bioterrorism of this magnitude and complexity. Thus, it lacked previous learning experiences upon which to base its response. Second, the CDC had "little scientific evidence to work with" (p. 3)[20] to evaluate the effects of anthrax in a highly refined aerosol form. Most previous research had focused on cutaneous (skin), rather than inhalation anthrax cases. Thus, at the onset of the crisis, the CDC faced a particularly intense level of uncertainty.

*Misconceptions*

Freimuth explains that the CDC's public communication about the anthrax crisis was also hampered by three false assumptions held by scientists and communication specialists representing the agency. First, many feared that "acknowledging uncertainty leads to panic" (p. 3).[20] This is a pervasive belief about crisis communication, which is generally not supported by the available research.[21] Research clearly indicates that widespread panic is very rarely a consequence of crisis. This misconception nevertheless influenced the CDC to issue statements at the onset of the crisis that downplayed the potential for anthrax sent through the mail to cause widespread infection. In retrospect, these statements were misleading, if not incorrect. Second, the agency's recommendations for "changing practices based on evolving knowledge" were "treated as mistakes" by the public.[20] As the crisis evolved, the CDC's ongoing investigation yielded an increased understanding of the form of anthrax used in the attack and of the process used to increase the spores' potency. Third, Freimuth noted a "reluctance of scientists to make recommendations with inadequate evidence" (p. 3).[20] Clearly, no competent or responsible scientist would announce definitive conclusions without first considering an adequate level of evidence. Unfortunately, the anthrax crisis created an immediate need for advice in managing a crisis that intensified daily. The CDC's hesitation to offer recommendations was criticized in the media as insensitivity to those who were at risk.

*Spokespersons*

In addition to the challenges CDC personnel faced in communicating under the intense uncertainty of the crisis, the agency had difficulty selecting and managing its spokespersons during level five of the crisis. The anthrax crisis topped the media's agenda in October and November 2001. Daily reports portrayed an expanding crisis with uncertain boundaries. The urgency of the anthrax story created a need for daily, if not hourly, interviews with CDC spokespersons. In a content analysis of the print media's coverage of the anthrax crisis, Barrett and others identified eighty-one different spokespersons cited by major newspapers as being affiliated in some manner with the CDC.[22] The two individuals quoted most often were CDC director Jeffrey Koplan and the secretary of Health and Human Services, Tommy Thompson. Still, the comments of seventy-nine other self-identified spokespersons appeared in the print media. With so many individuals addressing the crisis, contradictions and inconsistencies were inevitable.

Freimuth indicates that the demand for spokespersons was overwhelming and dynamic.[20] She describes media interest that vacillated between spokespersons who were politicians and those who were scientists. She also observed conflicting demands among reporters, who sometimes sought reassurance and at other times candor; sometimes empathy, sometimes expertise. These changing demands, in addition to the sheer number of media inquiries, made consistency of message particularly challenging.

*Collaboration*

Another criticism of the CDC was its apparent reluctance to collaborate with professional groups, such as state health departments and physicians. This led to strained relationships nationwide between the CDC and state health departments. The crisis also forced the CDC to interact with the FBI and the U.S. Postal Service (USPS). Freimuth indicates that these interagency relationships raised struggles over "who's in charge" (p. 4).[20] The complexities of bioterrorism put the CDC in an unfamiliar position. Clearly, the terrorist nature of the crisis demanded a response from a legal perspective. Further, the anxiety fostered by the September 11 attacks, along with the fact that anthrax had been mailed to politicians, made the assault a political issue as well. Thus, the CDC was forced to balance these pressures with its normal approach as the nation's medical detective.

## New Normal

Jeffrey Koplan argues that "the calculus may have shifted forever with the anthrax attacks of 2001" (p. 144).[23] The shift Koplan describes represents a new normal for the CDC and its stakeholders. Central to this new normal is enhanced external communication. Koplan explains: "During the anthrax crisis as in no other, it became obvious that public communication had become in some sense fully as important as—if not even more important than—the line duties of senior decision makers" (p. 144).[23] For an agency that prides itself on scientific inquiry, discovery, and objectivity, and which is grounded in the long tradition of public health, this view of the escalated role communication plays in a crisis is a dramatic change.

The new normal described by Koplan is based on a detailed analysis of the agency's strengths and weaknesses, as revealed throughout the various stages of the anthrax crisis. As Freimuth explains, the "CDC is committed to an ongoing critical examination of the strengths and weaknesses of its emergency health communication systems" (p. 151).[24] This examination has produced both sweeping and subtle changes in how the organization prepares for and responds to crisis and risk. We discuss five communication-related changes undertaken by the CDC: acknowledging uncertainty, addressing an evolving communication environment, increasing spokesperson management, expanding an understanding of audience and audience needs, and expanding a view of communication training and readiness.

*Acknowledging Uncertainty*

The CDC scientists' perceived need to communicate certainty in an environment of unprecedented uncertainty created serious credibility problems for the agency during levels four and five of the crisis.[25] As Freimuth explains, the evolving knowledge of the event created a need for the CDC to repeatedly revise its position during the crisis.[24] The certainty with which the initial messages were delivered to the public created a perception that the agency was "making mistakes" (p. 3). In reality, CDC scientists were giving what they believed was the best advice available at that particular time. Koplan explains that, in the future, CDC must "balance the wish to reassure key audiences, especially the general public, against the need to convey the very real uncertainties, difficulties, and complexities inherent in all such investigations" (p. 145).[23] For Koplan, the lesson learned is that "candidly admitting 'we don't know' and acknowledging uncertainty is often the best way to earn long-term public confidence and acceptance of our eventual recommendations" (p. 145).[23] Although this lesson appears counterintuitive to those CDC specialists who have dealt with routine outbreaks in the past, the novel aspects of a bioterror event, or other unexpected crises with high levels of uncertainty, make recognition of this uncertainty essential. Simply stated, the CDC has learned to avoid making unequivocal statements about what is inherently an ambiguous situation. Part of this change is an acknowledgment that public-health crises, particularly those involving bioterrorism, are so complex and dynamic that they defy simple predictions. It is worth noting that during the recent outbreak of SARS, the new CDC director, Julie Gerberding, was forthright in acknowledging that the outbreak was complex and that not much is known about this disease.

*Evolving Communications*

Congruent with the unparalleled uncertainty and perceived threat of the anthrax crisis was the intense media scrutiny created by continuous cable television and Internet news and information services. The CDC was forced to address real-time, 24-hour news coverage every day during the crisis. Addressing this mammoth task overwhelmed CDC communication staff, which was admittedly unprepared. Recognizing this, the CDC has expanded its staff to include teams working with all forms of media communication. Koplan explains that the "management of all the various tools of communication in a 24/7, cable television, and Internet world demands an unprecedented degree of technical sophistication and attention to multiple, parallel channels of public access" (p. 145).[23] Freimuth notes that the CDC has addressed this demand by adding additional communication teams to "manage some channels such as the web and hotlines" (p. 149).[24] By recognizing and addressing the additional communication demands posed by these expanding channels of communication, CDC is now better prepared to manage the information demands of an urgent health crisis.

*Managing Spokespersons*

As described above, the CDC had little control over the myriad of individuals who spoke on behalf of the agency during the crisis. This situation is evident in the findings of an organizational ethnography focusing on CDC communication personnel conducted by Robinson and Newstetter.[25] Their study shows that the CDC lacked an adequate system to take advantage of available expertise on anthrax. Rather than funneling its public communication through predetermined spokespersons, individuals with varying expertise communicated directly to the media. The situation allowed an unwieldy number of spokespersons, many of whom were not directly affiliated with the CDC, to speak on behalf of the agency. Throughout the crisis, this cumbersome situation resulted in numerous leaks and the spread of misinformation. One of Robinson and Newstetter's interviewees explained that, in the absence of scientific information coming directly from the CDC, the press would discuss scientific data with governors, senators, and congressmen. As a result, "they would start talking about scientific issues for which they had no expertise and they would misspeak" (p. 27).[25] One interviewee explained simply, "There were a whole lot of people desiring to be in the know, and wanting to be the source of information" (p. 27).[25] On several occasions, such individuals provided information before it had been cleared by the CDC. In retrospect, another interviewee admitted, the agency "lost the opportunity to take control of the communication process" (p. 23).[25] This interviewee explained further that "what should have happened . . . was to sit everybody down and . . . find out what's already available, who needs to get what information, and what's been said about developing that information" (p. 23).[25] Robinson and Newstetter explain that the disorder caused by these unfettered spokespersons is unlikely to occur in the future because of the "tighter integration of communication teams with the CDC's investigation teams" (p. 33).[25] In other words, the new normal at CDC includes communication experts working directly with subject matter experts and agency decision-makers. In the future, rapid and responsible communication by the CDC is intended to fulfill the needs of the media. Thus, freelancing spokespersons are likely to find fewer outlets for their uninformed communication.

*Understanding Audiences*

Koplan observes that during the anthrax crisis, "the federal health establishment crossed the line, perhaps irreversibly, into becoming a fully functioning component of the U.S. government's national security defenses" (p. 145).[23] This redefinition of the CDC's role demanded an expanded view of the agency's audience. Koplan explains that in addition to the general public, elected officials and "professional groups with roles to play in solving health problems" are essential CDC audiences during crises (p. 145).[23] As Freimuth explains, the CDC was criticized for being inattentive to the demands of all three audiences.[20] At times, the general public saw the agency as equivocal on key matters. Congressional members accused the CDC of being inattentive to their demands. Some members of professional groups, such as state health officials and physicians, complained that they were not included in the CDC's external messages. In addition, postal workers from largely African-American neighborhoods in Washington, DC, felt their needs were overlooked during the crisis. In response to this concern, the CDC has both a heightened awareness and additional infrastructure to address the needs of its many diverse audiences. Freimuth explains that the agency has designed a new "emergency communication system" that "recognizes that CDC serves many audiences" (p. 149).[24] To address the needs of these audiences, this new system has adopted procedures that capitalize on opportunities to "speed new scientific information to the field in a public health crisis" (p. 149).[24] To maintain efficient communication relationships throughout the crisis, the CDC has developed several new communication teams to address the needs of policymakers, clinicians, the public-health workforce, and community-health education workers. These teams are designed to identify and satisfy the unique needs of each audience. In this manner, the CDC is prepared to provide a communication response flexible enough to meet the needs of its distinct and diverse audience groups.

*Expanding Communication Readiness*

The anthrax crisis vividly revealed a need for crisis-communication training. Courtney, Cole, and Reynolds, all members of the CDC's Office of Communication, explain that in crisis situations, effective communication is essential at both the federal and local levels.[26] This realization, too, is part of a new normal for the CDC. The agency is currently sponsoring crisis-communication training for public-health professionals throughout the United States. Courtney and others argue that in addition to public-health professionals, "governors, city officials, and respected community leaders could improve rapport and cooperation and minimize potential panic and confusion by learning and adhering" to the principles of effective crisis communication (p. 133).[26] The ultimate goal of this training for health professionals and other leaders is to enable them to "communicate complex issues quickly, accurately, and credibly in extreme and uncertain situations" (p. 133).[26]

In addition, the CDC helped establish a variety of new communication tools and structures that will allow for more rapid identification of risk and more effective communication during crisis. One of these tools is the national and state Health Alert Networks (HAN), a computerized system that connects public-health processionals via the web. Notices of disease outbreaks and updates on issues of public health can be rapidly disseminated to pubic-health officials. The CDC also produced and disseminated a state-of-the-art compact disk (CDCynergy) with crisis-communication templates, checklists, worksheets, message maps, and related crisis-communication resources. Included are elaborate models of communication strategies appropriate for before, during, and after a crisis; outlines of the principles of risk communication and the psychology of crisis; an outline for audience analysis; and an overview of the role public health would play in a major event. Moreover, the CDC has offered crisis-communication training to public-health departments throughout the nation. This CDC and associated training have helped create a much broader crisis-communication response capacity at state and local levels.

## DISCUSSION AND IMPLICATIONS

Clearly, the CDC is not the same agency it was before the anthrax crisis. It has undergone extensive changes in personnel, function, emphasis, training, and structure. Following the anthrax episode, the agency conducted an extensive critique and self-examination and as a result, made strategic changes based on lessons learned. This process has created a new normal that has better equipped the CDC to remain vigilant and maintain effective communication, despite the tremendous uncertainty produced by crises such as bioterrorism. Other organizations may benefit from the CDC's example. We distill these generalized lessons from CDC in the following paragraphs.

As officials at the CDC learned from the anthrax crisis, uncertainty is an inherent element of crisis situations. Terrorism serves to intensify this ambiguity well beyond that associated with most naturally occurring public-health crises. Organizations need to ensure that as they approach crisis situations, they are sensitive to the unique circumstances of the case and do not rely fully on their past experiences. The new normal at CDC involves identifying, accepting, and acknowledging uncertainty. As Koplan asserts, admitting uncertainty will, in the long run, actually enhance credibility and public trust.[23] This observation can be applied to other organizations facing crisis. An organization that tries to convey complete control and certainty in the midst of the typically chaotic acute stages of a crisis is likely to only diminish its long-term credibility. Moreover, enacting certainty in response to a crisis may reduce an organization's flexibility.

A larger lesson is also evident for the CDC's stakeholders, including the general public. Crises are by definition complex and dynamic, and even the most vigilant organization can be taken by surprise by events such as terrorism. The general public, therefore, should not expect agencies such as the CDC to have all the answers. Nor can agencies such as CDC anticipate all crises. Expecting immediate and accurate responses to every crisis is unrealistic, especially when terrorism is involved. The anthrax case and 9/11 demonstrated vulnerabilities that had heretofore been largely overlooked and ignored. While much can and has been done to bolster crisis avoidance and response capacity, this vulnerability is also part of the new normal.

The CDC, as part of its lessons learned, has granted communication a more central role in its larger mission. Public-relations scholars have consistently called for the inclusion of communication personnel in strategic organizational decision-making.[27] The CDC is wise to expand its communication focus and to involve communication specialists in all phases of its decision-making and public communication. This decision will improve the chances of the agency communicating more effectively at all stages of crises. Too often, communication specialists are called upon to repair the damage created by subject-matter experts who have little knowledge of public communication. Research suggests that communication specialists can help organizations identify the onset of crises as well as manage the complexities of uncertainty during and following them.[27,28] Any organization that faces the threat of a highly public crisis should consider making communication part of its larger strategic management decisions.

During the anthrax case, the CDC learned the importance of cooperative relationships with other groups and agencies. Research has argued that pre-event relationships are particularly important to successful crisis management.[29] The connection the CDC is fostering with its related agencies will likely prove particularly valuable in managing future crises in several ways. By enhancing its relationships before a crisis event occurs, the agency is likely to have more efficient communication with its cooperating agencies. Similarly, the training that the CDC is sharing with its affiliated agencies is likely to help reduce communication errors on the local level during future crises. Establishing relationships also builds trust and credibility, which may translate into heightened cooperation and credibility during a crisis.[15] This proactive effort to cultivate relationships with key affiliates is advisable for any organization as it engages in crisis-management planning. It has been shown that effective crisis response can involve many groups, including community groups, local agencies such as the Red Cross, faith-based organizations, service clubs, and local businesses and industries. During the Exxon Valdez oil spill, local fisherman organized to help divert oil from sensitive fish hatcheries. During the North Dakota floods of 1997, community groups helped lay sandbags. The terrorist attacks on the WTC and Pentagon induced a number of community groups and agencies to assist in the response, search for victims, feed rescue workers, provide support to families, and help persons stranded by the air-travel ban. Not only are these groups usually first on the scene because they are part of the local community, but they also have a more detailed understanding of the community. Their response activities, therefore, are often more immediate and effective.

A final implication concerns the willingness to learn and the process of learning. The CDC engaged in a systematic, detailed, and critical review of its response to the anthrax episode. The agency invited critiques from a number of experts. Open debate and candid criticism were encouraged. Lessons were encoded in structures and procedures, and these were disseminated broadly throughout the agency and to other stakeholders. Learning through critique and dissemination is inherently tied to the processes and tone of post-crisis communication. More often than not, post-crisis communication is about avoiding blame, diffusing responsibility, and returning to the pre-event status quo as quickly and with as little cost as possible. Leaning, in contrast, is about using the crisis to construct a new, more robust, and resilient notion of normal. In order to learn, therefore, organizations must find ways to move beyond limited questions of blame and responsibility and embrace the crisis as a form of feedback and as an opportunity to correct deficiencies. Lessons should be communicated broadly, institutionalized in the organization's collective memory, and reified even when the risk no longer seems immediate. In this way, organizational crisis is at once a time of loss, uncertainty, and suffering, and also an opportunity for growth, development, and renewal.[30]

## CONCLUSION

The terrorist acts of 9/11 and the subsequent anthrax attack demonstrated vulnerabilities, pointed out weaknesses, challenged assumptions, and dispelled long-held beliefs that such attacks were unlikely. In doing so, they created high levels of uncertainty and learning opportunities. Learning requires that organizational participants consider alternative explanations and interpretations, and assess these interpretations in terms of their utility. Learning also requires that lessons be widely disseminated.

No organization wishes to endure a crisis of any kind—especially one involving terrorism. By its own admission, the CDC was not prepared for the crushing media attention, public scrutiny, and uncertainty it faced during the anthrax crisis. Although some of its actions during the crisis were regrettable, the agency persevered and ultimately fulfilled its role as the crisis was resolved. Most importantly, however, the CDC serves as an excellent example of how organizations can learn from crises and emerge with a more robust and vigilant crisis-response capacity.

## NOTES

1. Gouran DS. Making decisions in groups: choices and consequences. Glenview, IL: Scott, Foresman, & Company; 1982.

2. Hermann CF. Some consequences of crisis which limit the viability of organizations. Adm Sci Q 1963;8(1):61–82.

3. Weick KE. Enacted sensemaking in crisis situations. J Manage Stud 1988;25(4):305–17.

4. Lerbinger O. The crisis manager: facing risk and responsibility. Mahwah, NJ: Lawrence Erlbaum; 1997.

5. Seeger MW, Vennette S, Ulmer RR, Sellnow TL. Media use, information seeking, and reported needs in post crisis contexts. In: Greenberg BS, editor. Communication and terrorism: public and media responses to 9/11. Cresskill, NJ: Hampton Press; 2002. p. 53–63.

6. Sandman PM. Bioterrorism risk communication. J Health Commun 2003;8:146–7.

7. Covello VT. Communication. J Health Commun 2003;8:5–8.

8. Seeger MW, Sellnow TL, Ulmer RR. Communication and organizational crisis. Westport, CT: Praeger; 2003.

9. McKie D. Updating public relations: "New Science," research paradigms and uneven developments. In: Heath RL, editor. Handbook of public relations. Thousand Oaks, CA: Sage; 2001. p. 75–92.

10. Murphy P. Chaos theory as a model for managing issues and crises. Public Relations Rev 1996;22(2):95–113.

11. Seeger MW, Ulmer RR. Virtuous responses to organizational crisis: Aaron Feuerstein and Milt Cole. J Bus Ethics 2001;31:369–76.

12. Weick KE. The social psychology of organizing. 2nd ed. New York: McGraw-Hill; 1979.

13. Weick KE. Sensemaking in organizations. Thousand Oaks, CA: Sage; 1995.

14. Weick KE. The collapse of sensemaking in organizations: the Mann Gulch disaster. Adm Sci Q 1993;38:628–52.

15. Sellnow TL, Seeger MW, Ulmer RR. Chaos theory, informational needs, and natural disasters. J Appl Commun Res 2002;30:269–92.

16. Cohen MD, Sproull LS, editors. Organizational learning. Thousand Oaks, CA: Sage; 1996.

17. Turner B. The organizational and interorganizational development of disasters. Adm Sci Q 1976;21:378–97.

18. Billings RS, Milburn TW, Schaalman ML. A model of crisis perception: a theoretical and empirical analysis. Adm Sci Q 1980;25:300–16.

19. Allen WM, Caillouet RH. Legitimation endeavors: impression management strategies used by an organization in crisis. Commun Monogr 1994;61:44–62.

20. Freimuth V. Managing the anthrax attacks at CDC. [unpublished manuscript]; 2003.

21. Quarantelli EI. Disaster crisis management: a summary of research findings. J Manage Stud 1988;25:273–385.

22. Barrett S, Berg MP, Grand S, Hasbargen K, Markey V, Ocana A. The CDC and anthrax: a communication study. Proceedings of the National Communication Association; 2002 Nov; New Orleans, LA.

23. Koplan JP. Communication during public health emergencies. J Health Commun 2003;8:144–5.

24. Freimuth V. Epilogue to the special issue on anthrax. J Health Commun 2003;8:148–51.

25. Robinson SJ, Newstetter WC. Uncertain science and certain deadlines: CDC responses to the media during the anthrax attacks of 2001. J Health Commun 2003;8:17–34.

26. Courtney J, Galen C, Reynolds B. How the CDC is meeting the training demands of emergency risk communication. J Health Commun 2003; 8:128–9.

27. Seeger MW, Sellnow TL, Ulmer RR. Public relations and crisis communication: organizing and chaos. In: Heath RL, editor. Handbook of public relations. Thousand Oaks, CA: Sage; 2001. p. 155–66.

28. Coombs WT. Ongoing crisis communication: planning, managing, and responding. Thousand Oaks, CA: Sage; 1999.

29. Ulmer RR. Effective crisis management through established stakeholder relationships: Malden Mills as a case study. Manage Commun Q 2001; 14(4):590–615.

30. Seeger MW, Sellnow TL, Ulmer RR. Communication, organization and crisis. In: Roloff ME, editor. Communication Yearbook. Thousand Oaks, CA: Sage; 1998. p. 231–275. (vol 21).

# 9 The Critical Role of Communication to Prepare for Biological Threats: Prevention, Mobilization, and Response

*Gary L. Kreps, Kenneth Alibek,
Charles Bailey, Linda Neuhauser,
Katherine E. Rowan, and Lisa Sparks*

Communication is central to the effective prevention of, preparation for, and response to biological threats and hazards because it is the primary social process for sharing relevant information among the key policymakers, security personnel, healthcare providers, and members of the general public who need to coordinate efforts in times of crisis.[1] Effective communication for biodefense involves multiple challenges and competences in information gathering and dissemination.[2] Successful biodefense communication includes the following primary principles:

- gathering risk information about potential threats
- communicating risk information to health and safety professionals and to the media
- crafting effective messages for diverse audiences
- selecting appropriate channels to disseminate information to multiple audiences
- assessing feedback from groups who receive communication
- updating risk and crisis communication

There is a tremendous need for interdependent groups of policymakers, security forces, healthcare workers, and members of the public to gather relevant information to discover any potential risks for biological contamination, understand the nature of such threats, identify any incidences of contamination, and guide development of the best strategies for responding to and minimizing harm from such problems.[3,4] As a result, appropriate information about biological threats must be made available to these diverse groups of people. This information must be carefully crafted into messages that key groups can clearly understand and use. The messages also must be strategically disseminated via communication channels that these groups can easily access, and by sources the specific intended audiences trust.[5,6]

## THE NEED FOR RELEVANT INFORMATION

Teich, Wagner, Mackenzie, and Schaefer emphasize that carefully gathered and interpreted information is of utmost importance in times of emergency.[7] Such information is needed to quickly and accurately gauge the nature and intensity of potential threats, and to determine the best strategies for response. In the case of biodefense efforts, information must be presented quickly and meaningfully to a broad range of unique groups of people who possess differing levels of education, expertise, and capacities to understand and act upon complex health threats. The need for rapid dissemination can present many problems if handled inappropriately. For example, Moscrop claims it is vitally important to combat the psychological threat of bioterrorism by providing the public with "sound, sensible information" that is "accurate and reassuring."[8] The author suggests that biological weapons often are weapons of mass hysteria rather than destruction, with high potential to incite public panic and loss of confidence in the authorities. Therefore, information must not only be presented in understandable and accessible messages, but also in ways that will motivate strict compliance with important life-preserving recommendations and encourage broad collaboration with community representatives, and health and safety workers. In response to these needs, there have been many calls for developing national health-information systems to respond effectively to national health threats.[9]

It is critically important that biodefense information be both accurate and up-to-date. Otherwise such information can lead to actions that exacerbate biodefense problems and increase, sometimes fatally, the risk of harm. One example of inaccurate or misleading information released to the press occurred after the first inhalation anthrax case in 2001, when Secretary of Health and Human Services Tommy Thompson suggested the anthrax contamination was probably of natural origin and picked up while drinking from a South Carolina stream. People who understand this form of the disease knew, however, that anthrax is not a water-borne organism, and it is impossible to contract inhalation anthrax by participating in these types of outdoor activities.[10] Moreover,

Thompson, a former Wisconsin governor with no in-depth scientific or medical training, issued orders that all anthrax-related information to the public and media come directly from his office, barring government scientists and health experts from providing expert advice or information.[10] The secretary's errant comments haunted his department's reputation and that of the Centers for Disease Control and Prevention (CDC) as credible sources of health information concerning anthrax (see Sellnow, Seeger, and Ulmer,[11] in this volume).

Because emergency biodefense information is frequently updated, care must be taken to present new information in a manner that avoids confusion and frustration. This is difficult, given that many people are resistant to changing their views and actions. For example, during the anthrax scare, evidence became available that new medications like doxycycline could replace ciprofloxacin, which has negative side effects. However, when postal workers were informed they were going to be provided with access to the new medication, there were deep concerns that they weren't being given the best medication, and there was an outcry among many postal workers for access to ciprofloxacin. These fears could have been avoided by better communication about the advantages of doxycycline and the dangerous side effects of ciprofloxacin.[12]

## Information Credibility

A basic tenet of successful risk communication is that information must be presented in a credible manner to be believable. This means that biodefense messages have to be presented by trusted, expert, and credentialed information sources.[5] For example, public-health information may need to be presented by important health professionals who represent major public health agencies (such as the Surgeon General, the director of the CDC, or local public-health officials). Similarly, security information may be best presented by leading security officials (such as the director of the FBI, local police chiefs, or military leaders). The believability of key messages is often dependent on how expert and trustworthy the message sources are believed to be. To further complicate this issue, different audiences often perceive different people as being credible. For example, new Asian immigrants may have much less trust in unfamiliar Western medical systems than second-generation Asian-Americans.[13] Therefore, biodefense information sources must be selected based on their perceived credibility by the intended audiences for the messages. Blendon, Benson, Desroches, and Weldon advise that opinion surveys designed to find out who people trust can help guide official communication strategies.[14] Evidence suggests that in times of disease outbreaks most Americans prefer to receive health advice from their physicians.[15,16] This implies that it would be important to enlist primary-care physicians as essential distributors of health information in biodefense efforts.[16] Indeed, most county health departments in the United States have now established biodefense information networks for local physicians.

Another way to enhance the credibility of messages is to support stakeholders' efforts to understand warning messages. According to research in disaster settings, people give considerable attention to such tasks. Though initially they often respond with denial, later efforts are devoted to "confirming the message, arriving at a warning belief, and assessing personal risk" (Drabek,[17] quoting Perry and Mushkatel,[18] p. 21). For example, many people told of an impending tornado near their homes walk outside and look for funnel clouds (confirmatory behavior) before they attempt to locate and inform others or seek cover themselves (functions of assessing personal risk). Research shows that people's efforts to interpret and confirm warning messages can and should be supported.[19-23] Community members are more apt to interpret warnings constructively when their confirmatory efforts are assisted. To provide such assistance, officials can take steps, such as creating hot lines to answer questions and providing background information online that discusses emergent risks. In nonemergency times, hosting open houses at facilities perceived as threatening can help community members identify local individuals whom they perceive as credible.[23,24] Heath offers a thoughtful account of how crisis spokespersons can analyze and respond to the stories ordinary people develop as they attempt to make sense of crises.[25] One current credibility challenge thwarting people's confirmatory efforts is the vagueness of the U.S. Department of Homeland Security's color-coded warning system for terror alerts.[26] Official acknowledgment that the system is vague may enhance its credibility while improvements are developed.

Consistency is another important feature that enhances message credibility. Biodefense information, while tailored to key audiences, must remain consistent across the range of messages and communication channels. Conflicting messages lead to confusion, frustration, and misinformation. While it may be necessary to provide different groups with information specific to their unique situations (perhaps due to pertinent regional or occupational factors), it must be clear which guidelines apply to which groups and situations. These requirements can become complex because biological threats often require multiple responses. If such is the case, it may be advisable to reinforce and clarify key messages repeatedly, using different strategies, and employing different, familiar communication channels. An optimal level of message redundancy must be established to clarify key biodefense messages, without overwhelming or irritating key audiences. If too many messages are sent, recipients may block out or trivialize the messages as a way of coping with information overload.

## Communication Channels

It is of utmost importance to carefully select appropriate communication channels for disseminating biodefense information. Just as audiences perceive the credibility of information sources differentially, they are also likely to have preferences for specific channels of communication. For example, it has been suggested that new information technologies can provide important functions in communicating biodefense information and protecting public health in times of crisis.[27-29] Some technologically sophisticated groups of people might prefer to receive biodefense updates via e-mail, since they check their e-mail several times each day.[13] On the other hand, e-mail would be a terrible communication channel for audiences who rarely or never use e-mail. Moreover, different information channels have unique communication advantages and disadvantages for disseminating complex and pertinent information. While presentations of emergency information via radio and television can be very dramatic and are accessible by a large audience, the messages are often presented fleetingly and information can be missed.[30] It is difficult to know which audiences were exposed, and to gauge the effect of radio and television messages. Because such a large and diverse audience has access to these communication channels, they may be best for providing general information, as opposed to unique messages appropriate only to specific groups. At other times, due to concerns about privacy and the need to provide very specific information, more personalized channels of communication, such as mail, telephone, and even face-to-face personal communication may be warranted.[31]

The most successful risk and crisis communication permits two-way interaction between the sender and receiver.[32] For this reason, it is important to establish usable feedback channels for different groups of people. These channels will help gauge the effectiveness of biodefense communication by illustrating how well it is understood. Moreover, feedback serves to clarify misunderstood information among different audience members by answering people's questions. For example, telephone hot lines, interactive web pages, and e-mail contacts can be employed as accessible communication channels for feedback. Once again, these feedback channels must be familiar and easy to use for their intended audiences. In summary, it is important to carefully analyze the different audiences for biodefense messages to determine the best message strategies, information sources, and channels for communicating effectively with these unique groups of people.

## Message Content and Comprehension

One of the biggest challenges to effective biodefense communication is making relevant information accessible and understandable to highly varied subgroups in society. Several critical communication issues related to language, culture, literacy, disability and information connectivity must be taken into consideration when disseminating health information to diverse populations.[33-35] Currently, most health and safety information in the United States is presented in English, and secondarily in Spanish. Such information, of course, is not adequate for millions of people with a different language preference. For example, only an estimated 2 percent of U.S. websites are in a language other than English,[36] but because biodefense information must often be quickly updated, websites are a preferred communication channel. There is some evidence that state agencies are addressing the issue of translation. The Public Health Preparedness Survey conducted by the U.S. Association of State and Territorial Health Officers (ASTHO)* found that 73 percent of officials in charge of state risk-communications plans were addressing language differences in 2002, up from 38 percent.

Differences in culture are particularly important in the communication of biodefense information, which can invoke strong feelings of vulnerability and mistrust. For example, cultures vary greatly in their responses to death and expressions of grief.[13] If communication is not culturally appropriate, it can provoke distrust or hostility toward the official communicators and even cause a setback in emergency efforts.[32] In the 2003 ASTHO report on public health preparedness, U.S. health officers voiced their need for help in communicating with special populations. Health and safety communicators often lack guidance on principles and practical processes for developing communication for multiple audiences.

*ASTHO (Association of State and Territorial Health Officers). Public Health Preparedness: A Progress Report—The First Six Months. 2003. Available from: http://www.astho.org/?template=public_health_preparedness.html. Accessed January 15, 2004.

According to the results of the National Adult Literacy Survey, an estimated one-half of Americans are functionally or marginally illiterate.[37] Research during the past thirty years has found that most health-related materials require high school, college, or even graduate reading levels,[38] thus putting this information out of the skill levels of half of all Americans, especially those in vulnerable populations. Lundgren and McMakin point out that risk communication often involves complex vocabularies that are not familiar to the average person.[32] Although online information is often used for crisis communication, Lazarus and Mora estimated that only 1 percent of this information is usable by people with low literacy.[36] Internet communications pose further barriers because they require "multiple literacies," such as using browsers, spelling, selecting from a large database, and even typing.

A variety of disabilities also can pose barriers to effective information dissemination. Learning and cognitive disabilities may limit reading abilities to an elementary school level. Likewise, much information is inaccessible to people with eyesight limitations. People who are deaf or hard of hearing may have difficulties with emergency communication that is directed to them by automated phone calls from health and safety agencies. Internet communication may also be of limited use for many people with disabilities that prevent typing and using a mouse. The U.S. Department of Commerce found that people with disabilities were much less likely to use computers or the Internet.[39] Tremayne, Dunwoody, and Tobias estimate that 30 million Americans with disabilities have restricted access to Internet information.[40]

Lenhart estimates that 42 percent of Americans lacked access to the Internet in 2002.[41] The "digital have-nots" are primarily from low-income, minority, older, and disabled populations who are the hardest to reach for preparedness and crisis response. For this reason, other media channels for biodefense communication are required for these groups. A fundamental factor that contributes to the weaknesses of communication for diverse and vulnerable populations is that members of these groups are rarely involved in the design and testing of communication.[42] We advocate community-based approaches involving key audiences in risk communication biodefense efforts.[2]

## THE STRATEGIC BIODEFENSE COMMUNICATION MODEL

To structure our analysis of the multifaceted roles for strategic communication in biodefense efforts, we describe a three-stage "strategic

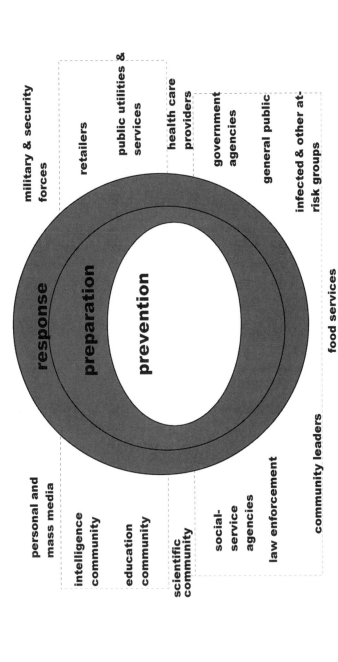

Figure 9.1
Strategic Biodefense Communication Model

biodefense communication model" of *preventing, preparing* for, and *responding* to biological threats. According to Dudley, effective biodefense efforts depend on coordinating communications to promote awareness, surveillance, mobilization, and response.[43]

In this model, prevention of biological threats is the central and constant communication activity for biodefense efforts. Our very best options for avoiding biohazards and protecting health and welfare are to learn about and divert biological threats before they are introduced. All other biodefense communication efforts are built upon these initial prevention efforts. Even the best prevention efforts, however, are not likely to help us avert all biological threats, and communication activities must also prepare key groups to respond effectively to any biological threats that might enter our ecosystems. It is untenable to develop complex and interrelated strategies for coping with biological hazards as they occur. Systematic preparations for key groups of people are required well ahead of the advent of any biological emergencies. (See the excellent website developed by the CDC concerning emergency preparedness and response for an example of in-depth planning and coordination efforts for biodefense at www.bt.cdc.gov/planning/index.asp.)

The outer circle of our model describes the critical communication activities needed for an effective response to biological hazards once such problems occur (see figure 9.1). To a large extent, these response activities are designed to implement plans developed in the preparation phase of the model. However, emergency-response communication must be adaptive and adjust to changing conditions and unforeseen issues. In fact, scholars of chaos theory suggest that in times of crisis, logical advance planning does not always reflect the unpredictable and equivocal nature of crises. Crisis communications must take into account unexpected events and suggest novel strategies for responding to crises.[11]

Surrounding the concentric circles of the model are examples of the many interdependent groups of people who must coordinate activities and share relevant information in biodefense efforts.

### Prevention

Biodefense prevention efforts begin with coordinated in-depth intelligence-gathering activities to identify potentially significant health risks before the risks are imminent.[44,45] By gathering such information ahead of time, efforts can be mounted to defuse dangerous situations before they occur. This is the best and most effective strategy for reducing potential harm, by nullifying biological threats before they occur.

Intelligence-gathering activities occur on many levels of communication and employ numerous communication media and technologies.[46] Intelligence efforts involve actively seeking regular updates from far-reaching networks of informants and organizational contacts to uncover threatening plans and activities. In addition to seeking information from respondents, biohazard intelligence is gathered through close (and often unobtrusive) surveillance of group activities and environmental conditions that might identify risk factors and indicators, including monitoring communications among terrorist groups, tracking any unauthorized or suspicious access to contagious substances, and identifying epidemiological evidence of biological contagion and disease from around the world.[47,48]

Prevention also involves efforts to increase public safety by monitoring information about ways that biohazards might be delivered to citizens, carefully identifying and closing down any potential access points for introducing contagious elements. Access points might include, for example, food sources and distribution sites, the water supply, air and ventilation sources, various modes of transportation, with particular attention to border crossings, airports, and other transportation centers. Information gathered can inform the development and refinement of security measures to minimize opportunities for the introduction of biohazards.

### Preparation

While it is worth our best efforts to prevent the introduction of biohazards, such efforts are certainly not foolproof, and risks remain such that we must develop strategies and procedures for an effective response if necessary.[49,50] In the face of potential health hazards, medical personnel need to have adequate medical supplies, equipment, and services available to respond to the needs of consumers.[51,52] Infection-control personnel have to be educated about the etiology of specific contagious substances and the best responses to them.[53] This takes concerted planning and preparation.[54] Communication is the primary tool for disseminating information to these groups of professionals about the best strategies for protecting the public from biocontamination.

Guidelines for a rigorous response to biological threats need to be developed, refined, and disseminated to key health and safety personnel or they face underpreparation. For example, a study by M'Ikanatha, Lautenbach, Kunselman, Julian, Southwell, Allswede, and others, found that during the 2001 anthrax outbreak, emergency physicians had inadequate knowledge about anthrax and smallpox diagnosis.[55] Community planning for emergencies, including simulated response drills, must be developed to aid rapid, appropriate responses to biological emergencies.[56,57] Likewise, the public needs to be educated about potential bio-threats so they can be prepared if such events occur.[58] Public education and preparation is particularly important due to heightened public fears of bioterrorism after the events of September 11, 2001, and the anthrax scare of 2001.[59] Unfortunately, public understanding of biodefense information is often faulty. A national survey conducted in November and December 2002 found that nearly half of all U.S. adults erroneously thought that anthrax is contagious and that smallpox vaccination is not effective after exposure.[60] Federal agencies, such at the CDC and the Federal Emergency Management Association have developed plans for guiding coordinated responses to biological emergencies.[15,61]

In order to respond to biohazards, more research into infectious-disease detection, vaccination, and treatment, must be undertaken and its results quickly and effectively disseminated to those that can put them into practice.[62] The latest information about infectious diseases should be made available to key health and safety communities, perhaps via websites that can be easily updated as new information becomes available.[63] The best research information must be included in what Rosen, Koop, and Grig describe as "cybercare," an information "system that will enable us to mobilize all our health care resources rapidly wherever they are needed."[64]

The Center for Community Wellness at the University of California, Berkeley (www.ucwellness.org), is experimenting with an approach to reach diverse audiences with preparedness information. The intervention incorporates emergency preparedness advice and community, state, and national referrals into general health guides that go to millions of households each year. The groups that have collaborated on developing and testing the guides include people from multiple socioeconomic, cultural and linguistic backgrounds, and disability conditions. Some of this information is also in an online format (ContraCosta.networkofcare.org/kids/home/index.cfm) as well as in Braille and audio.

## Response

Just as preparation for biodefense communication builds upon prevention, response communications builds upon planning efforts. Planning efforts are used to develop the guidelines and partnerships that key groups of health and safety professionals need to follow to effectively confront biological hazards. After significant biological hazards have entered human ecosystems and threaten the public, communication is essential to effectively mobilize efforts and implement coordinated responses among interrelated health and safety officials and affected individuals and groups.[52] It is important to identify the people most at risk from the biohazards, and who may need different forms of intervention based upon the interpretation of specific geographic, epidemiological, and health information.[65] Early warning systems, like automatic infectious-disease surveillance systems and electronic sensors to detect biological hazards, can quickly detect cases of biological emergency.[66,67]

The smallpox vaccinations conducted in response to perceived terrorist threats provide an example of methods to improve risk communication. For example, after 9/11, the San Francisco Department of Health developed an analysis of estimated risks versus benefits for smallpox vaccination.[68] People considering vaccination were presented with these potential risks and benefits, tailored to each person's situation. This balanced approach helped demystify the conflicting views, and also engendered trust, and helped individuals make an informed decision.

An obvious limitation to response communication is that it cannot usually be pre-scripted and thus is not easily tailored to the needs of multiple audiences. Rudd, Comings, and Hyde compared a 1988 AIDS mailing to the general public with that of a 2001 anthrax mailing.[34] Because of its urgency, there was inadequate time to craft the anthrax communication to audience needs. For example, the anthrax mailing was written at a tenth- or eleventh-grade level, posing significant literacy problems for its readers. The problems of poorly constructed communication materials are often magnified when coupled with the problem of audience anxiety and information overload from other media.

Although "urgency" is often cited as the reason for poor communication, another view is that crisis situations highlight underlying weaknesses in communication development. Thus, even after the anthrax scare ended, health officials were unable to prepare an effective risk communication.[69] Many physicians, scientists, and researchers continue to use specific, technical language that simply fails to communicate the importance of a message that must be understood—immediately. For instance, Preston describes a briefing, during the 2001 anthrax outbreaks, in which a scientist characterized the anthrax powder contained in anonymous letters as "energetic," meaning that they were likely to become airborne and cause significant harm.[70] Members of his audience, which included government officials, misunderstood his terminology, and thought he was minimizing the possibility for harm.

Similarly, Benjamin finds that the healthcare community and the general public received inconsistent messages from numerous sources for almost four weeks after the first anthrax attacks.[71] Often, the misinformation resulted when the media turned to any available source, qualified or unqualified, to answer questions about anthrax, terrorism, and health-related issues. For example, a study by researchers at the ANSER Institute for Homeland Security and the Johns Hopkins Center for Civilian Biodefense Strategies demonstrates that when journalists found public-health officials unwilling to respond to their inquiries, they turned to other sources of information. Some of these sources, including websites and other so-called experts, lacked credibility.[72] Additionally, in attempts to reassure the public, officials frequently made erroneous statements, projecting an appearance of confusion. For instance, concerned U.S. postal workers were originally told by the CDC that envelopes containing anthrax posed no threat and would not contaminate other pieces of mail. This was later found to be false.[73] In hindsight, officials recognized that a single, accurate message from credible sources can calm fears and forestall panic. Clearly, better training would help public-health professionals to respond to media inquiries, educate the public, and improve information resources that support communication needs.[72]

Precise language does matter. Many officials claimed the anthrax was "weaponized," which has a different meaning for the general public and public-health officials than for scientists and experts in offensive biowarfare. Scientists use the term to describe the composition and formulation of a substance like anthrax. Technically, weaponized anthrax has been processed to increase its survival and viability during an explosion, as opposed to the more common public assumption that "weaponized" anthrax refers only to the use of anthrax as a weapon. Communication is a two-way street. It is not only important that scientists begin to understand the responsibility of translating specific and technical messages in ways their audience can understand, but it is equally important that interactants (in this case public-health officials) learn to probe with further questions.

A major task of biodefense response communications is developing a coordinated plan for media relations to promote the most accurate and strategic coverage of biological emergencies.[73] Such a plan involves coordinating media coverage via numerous news channels, including television, radio, newspapers, the Internet, magazines, news-wire services, and many other news information sources.[2] Effective news coverage can provide basic information, identify key communication channels for follow-up information, and help to reassure the public in emergencies. As noted earlier, ineffective news coverage can cause confusion, spread misinformation, and even incite public panic. For instance, the media often provide inaccurate reports of scientific information and data. In an effort to get information on the air as soon as possible, the media may interview any so-called expert who is willing to talk. Sometimes these sources possess credentials that don't pertain to the current problem at hand. The media, public officials, and the general public must begin to distinguish the subtle differences between experts in offensive biowarfare, experts at U.S. Army Medical Research Institute of Infectious Diseases, and scientists who have conducted research to develop vaccines and therapeutics, but who have little experience with offensive biowarfare agents such as anthrax. Often, news sources discuss subjects outside their area of expertise based on relatively little knowledge. These judgments can result in vast amounts of misinformation.

Local, regional, national, and even international media can be effective at disseminating relevant information if key media representatives (such as reporters) are provided with the latest and most accurate information and are treated as important and respected partners in biodefense efforts.[74] In the United States, the CDC has taken the lead to provide accurate and quickly updated information about biodefense and other health emergencies directly to state health-and-safety agencies through its Health Alert Network (www.cdc.gov and www.bt.cdc.gov). In addition, it is a trusted information source for the general public. Some states have also developed their own sites for professionals and the public. However, as discussed earlier, there is still much to do to make this information accessible to people who are not digitally connected or who have barriers related to literacy, language, culture, or disability.

Research on science, health, risk, and crisis communication can guide efforts to build effective media relations.[40,61,74-78] One useful resource is a government publication offering research-based tips for crisis and risk spokespersons.[79] Still other resources are websites offering reporters in-depth, accessible explanations of the science behind news events. For example, the University of Wisconsin maintains the Why Files: Science behind the News (whyfiles.org), which offers explanations of "dirty bombs," "Mad Cow" disease, and other current topics of daily news coverage. Research on the Why Files and other interactive sources designed to help journalists suggests that these resources deepen users' understanding of complexities and may enhance coverage quality.[42,80]

## CONCLUSIONS

Communication is a critical part of biodefense efforts and must be carefully planned and executed to be effective. Multiple channels of human and mediated communication (including the use of new information technologies) must be strategically coordinated to help prevent biological threats, identify the risks of such threats, prepare for biological hazards, and coordinate effective, evidence-based responses to biological emergencies. Careful audience analyses help communications professionals to craft the most effective messages for diverse audiences and to disseminate these messages via credible sources across the most appropriate and accessible communication channels. Care must be taken to work cooperatively with media representatives to make sure the most accurate and timely information reaches those individuals most affected. Communication also provides essential support in coordinating groups of health and safety professionals affected by biological threats.

Communication plays a vital role in identifying and mitigating risks at the "prevention core" of biodefense efforts. Prevention efforts also link with biodefense preparation: gathering information that informs planning efforts and developing guidelines for effective responses. Finally, communication is critical in mobilizing key groups of health and safety professionals, as well as the media and the general public to respond during and after a biological emergency. By identifying the critical roles that communication performs in biodefense efforts, we hope to encourage a concerted investment in biodefense communication prevention, planning, and response activities.

## NOTES

1. Riley, B. Information sharing in homeland security and homeland defense: how the Department of Defense is helping. J Homeland Secur [serial online] 2003. Available from: www.homelandsecurity.org/journal/articles/displayArticle.asp?article=97. Accessed January 15, 2004.

2. Covello VT. Best practices in public health risk and crisis communication. J Health Commun 2003;23:164-93.

3. May T, Silverman R. Bioterrorism defense priorities. Sci 2003; 301(5629):17.

4. Talbot LA. Biological threats to America's health. Biol Res Nurs 2003; 4(4):241–3.

5. Pollard WW. Public perceptions of information sources concerning bioterrorism before and after anthrax attacks: an analysis of survey data. J Health Commun 2003;8:93–103.

6. Shore DA. Communicating in times of uncertainty: the need for trust. J Health Commun 2003;8(23):13–4.

7. Teich JM, Wagner MM, Mackenzie CF, Schaefer KO. The informatics response in disaster, terrorism, and war. J Am Med Inform Assoc 2002;9(2): 97–104.

8. Moscrop A. Mass hysteria is seen as main threat from bioweapons. Br Med J 2001;323(7320):1023.

9. Tangm PC. AMIA advocates national health information system in fight against national health threats. J Am Med Inform Assoc 2002;9(2):123–6.

10. Garrett L. Questions linger a year after anthrax mailings: unknown dominates probe. Newsday 2002 Oct 7. Available from: www.ph.ucla.edu/epi/bioter/ questionslingeranthrax.html. Accessed January 15, 2004.

11. Sellnow TL, Seeger MW, Ulmer RR. Chaos theory, informational needs, and natural disasters. J Appl Commun Res 2002;30(4):269–92.

12. Vanderford ML. Communication lessons learned in the emergency operations center during CDC's anthrax response: a commentary. J Health Commun 2003;8(23):11–2.

13. Centers for Disease Control and Prevention. Crisis and emergency risk communication 2003. Available from: www.cdc.gov/communication/emergency/ cerc.htm. Accessed January 15, 2004.

14. Blendon RJ, Benson JM, Desroches CM, Weldon KJ. Using opinion surveys to track the public's response to a bioterrorist attack. J Health Commun 2003;8(23):83–92.

15. Blendon RJ, Benson JM, DesRoches CM, Pollard WE, Parvanta C, Herrmann MJ. The impact of anthrax attacks on the American public. MedGenMed [serial online]. 2002;17(4):1.

16. Hobbs J, Kittler A, Volk L, Kreps GL, Bates D. The internet as a vehicle to communicate health information during a bio-terrorist emergency: a survey analysis involving the anthrax scare of 2001. J Med Internet Res 2004; forthcoming.

17. Drabek TE. Disaster warning and evacuation responses by private business employees. Disasters 2001;25:76–94.

18. Perry RW, Mushkatel AH. Disaster management: warning response and community relocation. London: Quorum; 1984.

19. Dynes RR, Drabek TE. The structure of disaster research: its policy and disciplinary implications. Int J Mass Emergencies Disasters 1994;12(20): 5–23.

20. Perry RW, Lindell MK. Understanding citizen response to disasters with implications for terrorism. J Contingencies Crisis Manag 2003;11(2):49–60.

21. Rowan KE. Goals, obstacles, and strategies in risk communication: a problem-solving approach to improving communication about risks. J Appl Commun Res 1991;19:300–29.

22. Rowan KE, Sparks L, Pecchioni L, Villagran M. The "CAUSE" model: a research-supported guide for physicians communicating cancer risk. Health Commun 2003;15:239–52.

23. Sandman PM. Responding to community outrage: strategies for effective risk communication. Fairfax, VA: American Industrial Hygiene Association; 1993.

24. Heath RL. Corporate environmental risk communication: cases and practices along the Texas Gulf Coast. In: Burleson BR, editor. Communication yearbook. Thousand Oaks, CA: Sage Publishing; 1995. p. 255–77. (vol 18).

25. Heath RL. Telling the story: a narrative approach to crisis. In: Millar DP, Heath RL, editors. Responding to crisis: a rhetorical approach to crisis communication. Mahwah, NJ: Lawrence Erlbaum; 2004. p. 167–88.

26. U.S. Department of Health and Human Services. Remarks by U.S. DHS Secretary. 2003 Dec 21. Available from: www.dhs.gov/dhspublic/. Accessed January 15, 2004.

27. Eysenbach G. SARS and population health technology. J Med Internet Res 2003;5(2):e14.

28. Mastrangelo MJ. Biodefense communications. J Homeland Secur [serial online] 2001. Available from: www.homelandsecurity.org/journal/articles/displayArticle.asp?article=23. Accessed January 15, 2004.

29. Ortiz E, Clancy CM. Use of information technology to improve the quality of health care in the United States. Health Serv Res 2003;38(2):xi–xxii.

30. Neuhauser L, Kreps GL. The advent of e-health: how interactive media are transforming health communication. Medien Kommunikationswissenschaft 2003;51:541–56.

31. Bruce J. Bioterrorism meets privacy: an analysis of the Model State Emergency Health Powers Act and the HIPAA privacy rule. Ann Health Law 2003;12(1):75–120.

32. Lundgren R, McMakin A. Risk communication: a handbook for communicating environmental, safety and health risks. Columbus: Battelle Press; 1998.

33. Parker RM, Gazmararian JA. Health literacy: essential for health communication. J Health Commun 2003;8(15):116–8.

34. Rudd RE, Comings JP, Hyde JN. Leave no one behind: improving health and risk communication through attention to literacy. J Health Commun 2003;8(15):104–15.

35. Zarcadoolas C, Pleasant A, Greer D. Elaborating a definition of health literacy: a commentary. J Health Commun 2003;23(15):164–93.

36. Lazarus W, Mora F. Online content for low-income and underserved Americans: the digital divide's new frontier. 2000. Available from: www.childrenspartnership.org/. Accessed January 15, 2004.

37. Association of State and Territorial Health Officers. Public health prepared-ness: a progress report—the first six months. 2003. Available from: www.astho. org/?template=public_health_preparedness.html. Accessed January 15, 2004.

38. Logan R, Kirsch JS, Junegeblut A, Jenkins L, Kolstad A. Adult literacy in America: a first look at the results of the National Adult Literacy Survey (NALS). Washington DC: U.S. Department of Education; 1993.

39. Rowan K, Rudd RE, Moeykens B, Colton T. Effective explanation of uncertain and complex science. In: Friedman S, Dunwoody S, Rogers SL, editors. Communicating new and uncertain science. Mahwah, NJ: Lawrence Erlbaum; 1999. p. 201-33.

40. U.S. Department of Commerce. A nation online: how Americans are expanding their use of the internet. National Telecommuncations and Information Administration, Economics and Statistics Administration, Washington DC: U.S. Department of Commerce; 2002.

41. Tremayne M, Dunwoody S, Tobias J. Interactivity, information processing, and learning on the World Wide Web. Sci Commun 2001;23:111-34.

42. Lenhart A. The ever-shifting Internet population. Washington, DC: The Pew Internet & American Life Project. 2003. Available from: www.pewinternet. org/reports/toc.asp?Report=88. Accessed January 15, 2004.

43. Neuhauser L. Participatory design for better health communication: a statewide model in the USA. Electron J Commun [serial online] 2001;11(3-4). Available from: www.cios.org/www/ejc/v11n3.htm#design. Accessed January 15, 2004.

44. Dudley JP. New challenges for public health care: biological and chemical weapons awareness, surveillance, and response. Biol Res Nurs 2003;4(4):244-50.

45. Mortimer PP. Anticipating smallpox as a bioterrorist weapon. Clin Med 2003;3(3):255-9.

46. Rotz LD, Koo D, O'Carroll PW, Kellogg RB, Lillibridge SR. Bio-terrorism preparedness: planning for the future. J Public Health Manag Pract 2000;6(4):45-9.

47. Sawyer M. Connecting the dots: the challenge of improving the creation and sharing of knowledge about terrorists. J Homeland Secur [serial online] 2003. Available from: www.homelandsecurity.org/journal/articles/displayArticle. asp?article=93. Accessed January 15, 2004.

48. Fisher U. Information age state security: new threats to old boundaries. J Homeland Secur [serial online] 2001. Available from: www.homelandsecurity. org/journal/articles/displayArticle.asp?article=25. Accessed January 15, 2004.

49. Stephenson, WD. Homeland security requires Internet-based thinking—not just technology. J Homeland Secur [serial online] 2002. Available from: www.homelandsecurity.org/journal/articles/displayArticle.asp?article=28. Accessed January 15, 2004.

50. Haas JM. Addressing bioterrorism: what ethical issues and questions surround potential responses to bioterrorist attacks? Healthc Exec 2003;18(3):76-7.

51. Heightman AJ. The need to address new threats. J Emerg Med Serv 2003; 28(4):12.

52. Bartlett JG. Mobilizing professional communities. Public Health Rep [Suppl 2] 2001;116:40–4.

53. Rippen HE, Gursky E, Stoto MA. Importance of bioterrorism preparedness for family physicians. Am Fam Physician 2003;67(9):1877–8.

54. Shadel BN, Rebmann T, Clements B, Chen JJ, Evans RG. Infection control practitioners' perceptions and educational needs regarding bioterrorism: results from a national needs assessment survey. Am J Infect Control 2003;31(3):129–34.

55. Manassaram DM, Orr MF, Kaye WE. Counterterrorism planning using the Hazardous Substances Events Surveillance system. Disaster Manag Response 2003;1(2):35–40.

56. M'Ikanatha NM, Lautenbach E, Kunselman AR, Julian KG, Southwell BG, Allswede M, et al. Sources of bioterrorism information among emergency physicians during the 2001 anthrax outbreak. Biosecurity Bioterrorism: Biodefense Strategy Pract Sci 2003;1(4):259–65.

57. Ashford DA, Kaiser RM, Bales ME, Shutt K, Patrawalla A, McShan A, et al. Planning against biological terrorism: lessons from outbreak investigations. Emerg Infect Dis 2003;9(5):515–9.

58. DiGiovanni C Jr, Reynolds B, Harwell R, Stonecipher EB, Burkle FM Jr. Community reaction to bioterrorism: prospective study of simulated outbreak. Emerg Infect Dis 2003;9(6):708–12.

59. Brooks KL, Dauenhauer SA. The anthrax team: a novel teaching approach to increase anthrax and bioterrorism awareness. Am J Infect Control 2003;31(3):176–7.

60. Dworkin MS, Ma X, Golash RG. Fear of bioterrorism and implications for public health preparedness. Emerg Infect Dis 2003;9(4):503–5.

61. Fischhoff B, Gonzales RM, Small DA, Lerner JS. Evaluating the success of terror risk communications. Biosecurity Bioterrorism: Biodefense Strategy Pract Sci 2003;1(4):255–8.

62. Fiedelholtz G. Responding to biological terrorist incidents: upgrading the FEMA approach. J Homeland Secur [serial online] 2003. Available from: www.homelandsecurity.org/journal/articles/displayArticle.asp?article=91. Accessed January 15, 2004.

63. Fauci AS. Bioterrorism: defining a research agenda. Food Drug Law J 2002;57(3):413–21.

64. Yu VL. Bioterrorism web site resources for infectious disease clinicians and epidemiologists. Clin Infect Dis 2003;36:1458–73.

65. Rosen JM, Koop CE, Grigg EB. Cybercare: A System for Confronting Bioterrorism. The Bridge [serial online] 2002;32(1). Available from: www.nae.edu/nae/naehome.nsf/weblinks/CGOZ-58NLKL?OpenDocument. Accessed January 15, 2004.

66. Slezak T, Kuczmarski T, Ott L, Torres C, Medeiros D, Smith J, et al. Comparative genomics tools applied to bioterrorism defence. Brief Bioinform 2003;4(2):133–49.

67. Higgins JA, Nasarabadi S, Karns JS, Shelton DR, Cooper M, Gbakima A, et al. A handheld real time thermal cycler for bacterial pathogen detection. Biosens Bioelectron 2003;18(9):1115–23.

68. Popovich ML, Henderson JM, Stinn J. Information technology in the age of emergency public health response: the framework for an integrated disease surveillance system for rapid detection, tracking, and managing of public health threats. IEEE Eng Med Biol Mag 2002;21(5):48–55.

69. Aragón TJ, Fernyak SE. The risks and benefits of pre-event smallpox vaccination: where you stand depends on where you sit. Ann Emerg Med 2003;42(5):681–4.

70. Marmagas SW, Rasar King L, Chuk MG. Public health's response to a changed world: September 11, biological terrorism, and the development of an environmental health tracking network. Am J Public Health 2003;93(8):1226.

71. Preston R. The demon in the freezer: a true story. New York: Random House; 2002.

72. Benjamin GC. Managing terror: Public health officials learn lessons from bioterrorism attacks. Physician Exec 2002;28(2):80–3.

73. Gursky E, Inglesby TV, O'Toole T. Anthrax 2001: observations on the medical and public health response. Biosecurity Bioterrorism 2003;1(2):97–110.

74. Garrett L. Understanding the media's response to epidemics. Public Health Rep [Suppl 2] 2001;116:87–91.

75. Coombs WT. Ongoing crisis communication: planning, managing, and responding. Thousand Oaks: Sage; 1999.

76. Friedman SM, Dunwoody S, Rogers CL, editors. Communicating new and uncertain science. Mahwah, NJ: Lawrence Erlbaum; 1999.

77. Logan RA. Science mass communication: its conceptual history. Sci Commun 2001;23:135–63.

78. Sparks, L. Social identity and perceptions of terrorist groups: how others see them and how they see themselves. In: O'Hair HD, Heath R, Ledlow G, editors. Communication, Communities, and Terrorism. Westport, CT: Praeger Publishers; 2005. p. 13–28.

79. Weigold MF. Communicating science: a review of the literature. Sci 2001;23(2):164-93.

80. U.S. Department of Health and Human Services. Communicating in a crisis: risk communication guidelines for public officials. Washington, DC: Substance Abuse and Mental Health Services Administration [pub. SMA02-3641]; 2002. Available from: www.samhsa.gov. Accessed January 15, 2004.

# 10 The Terrorist Threat: Shifts in Crisis-Management Thinking and Planning Post-9/11

## W. Timothy Coombs

Every organization must face the threat of risks and the potential of exposure to loss. As a result, risk is a driving force of crisis management, which includes measures to identify and mitigate risk, as well as measures that prepare for a time when a risk becomes an actual crisis.[1,2] The tragic events of 9/11 changed how American organizations view risk. In turn, the risks associated with a terrorist threat have altered many facets of crisis management, as organizations seek to protect their personnel, physical infrastructures, and financial assets.

This chapter seeks to document, explain, and evaluate the post-9/11 shifts in crisis-management thinking and planning. The first section provides an overview of what crisis management is and identifies the post-9/11 shifts. The second section explains the reasoning behind the shifts and evaluates whether the shifts are warranted or an overreaction.

### CRISIS MANAGEMENT: FRAMEWORK AND POST-9/11 CHANGES

Crisis management provides a useful framework for analyzing and understanding the effects of the terrorist attacks of 9/11 on organizational practices. This section provides a brief overview of crisis management as a framework for identifying and analyzing post-9/11 changes. Crisis management is defined, the basic process identified, and related planning elements discussed. This framework is then used to document post-9/11 changes in crisis management.

### Overview of Crisis Management

Crisis management is a set of factors used to combat crises and lessen their damage.[2] Crisis management is a four-step process: prevention, preparation, response, and learning. Prevention involves actions taken to reduce risks and vulnerabilities to crisis. Vulnerabilities are weaknesses. A risk represents the potential of a vulnerability to develop into a crisis and create a loss for an organization.[3] Preparation involves creating a crisis-management plan (CMP), designating and training a crisis-management team, and rehearsing the CMP. Response is the actual measures taken when a crisis occurs, including the task of communicating with various stakeholders affected by the crisis. Learning is a review of what went right and wrong in the crisis-management effort, to understand which aspects of crisis management are working and which need to be refined. Terrorism has altered how organizations approach prevention and preparation for crisis management.

Crisis management is inextricably linked to business-continuity planning and emergency preparedness. Business-continuity (BC) planning refers to the actions an organization takes to maintain or reestablish normal operations. Examples include using alternative facilities for data processing or production, or renting replacement equipment. The BC plan works in concert with the CMP. For instance, if the BC plan identifies a "hot site" (alternative location where an organization can function), the CMP should have procedures for notifying employees, suppliers, and customers of that change. Because crises may require evacuation or so-called shelter-in-place, emergency preparedness addresses these issues, including how people exit, how they're accounted for, and who is responsible for various duties during an evacuation or shelter-in-place. Hence, emergency preparedness is often part of crisis management.

Terrorism has become a salient topic in crisis management after 9/11. Organizations have always been vulnerable to terrorism—it has been a recognized threat. However, planning for terrorism was largely restricted to overseas operations and the security of personnel traveling abroad. Terrorism was not prominent in crisis planning for facilities in the United States. The 9/11 terrorist attacks significantly changed how organizations perceive and utilize the terrorist risk in both prevention and planning.

*Prevention: Terrorism as Risk*

Prevention seeks to eliminate or reduce risks by strengthening an organization against vulnerabilities. Vulnerabilities may create risks that can develop into a crisis when they are exploited. For instance, relaxed safety procedures can develop into an industrial accident; weak security procedures can leave an organization open to a terrorist bombing. Every organization has inherent vulnerabilities (weaknesses that naturally exist) on which mitigation (efforts to reduce risks) will have little effect. Inherent vulnerabilities include the visibility of a facility, accessibility, presences of hazardous materials, potential for collateral damage (impact on surrounding areas), and the number of people at the facility (potential for mass casualties). A few examples will illustrate inherent vulnerabilities. A shopping mall has high visibility, is easily accessible, and contains large numbers of people. Naturally, management would not want to hide the mall, limit access, or reduce the number of people inside. A manufacturing facility that uses hazardous chemicals could limit access (employ mitigation) but would find it difficult to reduce visibility. In addition, a facility that uses and stores hazardous materials as part of its operation has the potential to create collateral damage.[3]

Preventative actions are tied to the perceived importance of a risk. Crisis managers identify and prioritize risks. A risk is assessed for the impact it can have on the organization (the strength of the hazard) and the likelihood of the risk occurring (the threat it poses).[3] The crisis team analyzes the organization for risks and then rates the likelihood and impact of each risk. One formula that is employed in such ratings is "risk = likelihood × impact" with likelihood and impact both being rated on a 1 to 10 scale, 10 being the highest score.[2] Some risks are easier to quantify than others. Weather data, for instance, can help determine the likelihood and impact of tornadoes in a particular geographic area. For terrorism, however, there is an element of subjectivity to risk assessment. "Terrorism . . . is the result of human behavior that often lies outside conventional ideas of appropriateness and rationality and is thus difficult to predict" (p. 2–16).[3] The crisis team can only generate estimates (educated guesses) about how likely terrorism is to occur and the impact it might have on the organization, based on the very limited information the U.S. government has about terrorist threats.

Three factors that affect the risk of terrorism for a given facility are its location, the types of materials stored there, and its strategic importance.[3,4] Another is its proximity to nearby targets. The 9/11 attacks made planners realize that another organization's crisis can be their crisis. Attacks on a nearby organization could affect your facility by restricting access or requiring evacuation. The attack could destroy transportation routes or create hazards, such as fires or chemical releases, that require evacuation at nearby facilities. Organizations must consider if their neighbors might be an attractive target. Specifically, transportation centers, locations where large numbers of people gather (e.g., parks), historical sites, and government offices are all vulnerable.

Moreover, an organization is at great risk for attack if it stores chemical, biological, or radiological hazards. FEMA's training materials acknowledge that risk increases for facilities that manufacture or store chemicals such as pesticides, swimming pool treatments, petrochemicals, or fertilizer; as well as facilities that store infectious waste, low-level radioactive waste, or munitions.[5] A list of such places in the United States includes a wide range and number of private facilities. A terrorist attack could cause significant collateral damage through the release of chemical, biological, or radiological hazards into the environment. Therefore, organizations must be cognizant that their operations could be the target of terrorist actions designed to spread hazardous materials to the general public.

Many chemical facilities are located near densely populated areas. It is estimated that there are 110 facilities in the United States, each of which could affect more than one million people in the event of a chemical release. These plants are dispersed through twenty-two states. Facilities in forty-four states could affect more than 100,000 people each with a release. Intelligence suggests that terrorists do consider economic assets, such as chemical facilities, as targets.[6] We see similar concerns expressed among vendors who specialize in business continuity and disaster management. Strohl Systems, a company specializing in data storage, recommends adding possible terrorist attacks aimed at facilities and personnel to any organization's hazard and vulnerability analysis.[7]

Since 9/11, chemical manufacturers have been urged to increase security, and the entire industry has done so.[8] In addition, legislation, namely the Chemical Security Act, has been introduced yearly to mandate improved security at chemical facilities. The Chemical Security Act parallels federal guidelines for crisis planning in the nuclear power industry. The act would require every chemical facility to develop a vulnerability analysis that includes terrorism.[6] Organizations with strategic relevance to an area or the nation, such as power generation or pharmaceutical supplies, face an increased risk. In such cases, an attack would cripple a strategic resource. Likewise, an organization is at greater risk when an attack would produce a significant amount of collateral damage or would create a greater incident of disruption.[3]

What we do know is that terrorism is possible and its impact can be catastrophic. FEMA cautions that any human-caused hazard, including terrorism, can occur at any facility. Possible terrorist actions include conventional bombs, biological agents, chemical bombs, nuclear bombs, radiological agents, arson, hazardous material releases, and "intentional accidents" at fixed facilities or on transportation networks.[3] After 9/11, organizations that had not considered terrorism a risk added it to their lists.[9] Moreover, in calculations of risk, terrorism was accorded a higher numerical value. Pinkerton Security conducts an annual survey of the top security threats and management issues facing corporate America. From 1997 to 2001, terrorism ranked in the teens, ranging from fourteen to seventeen. In 2002, terrorism rose to number three and held strong at number four in 2003.[10] A survey of crisis planners found that after 9/11, terrorism and biological hazards were rated significantly higher as threats.[11] In short, the evidence shows that corporate America changed its evaluation of the terrorist risk after 9/11.

Another sign of change is the increased emphasis on facility security after 9/11. A 2002 survey of health, safety, and environmental coordinators found security is now the top priority and budget item. As one coordinator reported, "We had never really stopped to think about a terrorist attack at our facility. We didn't have a plan where we could control access 100 percent."[12] The risk of terrorism has led to an emphasis on perimeter security and building access. Organizations want to be able to monitor their perimeters for suspicious activities as a means of preventing terrorist attacks. The same prevention mentality is behind the need to control building access.[4,12]

Similar results are reported in the 2003 Competitiveness and Security Survey conducted by the Council on Competitiveness. The survey of 317 business executives (top management personnel) found that 88 percent rated security a top or high priority. New security procedures and standards had been adopted by 65 percent of the companies in the past twelve months compared to 53 percent in the previous year. Of those changes, 35 percent were a result of internal company risk/vulnerability assessments.[13] In other words, increased security is viewed as a viable means to mitigate the terrorist threat, and U.S. corporations are altering their preventative practices to reflect this fact.

Prevention is a noble goal. However, any crisis manager knows s/he cannot eliminate all potential risks. This is especially true of terrorism. Human risks (terrorism is a human action) are the most unpredictable and most difficult to prevent.[3] Because prevention is never total, crisis managers know they must prepare for crises, especially those connected to human risk.

*Preparation: Terrorism and Planning*

Preparation in crisis management is composed of two primary components: (1) the CMP, and (2) training/exercises using CMP. Current evidence indicates that post 9/11, organizations have changed or intend to change plans and training, in order to include a stronger focus on terrorism.

### CMPs

The creation of CMPs is guided by the risks an organization faces. According to the American Marketing Association, which tracks the creation of CMPs, the number of organizations with CMPs rose from 49 percent in 2002 to 64 percent in 2003. Of those with CMPs, 45 percent included terrorism. There is no data to indicate if the terrorism component of CMPs has risen, but given the limited consideration of terrorism prior to 9/11, it is a safe assumption that it has.[14] A survey of crisis managers immediately following 9/11 found only 15.5 percent had plans that included terrorism. However, in this same sample, 97 percent said their plans must be altered after 9/11, with 39 percent indicating the need for significant changes.[11] CMPs are changing to reflect the need to include terrorism. This change is to be expected because the methodology in crisis management is for the CMP to reflect the organization's risk assessment. If risk assessments are increasing the salience of terrorism, the CMPs should reflect that change.[2,15]

### Crisis Drills and Exercises

A consistent recommendation is that any CMP should be practiced at least once a year.[1] FEMA requires practicing of community disaster plans on a regular basis.[16] Practice drills or exercises allow for an evaluation of the thoroughness and accuracy of the CMP, as well as the ability of the crisis-management team to enact the CMP.[2] Organizations either create and run their own exercises or hire consultants who plan, execute, and evaluate the drill or exercise. Participants can include emergency responders (fire, police, and government and medical personnel) to test coordination with these agencies.

Crisis drills and exercises are now emphasizing terrorism-based crises. Consequently, there has been an increase in demand for consultants who can assist with terrorist-related exercise scenarios.[12] JS Consulting Services is one of the vendors who has witnessed increased demands for their terrorism-related exercise scenarios. Once again, there is a logical progression as terrorism becomes identified as a risk, is included in CMPs, and then is the subject of drills and exercises. Shortly after 9/11, organizations were urged to consider if they had conducted a terrorism-related drill or exercise.[7]

Terrorist attacks, especially those targeting facilities with hazardous materials, create the need to coordinate the organizational response with those of emergency responders. Every community is required to have a Community Emergency Operation Plan (EOP) that works much like an organization's CMP. Historically, organizations and communities have done little to integrate their crisis plans in order to coordinate responses. Experts now argue, however, that terrorist attacks are placing a premium on integration. The public-private boundary needs to dissolve. Corporations have many resources and responsibilities that should be integrated into community emergency-preparedness for terrorism. The key to seamless integration is to conduct coordinated exercises between public and private personnel.[9]

Not all employees are involved with traditional crisis management. Thus, CMPs are typically considered confidential material and are distributed to only those directly involved in the crisis-management process.[1] Similarly, the crisis drill or exercise would only involve the crisis-management team and other personnel, such as security personnel, germane to the practice sessions. Overall, employees at all levels have limited involvement with the CMP, and likewise with practice exercises. Another change triggered by the terrorist attack of 9/11 is a shift in emphasis to inclusive crisis/emergency planning.

*Emergency Planning*

In 2003, the U.S. government launched a public-information campaign intended to prepare citizens for future terrorist attacks. The campaign was designed to move beyond the confusing and maligned color-coded threat levels to individual preparedness. The campaign was run by the Department of Homeland Security. The advertisements featured Secretary Ridge and emphasized the need for emergency preparedness. Citizens were directed to a website, ready.gov, for more information. At the website, people can find advice on how to create family emergency kits, conduct fire drills, and how to shelter-in-place. The idea was to empower people and make them feel secure by explaining skills they could use to protect themselves. One unfortunate side effect was the East Coast run on duct tape and plastic in 2002. The two products are used to seal a room for sheltering-in-place. While problematic in execution, the idea behind the campaign is sound— preparation information and tasks should reduce anxiety about terrorism. A private organization, America Prepared Campaign, Inc., also has been formed to promote the message of terrorism preparedness. The focus of this private effort is on providing information about preparedness that can be used to save lives in the event of a terrorist attack.[17]

Organizations were targets for the preparedness campaign as well. Employers were told to prepare employees and the workplace for possible terrorist attacks. As with individuals, the messages focused on three points: evacuation, shelter-in-place, and equipment (kits).

Organizations were urged to review and practice their evacuation plans. Every organization was to have a site-specific evacuation plan and to practice it.[18] Data suggests organizations had already rediscovered evacuation drills. A 2002 survey found 74 percent of companies were using evacuation drills and others planned to implement them.[12] Evacuations are useful if the terror attack is a conventional explosive or arson.

Terrorist attacks, however, can be unconventional and involve the release of dangerous chemical, biological, or radiological elements into the air. As a result, organizations must be prepared to shelter-in-place. This means employees must be kept inside and the facility sealed off from outside air. The heating, cooling, and ventilation systems must be shut off, signs must be displayed indicating shelter-in-place is in effect, windows and vents must be sealed with plastic, doors must be sealed with duct tape, and sign-in sheets must be circulated and tallied.[19]

Organizations must be equipped for the emergency. The necessary equipment includes plastic sheets for windows and vents, preferably precut to size; duct tape; battery operated radios, flashlights, and fresh batteries; first-aid kits; water; and food. There should be designated rooms for sheltering, preassigned tasks for sealing the building, and procedures to account for those sheltering in it. Officials recommend running two full-scale, shelter-in-place drills per year.[19] Many organizations are also equipping employees with respirators including escape hoods or gas masks. The National Institute for Occupational Safety and Health (NIOSH) has produced guidelines for the selection of respirators. NIOSH documentation states that the need for respirators is a result of terrorist threats that could involve biological and chemical substances.[20] Disaster consultants likewise recommend the purchase of emergency equipment for employees.[21]

The primary difference between the CMP and emergency-preparedness plans is the level of involvement of employees. While the CMP has limited dissemination, the emergency-preparedness plan must include all personnel. Organizations cannot inform a select few about evacuation routes or steps to shelter-in-place. Everyone must know how to leave the facility safely, where to gather after an evacuation, and how to check-in for the accountability system. Preparing a facility to shelter-in-place takes many hands; all employees must be advised not to leave the facility, where to gather inside, and where the necessary equipment (first aid, water, flashlights, and food) is stored. While only certain personnel are involved in crisis drills and exercises, all employees must participate in evacuation or shelter-in-place drills.

*Initial Crisis Responses*

Anecdotal evidence suggests that 9/11 affected the basic information given after a crisis involving an accident. Generally, the crisis team expresses sympathy for victims, describes the event, and notes what is being done to correct the problem.[2,22] However, high profile accidents now include a disclaimer concerning terrorist activity, identifying that the accident was not staged by terrorists with the intention to harm. A fatal accident on Disneyland's Big Thunder Mountain; a chlorine gas leak in Festus, Missouri; the crash of a chartered airliner in Egypt; and the explosion at a West Pharmaceutical facility in North Carolina all included statements that indicated the events were not terrorist-related. There has been no systematic study of accident crisis responses post 9/11, hence only anecdotal evidence supports the need to deny terrorism during a crisis. However, the cases do illustrate that a need to combat terrorist fears in crisis responses may exist.

## NEW TERRORISM PREPARATIONS IN CONTEXT

It would be easy to dismiss the post-9/11 shift in crisis thinking and planning as overreaction, as many did when people on the East Coast made a run on duct tape and plastic. However, the professionals who plan for crises and disasters are not easily frightened. These are people accustomed to thinking about things many would choose to ignore. In fact, corporate management often has to be sold on crisis preparation and planning because management would prefer to ignore the potential problems.[1] While the salience of terrorism to crisis management may diminish over time, its addition to the mix of potential crises is warranted and yielding unintentional benefits.

### Rationale Behind the Shift

As figures cited earlier indicate, the number of organizations without CMPs has dropped radically over the past few years.[14] Perceptions of risk have been found to be the driving factor in the creation of CMPs.[1,5] Organizations do not craft CMPs unless they perceive a serious risk and realize they are susceptible to a crisis. The first step in developing a CMP is often convincing top management of the plan's worth.[1] One crisis consultant tells the story of running a two-day workshop on workplace violence as a crisis threat. Initially, management's inattention showed a lack of concern. Near the end of the first day, however, tragic news arrived. An employee at one of the company's facilities shot other employees. Suddenly the managers were very attentive, as the risk became real.

Similarly, the shocking events of 9/11 made terrorism real for organizations in the United States. As noted earlier, terrorism has been always in the mix of risk and vulnerability assessment, but management tended to see it as something that happened in other countries. Organizations realized they could no longer live under that delusion. The potential for terrorist attacks had always existed in the United States, and now it could not be ignored. In the methodology of crisis management, risk perception drives the need for and content of CMPs. Since 9/11, terrorism is recognized as a risk, rated highly as a concern, and included in many CMPs. The evaluation of the shift in post 9/11 crisis management hinges on two questions: (1) is this terrorist shift warranted? and (2) is the terrorist shift beneficial to U.S. organizations?

*Is the Shift Warranted?*

Crisis management should be a systematic process, progressing from risk assessment to prevention to preparation.[2] The events of 9/11 made crisis managers reevaluate the risk posed by terrorists, using a formula that posits risk as a function of likelihood and impact. Terrorist attacks remain low on the likelihood scale. However, by examining terrorist attacks, including new worst-case scenarios, crisis managers have come to recognize the major impact of such incidents. The situation is analogous to an airplane crash: The likelihood of any one airplane crashing is small, but the impact is massive. After 9/11, terrorism, as a risk, moved from the periphery to full consideration. It is a legitimate risk, and is now receiving proper, not undue, notice. The statistics support this increased attention. As noted, dozens of chemical facilities in the United States could affect populations of 100,000 or more with a chemical release.[6] By definition, such a significant release of hazardous chemicals is a weapon of mass destruction. Plans for the prevention and response to such events should be part of an organization's crisis-management process.

As a human-behavior crisis, terrorism is difficult to predict, and it is equally difficult to quantify its likelihood. Organizations face the same challenges with workplace violence crises. Like workplace violence, if the impact is major, terrorism belongs on the list of crises that require prevention and preparation. Furthermore, terrorist experts agree that more lethal attacks will take place on U.S. soil. The message crisis experts communicate seems to be when, not if. These attacks could involve bioterrorism or turning existing facilities into weapons of mass destruction.[23,24] In light of these facts, terrorism deserves the attention it is now receiving in crisis management. Prior to 9/11, terrorism was largely invisible to all but the most forward-thinking organizations. Today, terrorism is a mainstream crisis that is considered along with industrial accidents, product recalls, and organizational misdeeds. Is this shift warranted? The answer is yes, if we believe in and follow the methodologies of crisis management. Moreover, many of the government efforts to inform people about terrorist risks echo this message as well.

### Is the Shift Beneficial?

Skeptics might argue that the rise of terrorism as a threat has only helped the sale of plastic, duct tape, and gas masks. However, closer examination of shifts in crisis management driven by terrorism reveals a number of benefits including renewed interest in emergency preparedness and building security.

In 2002, I attended a regional Red Cross conference about crisis planning. In one session, the participants were asked how many of them planned an evacuation route as they entered the conference facility and how many could quickly identify the quickest route from the room. Very few hands were raised. At a national meeting of disaster planners in 2002, the participants were asked how many had or knew if their organization had first-aid kits. Again, very few hands were raised. In each case the audience, attending out of a motivation to learn more about crisis management, was ill prepared for emergencies or crises. While anecdotal, the examples illustrate how little organizational personnel knew about emergency preparedness even after 9/11. The intense interest in emergency plans, such as evacuations, being created or practiced after 9/11, is a positive step toward making organizations safer.

Employees have always needed clear evacuation and shelter-in-place plans. Heightened fears of terrorism alone did not create the need. Nonterrorist crises such as fires, chemical spills, and explosions can create the need to evacuate or shelter-in-place. Such emergency preparedness should be a part of crisis management, and organizations had simply let the importance of emergency preparedness slip. The terrorist attacks of 9/11 reminded them that having and practicing emergency plans saves lives. Many more lives would have been lost on 9/11 had not employees in the World Trade Center been planning and practicing evacuations following the earlier bombing of the WTC. Organizations across the United States now have a greater appreciation and respect for emergency planning. This knowledge is a very good thing that will save countless lives in the future.

The survey data also support a strong emphasis on building security. Again, security concerns were not born from 9/11 but simply were enhanced by it. Let us revisit the Pinkerton surveys of top security threats. Over the past seven years, workplace violence has been ranked first six times and second once. Enhanced security in response to this threat includes the control of entry and exit from a building, monitoring people in a building, and securing the perimeter.[3] These security precautions can help prevent terrorism as well as workplace violence. One form of workplace violence is when current or former employees attack current workers on site. With former employees, it is critical to control entry to a facility. Controlling entry and exit helps to prevent disgruntled, dismissed employees from returning and inflicting harm. In addition, building and perimeter surveillance can indicate if an attack or sabotage is about to happen. We may not like locks coded to identification badges, but the threats in modern organizations demand strong security measures. In other words, terrorism has helped organizations devote more time and resources to already needed security enhancements. Security can go too far, however. The courts support an employee's right to privacy. Surveillance should be limited to public areas such as entrances and hallways and not invade private areas such as restrooms or changing rooms.

Is the shift beneficial? The answer is yes. Organizations needed to emphasize evacuation and shelter-in-place plans prior to 9/11. Improved security was also an existing need. By emphasizing emergency preparedness and security, organizations are becoming safer places in which to work.

## CONCLUSION

The terrorist attacks of 9/11 changed how organizations think about and plan for crisis management. The risk of terrorist attacks on U.S. facilities has always been a possibility. However, only a few very progressive CMPs gave the terrorist threat full consideration. Too often, terrorist attacks were viewed as something that happens "over there." As a result, terrorism was low to nonexistent on most crisis risk evaluations. The events of 9/11 have raised awareness of this risk and the potential damage it can inflict. Organizations, especially chemical facilities, have been reevaluating the risk and vulnerabilities associated with terrorism.[8] The increased salience of terrorism as a risk has led to changes in security to prevent such crises, and revisions to CMPs and simulations to ready organizations for a terrorist-related crisis. The post-9/11 changes in crisis management are not a costly overreaction but rather a necessary correction. Terrorism always has been a risk for which organizations should prepare and will remain so. Chemical companies have included the effects of massive releases (one possible outcome of a terrorist attack on a chemical facility) for years. Now they and nearby communities are taking the threat more seriously in their crisis and disaster planning.

Much of the preparation and planning for terrorism involves basic emergency preparedness such as evacuation and shelter-in-place procedures. All organizations should have and practice such procedures. The simple fire drill is a lifesaving tool that many organizations seem to have forgotten. The reawakening to the needs of emergency preparedness as part of organizational life is a positive development. Employees should know what to do individually and collectively during an emergency. Even if terrorists do not attack, tornadoes and hurricanes do hit, fires do happen, and hazardous chemicals have been known to be released. Increased security yields dividends beyond terrorism prevention. Workplace violence continues to be an important issue for organizations. The security changes to meet the terrorist threats will also help to prevent workplace violence and to identify its occurrence more rapidly. As a whole, the changes in crisis-management thinking and planning post-9/11 have made work environments safer. The 9/11 tragedy was a wake up that facilitated many needed changes to how organizations perceive crisis risk, work to mitigate those risks, and how they respond to crisis events.

## NOTES

1. Barton L. Crisis in organizations. 2nd ed. Cincinnati, OH: College Divisions, South-Western; 2001.

2. Coombs WT. Ongoing crisis communication: planning, managing, and responding. Thousand Oaks, CA: Sage Publications; 1999.

3. Federal Emergency Management Agency. Toolkit for managing the emergency consequences of terrorist incidents. 2002. Available from: www. fema.gov/preparedness/toolkit.shtm. Accessed October 23, 2003.

4. Watson S. Buildings with bull's-eyes: assessing the risk and vulnerability of "soft" target facilities. Contingency Plann Manag 2003;8(5):32–35.

5. Federal Emergency Management Agency. Integrating human-caused hazards into mitigation planning: FEMA how-to guide number seven. 2002. Available from: www.fema.gov/fima/planning_toc6.shtm. Accessed October 16, 2003.

6. Chemical Security Act of 2003. S 157, 108th Congress. Introduced January 14, 2003.

7. Planning for the worst. Contingency Plann Manag 2001;6(5):16.

8. American Chemistry Council. Progress report: two years later significant security enhancements make chemical plants safer. 2003 Sep. Available from: www.accnewsmedia.com/site/page.asp?TRACKID=&VID=1&CID=361&DID=1313. Accessed October 23, 2003.

9. Ross, N. Terrorism: how will it impact contingency planning? Contingency Plann Manag 2001;6(5):14–7.

10. Pinkerton. Top security threats and management issues facing corporate America. New York: Pinkerton; 2003.

11. Chandler RC, Wallace JD. What disaster recovery experts were thinking just after the attacks. Disaster Recovery J 2002;15(1):26–31.

12. Nighswonger T. Threat of terror impacts workplace safety. Occup Hazards 2002;64(7):24–7.

13. Council on Competitiveness. 2003 competitiveness and security survey. 2003. Available from: www.compete.org/pdf/c_and_s_report.pdf. Accessed October 16, 2003.

14. American Management Association. 2003 AMA survey: crisis management and security issues. 2003. Available from: www.amanet.org/research/index.htm. Accessed October 12, 2003.

15. Wrigley BJ, Salmon CT, Park HS. Crisis management planning and the threat of bioterrorism. Public Relations Rev 2003;29:281–90.

16. Federal Emergency Management Agency. An orientation to community disaster exercises (IS-120). Washington, DC: Federal Emergency Management Agency; 1995.

17. America Prepared Campaign, Inc. America Prepared Campaign. 2003. Available from: www.americaprepared.org/pics/brochure.pdf. Accessed December 19, 2003.

18. U.S. Department of Homeland Security. Anti-terror checklist. 2003. Available at URL:http://www.contiuitycentral.com/news0246.htm. Accessed October 29, 2003.

19. Federal Emergency Management Agency. Are you ready? 2003. Available from: www.fema.gov/pdf/areyouready/areyouready_full.pdf. Accessed October 24, 2003.

20. National Institute for Occupational Safety and Health. Respirator fact sheet [brochure]. Atlanta, GA: National Institute for Occupational Safety and Health; 2003.

21. Rainey K. Workplace preparedness: the catalyst to a resilient community. Continuity e-guide. 2003 Nov 12. Available from: disaster-resource.com/newsletter/subpages/v7/meet_the_experts.htm. Accessed November 12, 2003.

22. Coombs WT. An analytic framework for crisis situations: better responses from a better understanding of the situation. J Public Relations Res 1998;10:177–91.

23. Propst R. New terrorists, new attack means? Categorizing terrorist challenges for the 21st century. J Homeland Secur 2002 Mar. Available from: www.homelandsecurity.org/journal/Articles/propstnewterroristprint.htm.  Accessed October 16, 2003.

24. Quinn S. We can do better than duct tape. The Washington Post 2003 Feb 13; Sect. A:3,1.

# 11  Incident Management System Network: Integrating Voice, Data, and Video Communications

## Paul Doute and Gary Green

A communication environment that is needed for any type of terrorism event, disaster, or serious incident that is part of the Incident Command (now Management) System must be based on providing real-time voice, video, and data over a secure, encrypted network that is flexible enough to send out an emergency vehicle with a remote camera to a chemical spill. With a Converged Asynchronous Transfer Mode (ATM) Network design this can be accomplished.

—Dr. Gerald Ledlow[1]

The Office of Homeland Security has mandated the key features of the communication network infrastructure required for federal, state, and local government agencies. The communication network infrastructure to interconnect these various agencies must be secure, scalable, reliable, flexible, and economical. The network must provide the highest quality communication capabilities for real-time applications like voice, video, and data. The network design must be reliable and flexible enough to allow diverse communication networks to interconnect both private and public networks, so that information can be exchanged in a timely manner in the event of an incident. Most importantly, security cannot be compromised to any degree.

In this chapter we will discuss these guidelines in terms of networking various types of agencies throughout our nation. A proposed solution with clear benefits will be presented: the Asynchronous

Transfer Mode (ATM). Finally, we will cover the MiCTA endorsed ATM solution for the convergence of applications specific to government agencies, educational institutions, and healthcare providers, and how this solution meets the transport requirements of the Office of Homeland Security.

## THE GUIDELINES

There are a number of network guidelines and standards that have been fostered by organizations like the Telecommunications Industry Association, the American National Standards Institute, the International Telecommunications Union, the Network Reliability and Interoperability Council, the National Airspace System Information Architecture Council, and the National Institute of Standards and Technology. The number of guidelines and standards is staggering, and sometimes their rules are contradictory. Standards in a communication environment serve to guide the network in terms of security, application interaction, protocol interaction, physical connectivity, session establishment, networking interaction, and data presentation.

Based on research at the websites of the National Institute of Standards and Technology website, (www.nist.gov), and the Office of Homeland Security (www.dhs.gov/dhspublic), the Homeland Security Network (HSN) must have the following characteristics:

Reliability: The HSN must have carrier-class. The network must provide 99.999 percent availability with less than 50 milliseconds of delay during a failover, or data transfer failure, whether the outage is due to a circuit failure (break in the "line") or physical card failure (technical component failure). The network must be designed on hardware components that support software upgrades and processor failover that will not affect service to the agency using the network. The network must be resilient in providing the greatest level of redundancy and survivability. In the case of an incident or national emergency, it must be able to support the prioritization and preemption of normal daily communications traffic to handle incident-related communications traffic.

Scalability: The network must be designed to be scalable to allow many users and nodes. The HSN must also be able to scale in terms of capacity. The network must allow for the growth in the total number of users, nodes, and services to insure equipment and network viability. The design must be hierarchical, allowing the network to scale to thousands of nodes.

Security: Of significant importance to the HSN is data and communications security. The HSN must be designed to protect management plane access, access to the system by those responsible for managing it, through a variety of methods. There are a number of methods to do so. Methods and system applications named by the organization of creation in some cases, for protecting the management plane include SecurID, Keberos or remote authentication dial-in user service, Secure Socket Layer, and Simple Network Management Protocol.

The HSN must be designed to also protect access to the control plan. In hierarchical network design, address filtering, a technique to stop system access by unknown or known systems to maintain security, must be used to restrict connections to specific network devices and services. Finally, the HSN must protect the data plane to ensure security is end to end with encryption.

Flexibility: The HSN must be able to carry various types of real-time and nonreal-time communication traffic including voice, video, and data. The network must support multiple services and multiple protocols to interface with the most prolific networking technologies used in the private sector today including Asynchronous Transfer Mode (ATM), Frame Relay, Multi-protocol Label Switching, Internet Protocol (IP), Time Division Multiplexing (TDM), Ethernet, and Packet over Synchronous Optical Networking (SONET (POS)). The network must be diverse in supporting the communications required during a national incident for command and control applications.

Economy: The HSN must be economical from a financial investment point of view. The HSN must be able to leverage many of the existing assets in the government, as well as the assets of the various agencies involved in the support of homeland security in order to control the overall cost of the network. Being able to utilize these assets in the network is essential in speeding up the deployment of the HSN. The Office of Homeland Security requires the network to be designed to prevent attacks on the economic, health, and educational development of the United States.

Obviously, these are not all of the required standards and guidelines. Only the most basic guidelines have been presented. Actually, networks by design are multifaceted with many applications, many protocols, and many components. The HSN is no different. Standards, guidelines, and recommendations are a necessary part of the national strategy to prepare various U.S. agencies to defend our country, our people, and our assets. Standards are ever changing and evolving.

## Convergence

In this chapter, convergence is used to describe the movement toward uniformity of voice, video, and data. Converged networks combine various applications and services over a single network. These networks can be based on many of the various protocols listed above.

Why does the HSN require convergence? It is very simple. Convergence is required to meet all the networking standards discussed above. The convergence of voice, video, and data applications over a single network will speed the deployment of the HSN. Convergence will reduce overall network costs though the consolidation of services. It will provide greater flexibility, faster application deployment, better performance, and allow the HSN to leverage many, if not all, of the existing agency communication assets deployed today. The convergence of network services is a great way to reduce ongoing hardware maintenance and management of communication devices associated with private lines and other types of communication lines. When resources are consolidated, various applications deployed over a converged network can produce significant savings in voice toll-bypass networking and video conferencing.

Convergence is one of the most important considerations today in the communications industry. One example of convergence is the Next Generation Network (NGN), a movement to consolidate traditional TDM voice services, data, video, and packet-switched services—voice over IP. The importance of the NGN is the bundling of multiple modes of data and communication over one secure and dynamic (the system is intelligent to know what bandwidth is needed for each mode) system rather than multiple and often contradictory systems. The NGN is advancing in the telecom industry. Telecoms are making daily announcements about the billion's of dollars being spent to upgrade their core infrastructures to integrate support for a packet-switched network, a more controlled and secure environment, to compliment their current Public Switched Telephone Network, an environment that lacks adequate security and control. For several years, many of the top carriers have made a commitment to packet-switched technology. So the technology is coming. It just a matter of time before this technology is part of the communication infrastructure and part of the HSN.

## ATM

The goal of this section is to provide basic, technical details about ATM and how it works, so an overall understanding is gained concerning the benefits of ATM technology. ATM is a high bandwidth, fast-packet switching technology based on fixed-length cells of 53 bytes. Simply put, the concept of ATM is to transmit all data in small, fixed-size packets, called cells. These small, fixed cells are perfect for the transmission of voice, video, data, and multimedia applications that are delay sensitive. ATM is a very fast broadband-networking technology that simultaneously supports voice, video, and data transmissions on a single network. ATM networks are connection oriented requiring logical connections between locations to communicate. To simplify, ATM benefits users by guaranteeing capacity providing constant and predictable transmission delay in order to support intermittent high volume users also known as traffic. Moreover, ATM is an international standards-based technology; this means communication networks are compatible across national boundaries (important for near or cross border incidents management). ATM supports multiple applications and multiple protocols. It is extremely flexible, scalable, and cost effective. Networking with ATM services will allow a homeland security agency to connect to other ATM locations, as well as to internetwork to frame relay sites, and/or the Internet/intranet.

Wide-area networking, based on ATM, will allow a homeland security agency to: (1) exchange information faster with transmission speeds ranging from T1 to OC-48 (this refers to the size of the bandwidth or data transmission "pipeline"), and (2) be able to, in real-time, collaborate better using the advanced Quality of Service (QoS) mechanisms in ATM.

Distinct QoS support both burstable or large volume transmission data traffic like IP and continuous stream traffic like voice or interactive video across the same network and access facilities. As mentioned, ATM will allow the consolidation of multiple networks to help reduce cost and management of resources. ATM will allow agencies to connect to sites in the United States, as well as to sites abroad, if so desired. ATM is very flexible and scalable in supporting expanded access for various applications. The migration of agencies to ATM is a seamless process. During the process, all agencies can communicate as usual with no service interruptions.

## The Benefits

The benefits of ATM to the various homeland security agencies are numerous. ATM provides scalability in terms of distance between locations, network topology size, and node/bandwidth capacity. ATM is designed to provide high-quality communications with added efficiencies in hardware, maintenance, application support, and bandwidth management in helping reduce the overall cost of the network. ATM will support multiple protocols, multiple media types, and multiple virtual connections. The system performs very well in terms of latency, loss of data, and data throughput. It is designed to ensure security, with mechanisms for controlling access, preventing data interception, and stopping disruptions.

ATM offers investment protection by allowing homeland security agencies to connect existing equipment through the network. It provides manageability with regards to the setup, network management, the setting of networking policies and the troubleshooting of problems. Applications can send traffic in bursts or steady rates. Flexibility is supported through bandwidth variations, meaning agencies use only the bandwidth that they need. ATM adapts to an application's needs instead of forcing the application to fit into a rigid bandwidth structure of a network. ATM provides a common network solution to meet the networking needs of the HSN of today and in the future.

Operating separate networks for the local area network, to include video conferencing, and other applications, increases the total cost of network ownership. With ATM, agencies will be able to transmit voice, data, and video information over a single network interface. ATM offers multiple categories of service with different performance characteristics allowing the agencies to transmit a variety of traffic types across the same access port. Consolidating applications can significantly reduce equipment, wiring, access, wide area network, administration, and operation cost for agencies and the HSN.

As a virtual private networking service, ATM provides connectivity options, network reliability, and resource efficiencies. Cells from independent applications and users may share the same physical facility. Users are able to define meshed or synchronized and connected and partially meshed logical networks for full connectivity between agencies. Logical connections have inherent reliability and security, being able to automatically reroute around network failures through alternate network facilities. The connections use only bandwidth when they have active traffic to carry. At other times, the bandwidth is available for other defined connections. Statistical sharing of resources amongst users and applications can result in significant network efficiencies. To simplify and speed up the handling of data, there is no processing of the data in the network above the cell level with ATM.

The industry-standards agencies have defined the standards to support the compatibility of ATM with existing LAN and WAN protocols, giving users a variety of options for migrating to ATM. Standard encapsulation or compartmentalization methods exist for wide-area networking protocols, such as frame relay and inter-networking protocols like IP.

Agencies can chose the wide-area service that makes the most sense for each site based on size, applications, existing equipment, and cost, while maintaining interoperability between all locations. New strategic business applications with very high-speed bandwidth or stringent QoS requirements may need the scalability or QoS support of ATM. An ATM implementation can meet HSN needs today while providing the HSN with a networking platform to build upon for the future.

## ATM TECHNOLOGY BRIEF: HOW DOES IT WORK?

ATM is based on fast-packet technology. ATM was developed by ANSI and ITU. Data information is transmitted in the form of cells with a short, fixed length. Each cell is 53 bytes long; 48 bytes are reserved for data and 5 bytes for overhead. Data and overhead are in the same place on each cell. ATM can transmit data up to 1 million cells per second.

From a user's PC, information destined for a remote location server over an ATM network will travel over the local area network to a router. The router will format the data packet and route the data packets out to the appropriate port to leave the network. The information is received by the local ATM switch. The ATM switch segments the data packets from the router into cells based on network standards and addresses them for their trip through the ATM wide area network. Virtual connection to the remote location will be built already or built on the fly as the cell prepares to leave the ATM wide area network port.

The information is delivered across the ATM core backbone to the remote destination. At the destination, information goes through the reverse process with end destination receiving the data packet.

The ATM switch combines the features of two types of multiplexing: TDM and statistical multiplexing. With TDM technology data is combined on a multiple channel link like a channelized T1 (sent through a communication pipeline with predetermined channels or partitions) and sent in channels/timeslots at fixed intervals. When data is received from a source, it is slotted alongside data from another source in a separate channel and sent to different destinations without affecting data in other channels. On the other hand, statistical multiplexing uses a high-speed link by assigning channels on the link only to user devices that have data ready to send. The statistical multiplexer assigns priorities to various types of information and allocates bandwidth on the high-speed link accordingly. If the allocations exceed the capacity of the high-speed link, the statistical multiplexer moves low-priority information into a buffer, where the data is held for later transmission. When data arrives at the ATM switch one or both of these multiplexing techniques is used to transmit and receive data. Obviously, there is much more technical detail in regards to ATM. Hopefully, an understanding has been gained.

## THE SOLUTION: CORE NETWORK

In its ongoing process to evaluate and influence technologies on behalf of its members, the MiCTA organization, a telecommunications and technology purchasing cooperative and education consortium, with a special interest in the communication security regulatory requirements mandated by the Health Insurance Portability and Accountability Act (HIPAA), and more recently, homeland defense security requirements, sought a product offering that had multiservice capabilities with the ability to assign quality of service to specific applications, and was built on a secure, reliable, and resilient network that was economical for MiCTA members. When the process was completed, MiCTA, with the help of Chris Marshall and Greg Robinson, engineers at Sprint, had developed a converged product that was dynamic, secure, reliable, resilient and economical for MiCTA members. The MiCTA solution, based on ATM, has been helping MiCTA members for the past three years converge voice, video and data securely.

From our earlier discussion on ATM one can tell that ATM is a very unique and dynamic protocol. An ATM solution has the ability to converge both applications and services together to meet the design requirements of HIPPA and the HSN. The MiCTA converged ATM solution is built on a superior network that has multiple transport layers to increase capacity, reliability, resiliency, and security. The solution is capable of virtually associating thousands of sites together through a network gateway that supports all customer-transmitted protocols.

As mentioned, the MiCTA solution is built in layers. MiCTA, through their evaluation process, found the best design to support their members' networking requirements is hierarchical design. MiCTA chose Sprint to support the design of their member networking requirements based on MiCTA's past collaboration with Sprint in the development of the World's first "dial-up, digitally compressed video network."

In particular, in recent years, MiCTA became aware of Sprint engineers's design and construction of a new Sprint backbone network. The first layer of the network is based on a growing deployment of thousands of miles of fiber-optic cable Sprint initially began to construct in the late 1980s. The fiber-optic cable network was deployed to provide users of the network the best clarity and quality of voice and data connections. Fiber optics is the most flexible, reliable, and fastest physical networking technology today. The fiber optics deployed in the core backbone has allowed Sprint to deliver a high quality, more scalable, more reliable communication product to MiCTA members's critical business applications.

From the beginning of its initial construction, Sprint Engineers had decided to deploy this network with an even more reliable and survivable design based on the World's first QUAD SONET (Synchronous Optical Networking) multiple ring topology. QUAD SONET was the first four-pipeline network with redirection and "self-adjusting" and "self-fixing" capability. Deploying SONET in this fashion provides the network with the capability of redirecting traffic in milliseconds to guarantee quality, reliable communications. This second layer of the design offered MiCTA members the resiliency necessary to provide communications on a nationwide basis. Just ask the FCC which carrier has had the least number of reportable outages for the past seven years? It is the network we are discussing.

The ability to provide the necessary capacity in the backbone network is accomplished with Dense Wavelength Division Multiplexing (DWDM), which allows the optical fibers to be divided in communications channels based on multicolor photo-optics to support the fast deployment of additional bandwidth when necessary. Again, this a great benefit to MiCTA members because backbone capacity is available to support all their communication needs.

The next layer in the network is the ATM. The ATM is the single network that can address all of the MiCTA members's voice, video, and data applications including wireless. ATM inherently provides QoS metrics to support multiple types of application, including delay sensitive applications like voice and video. The Sprint ATM network has the ability to connect to gateways to support various systems and applications such as Switched Digital Services for voice, Internet/intranet for Virtual Private Networking, and Frame Relay.

This addresses carrier network design. Another item worth noting that benefits MiCTA members is that each layer of the network is built on ubiquitous hardware. Why is ubiquitous hardware so important?

It may seem like a very trivial subject but it is an extremely important one. With each layer of the network, a single hardware platform is used to support the network infrastructure that is capable of being upgraded without affecting the daily networking operations of MiCTA members. The ubiquitous design of the various networks we've discussed allows for the deployment software patches, software upgrades, or hardware repairs faster with minimal to no service disruption.

## THE SOLUTION: THE MICTA CONVERGED ATM PRODUCT

The MiCTA Converged ATM product available to members extends the Sprint ATM Network directly to MiCTA member locations. The ATM service has a variety of connection speeds ranging from T1/ Multi-T1 to OC48. The ATM circuits terminate in a Marconi ATM Switch, which terminates all the wide-area network connections into a single high-speed data stream. Sprint is responsible for installing, configuring, managing, maintaining, monitoring and upgrading the Marconi hardware. The Marconi ATM switch will be configured to meet the MiCTA member networking needs. The hardware is monitored 7 days a week, 24 hours a day, and 365 days a year by Sprint. The Marconi ATM Switch hardware used at each location is designed to customer specifications including power redundancy and CPU redundancy. In a typical converged configuration the Marconi ATM Switch will directly connect to the members' router(s) or firewall(s), PBX, and video system(s). If security is required by the application in the form of encryption, the device attaching to the Marconi ATM Switch data port should provide this functionality in order to protect the data plane.

The preferred method of delivering these interconnecting services is to use a logical connection called a SPVC or SVC. By using one of these logical connections to deliver a service allows a connection to be rerouted in the case of a failure. Also, in the case of a SVC it provides an additional measure of security because the establishment of the virtual circuit is a dynamic process allowing for the connections to use a different path every time a virtual connection is established. No matter what type of virtual circuit is used, a QoS capability is associated with the virtual circuit. Why is this important? Certain applications have specific requirements. Each application can be prioritized to provide the type qualities specific to each application to run optimally. Also, it is important to note that priorities can be set based on the importance of an application. This functionality is extremely important to the network design. For example, voice from a PBX to the Sprint Switched Digital Service and to inter-networked PBX would have the highest priority. Video would have the next highest priority and the data applications would have the lowest priority. The design must be able to prioritize the most important traffic over least important traffic but still be able to provide the least impor-tant traffic with bandwidth for exchanging data. Please note that each Virtual Circuit is private. Data is not shared amongst Virtual Circuits. Data is shared between networking end points after an authentication process has completed to establish the Virtual Circuit. The services offered through the MiCTA Converged ATM product appear to the end application as a single hop away. An analogous network would be a point-to-point circuit with router communicating to a router, or a PBX connecting to a PBX. The Internet/intranet, Frame Relay, and Switched Digital Services networks are provided through gateways that intercon-nect with the ATM network at Sprint. Each gateway is responsible for converting ATM to the native service protocol (see figure 11.1).

## THE SOLUTION: MEETING THE REQUIREMENTS

The MiCTA Converged ATM product clearly meets the transport needs set forth by the Office of Homeland Security. The key features required are reliability, scalability, security, flexibility, and economical. How does the MiCTA Converged ATM product meet the require-ments of the HSN?

The MiCTA Converged ATM product is very reliable. The product is based on the best carrier network available in the United States. From a core backbone perspective the network has the ability to pro-vide 100 percent availability for the HSN. The core backbone network design is carrier class and is based on sound technology and engineer-ing. In the event of a failure the delay to reroute traffic is milliseconds. The hardware used in the core network is designed on hardware plat-form and components that support software upgrades and processor failover that will not affect service. The core backbone network is based on fiber optics, DWDM, and SONET redundant rings. The core back-bone network is very resilient providing the greatest level of redundancy and survivability. Finally, in the case of an incident or emergency, the network has the ability to support the prioritization and preemption of normal daily communications traffic to handle incident-specific com-munications traffic.

The MiCTA Converged ATM solution is built on a network and service that is very scalable. The network design allows the network to

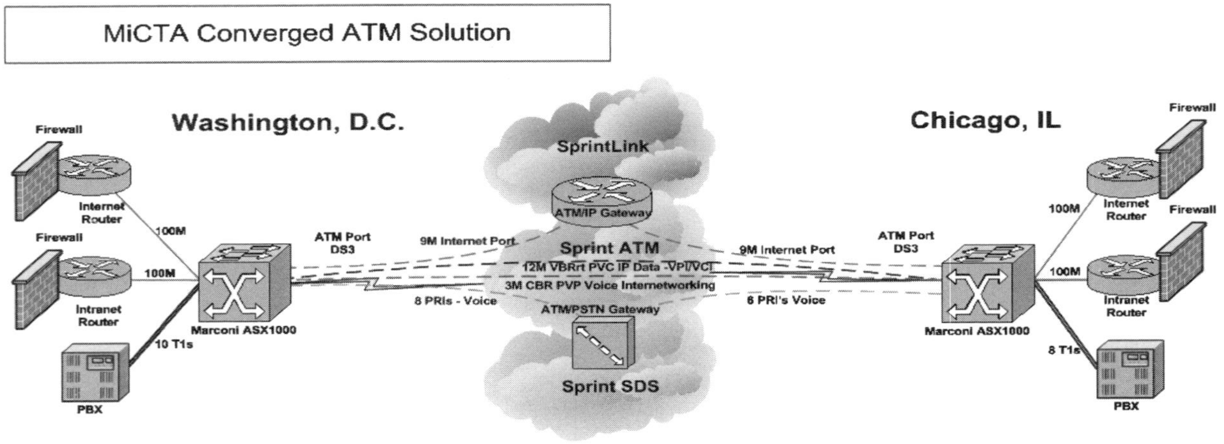

MiCTA Converged ATM Solution

Washington, D.C.

Chicago, IL

Firewall

Internet
Router

100M

Firewall

Intranet
Router

100M

PBX

10 T1s

Marconi ASX1000

ATM Port
DS3

9M Internet Port

8 PRIs - Voice

SprintLink

ATM/IP Gateway

Sprint ATM

12M VBR-rt PVC IP Data -Vpi/VCI

3M CBR PVP Voice Internetworking

ATM/PSTN Gateway

Sprint SDS

9M Internet Port

6 PRI's Voice

ATM Port
DS3

Marconi ASX1000

Firewall

Internet
Router

100M

Firewall

Intranet
Router

100M

PBX

8 T1s

Figure 11.1
Typical MiCTA Network Design for Internetworking Services

*Source*: Courtesy of Sprint Proprietary Information. Engineer Paul Doute, December 26, 2004.

scale as needed without interruption, providing for the capacity required by the HSN. The network has the capability to sustain and support the growth of the network in number of users, nodes, and services. The MiCTA Converged ATM product allows agencies to integrate their existing communications hardware. See figure 11.2 for a typical remote agency design. The design of the network is hierarchical allowing the network to scale to thousands of nodes.

Security in the MiCTA Converged ATM solution is built on a multi-layered defense. Each layer adds to the complexities, so an intruder is unable to intercept, eavesdrop, or spoof data on the network. Also, an encryption modem will be used for out-of-band management to access the management port on the Marconi switches. Sprint Managed services uses Simple Network Management Protocol (SNMP) to manage each device network over a virtual circuit to each device. Sprint will implement several access security mechanisms to control which users can place calls in the network and to whom, to discourage abusive or fraudulent use, both to protect network resources and to provide end user security.

For authentication to the network a valid calling party address (parties attempting to connect to the network) will be registered at the time of provisioning. This authentication consists of the customer-provided address or address ranges (a range of addresses could be another network made up of multiple parties). Any calling party address that matches the assigned address ranges is considered a valid address. Similar to Calling Party Address screening, Called Party Address will also validate the Called Party Address against a list of valid customer Called Party Addresses defined by the customer for the ATM user port. ILMI messages will be ignored by the Sprint network, preventing auto-discovery of other customers and other network elements by other ATM locations. The proposed network is a hierarchical design that uses employees' address filtering to restrict connections to specific network devices and services. The data plane security is handled by the external device(s) attaching to the Marconi switch insuring security is end to end with encryption.

The MiCTA Converged ATM Solution is an extremely flexible network design. The MiCTA Converged ATM solution provides home-land security agencies with the ability to carry multiple types of communications traffic. The network devices support multiple services and protocols to interface with Asynchronous Transfer Mode (ATM), Frame Relay, Multiprotocol Label Switching, IP, Time Division Multiplexing, Ethernet, and SONET (POS). Bandwidth can be upgraded and manipulated as necessary.

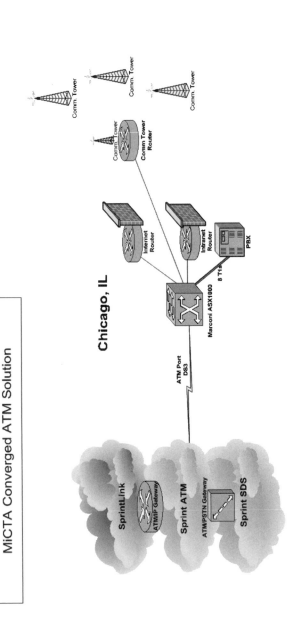

**Figure 11.2**
**Remote Agency Design to Support Day-to-Day Operations and First Responders**

*Source:* Courtesy of Sprint Proprietary Information. Engineer Paul Doute, December 26, 2004.

Virtual circuits can be reconfigured to support multiple environments like normal day-to-day operations and incident command and control operations. The MiCTA Converged ATM solution provides the diversity to implement multiple configurations in a short time frame in order to support the communications required during a national incident.

The HSN must be economical from an investment standpoint. With the MiCTA Converged ATM solution, agencies of the HSN will be able to leverage many, if not all, of their existing governmental assets. From economics standpoint it is important to control the overall cost of the network. With the MiCTA Converged ATM solution pricing has been already negotiated based on the 17,000 (plus) members of MiCTA. The member pricing negotiated represents some of the best rates available in term of access and services. Pricing is constantly being reviewed to provide MiCTA members with the best pricing for services. If the contract pricing is updated, MiCTA members with Sprint services automatically receive the reduced rates. Sprint carries the burden of maintaining, managing, installing, configuring, and upgrading the Marconi ATM switches that are deployed in the network. The economics of the MiCTA Converged ATM solution provides the HSN with untold benefits and savings. The MiCTA Converged ATM solution will allow the HSN to utilize the assets in the network to speed up the deployment of the HSN. Thus, the network solution from MiCTA is designed to support the economic, health, and educational development of the United States of America.

## CONCLUSION

In conclusion, the criteria discussed in the prologue of this chapter is met with the deployment of the MICTA Converged ATM solution based on Sprint's Network. Today Asynchronous Transfer Mode offers the Office of Homeland Security the security, scalability, reliability, flexibility, and economics required to network the multiple of agencies involved in homeland defense. First responders will be able to use wireless to deliver voice and video to command and control with an ATM while Emergency Operations Centers would have the ability to use wireless, line, and combinations of both to communicate in real time in multiple delivery modalities across the secure network.

## NOTE

1. Presentation to State of Michigan select members of the homeland security committee, House of Representatives office building, Lansing, MI, November 5, 2003.

# 12 Preparing for Terrorism: A Rationale for the Crisis Communication Center

## *Juliann C. Scholl, David E. Williams, and Bolanle A. Olaniran*

### INTRODUCTION

The terrorist attacks of September 11, 2001, sent a message to the American public in the clearest terms possible. We are at risk, and preparation is the key to our continued safety and way of life. Significant steps have been taken since the attacks, the most prominent being the creation of the Department of Homeland Security. However, despite a proactive approach to fighting terrorism abroad and increased security at home, the country still struggles with the fear of future attacks. Public concern escalates when the terror alert level is increased or when significant national holidays or events approach, including the anniversary of 9/11. In addition to these occasions, certain areas of the country suffer anxieties stemming from the proximity of a range of potential terrorist targets.

This chapter will explore those risks in terms of the national and local crises that they represent. We will suggest the creation of local Crisis Communication Centers (CCCs) that will disseminate information to local communities regarding terrorist risk, threat, or attack on specific geographical communities throughout the country. The generation of CCCs will be based on traditional approaches to crisis management and the formation of crisis-management teams. More specifically, we will outline the elements of crisis management and communication most useful in creating CCCs. The centers are proposed here with the belief that while nationwide terror alerts and warnings are useful, greater benefit can be derived from information generated and disseminated at the local level. The CCCs will research local terrorist targets as well as the best means of information dissemination for their particular community. These activities would be conducted with the belief that anticipation of terrorist attacks and preparations for their occurrence at the local level can supplement national efforts to keep our country safe. Following a brief review of the risks of terrorism, this chapter will establish the fundamental key to CCCs: anticipation of terrorist crises and the role of the media and public communication in managing such crises.

## THE TARGETS

Several types of potential targets of terrorism exist in the United States. Perhaps at highest risk for attack are the nation's 361 commercial ports[1] through which $750 billion in goods flow each year.[2] Bender reports that the United States is more likely to be attacked with a weapon of mass destruction smuggled into a port than with a missile.[2] Other devices easily smuggled include radioactive or biologically malignant material.[1] With security heavily focused on air travel, the lack of funding to bolster seaport security makes our ports especially vulnerable.[3] Besides the danger of smuggled weapons, an attack that temporarily shuts down port operations could restrict access to such things as spare parts for major industries and heating oil needed in winter.[2]

Locations known for marquee events or tourist attractions are also at risk. For example, New Orleans, with its Mardi Gras festival and other frequent celebrations could be a tempting terrorist target.[4] Tourist spots, such as Disneyland and Las Vegas, have been targeted by "sleeper cells" whose members collected intelligence on these areas[5] as targets of future terrorist attacks. Famous landmarks, such as the Golden Gate Bridge, and other high-traffic areas, might also be significant targets.[6]

It is noteworthy that while some targets may seem obvious to the public, any location containing government facilities, energy and transportation infrastructures, and agricultural interests are potential targets.[7] Widely dispersed chemically based threats, such as bioterrorism and environmental terrorism, mean that highly populated states, such as California, New York, and Texas, are not the only terrorist targets. Seemingly unlikely states, such as Wisconsin[8] and Rhode Island,[9] are especially vulnerable because of nuclear power plants and factories within their state borders.[10] In actuality, no community should consider itself immune or too underpopulated to be at risk of a terrorist attack, particularly considering the ease with which perpetrators can target the general public by using a gas attack, poisoning a food supply, disrupting an energy grid, killing large numbers of livestock, or contaminating a natural resource.[7,11]

## ANTICIPATORY MODEL OF CRISIS MANAGEMENT AND TECHNOLOGY

The times in which we live require that we need to be prepared for disaster, terrorism, and other crises. It is no longer a question whether terrorism will happen, but when. Therefore, it is the responsibility of key decision-makers and leaders to be prepared for the inevitable because the cost of unpreparedness is significantly greater. To this end we offer the anticipatory model of crisis management[12,13] as a pragmatic tool for those charged with the task of terrorism and disaster prevention and management. The model includes several distinct components, which are outlined below.

### The Anticipation Factor

The anticipation model focuses on prevention as a primary concern in managing crises and disasters. The anticipatory model is anchored in an "enactment perspective,"[14] which suggests that a prevention focus can not only thwart acts of terror, but can reduce their magnitude when they do happen. In essence, the anticipatory model focuses on predicting unpredictable crises and implementing programs that safeguard against their occurrence.

The model suggests the need for crisis team members and practitioners to pay attention to technologies.[12] However, when applying the model to terrorism, it is necessary to understand the concept of first- and second-order effect of technology. The first-order effect of technology describes technology being used as designed (e.g., an airplane as a means of transportation). The second-order effect of technology describes adapted and often negative uses of technology (e.g., e-mail being used to send viruses over computer networks). For the most part, an act of terrorism mirrors the latter. A case in point is 9/11, when terrorists used airplanes as high-explosive bombs. In essence, the very technology designed to foster better living standards can be used to disrupt lives. Consequently, it is argued that more attention should be devoted to understanding technologies and the potential negative consequences they hold in an attempt to prevent escalation. Furthermore, it has been argued that technologies, by nature, are fallible because they are designed by humans and are subject to both human error and deliberate attempts to cause disaster. Evidence suggests that a majority of industrial disasters are linked to a combination of both human and technological errors.[12,14-17]

### Understanding

The term "understanding" is used in this context to suggest having a thorough knowledge of conditions, situations, or events that could signal potential for danger. It is believed that understanding cannot be complete without two relatively similar concepts: enactment and expectations. Enactment is defined as a process in which a specific form of action is brought about.[18] Weick extends enactment to include consequences imposed by a given action.[14] Olaniran and Williams, moreover, contend that "anticipation" of crisis in itself is action because it constrains the choice an organization makes, based on given information.[12] They argue that decision-makers must look ahead to anticipate opportunities, threats, and weaknesses in their environment and then take appropriate actions. Furthermore, both action and inaction result in different outcomes during a crisis.

Expectation represents assumptions people make about certain events or objects. Assumptions about a given situation, environment, or technology, or their combination, can influence whether or not tragedies occur and moderate their magnitude. In essence, assumptions by decision-makers about technologies represent a critical element and a starting point for preventing terrorism and crisis in general. Olaniran and Williams note that assumptions sometimes bring about self-fulfilling prophecies.[12] For example, they argue that when organizations assume that a technology is fail-safe, they often relax safety measures. As a result, the crisis potential increases as decision-makers engage in actions that are consistent with false assumptions.[14,19]

While the anticipatory model emphasizes pre-crisis management activities, other components within the model address the importance of active engagement during crisis. This includes the concept of "control." A multifaceted term, it is used in this context to describe how well institutions and decision-makers are in command of crisis situations. Control, however, is measured in relative terms, which include the perceptions of stakeholders and relevant environments (e.g., the public). The notion of control in communication fosters the ability to prepare and implement effective crisis-management programs, including information dissemination, media relations, flexibility to make changes when necessary (i.e., rigidity), and so on.

## Anticipation as a Vigilant Response to Crisis

Enactment and expectation in an anticipatory model are crucial in any crisis prevention, but do not automatically represent a vigilant response. Expectation and enactment processes are interdependent. Expectations promulgate actions that specify where one places decision emphasis (e.g., preventive or post-crisis mode).

The vigilant decision-making process also requires that decision-makers move through the process in an efficient manner by carefully analyzing the situation, setting goals, and evaluating the outcomes.[20,21] Thus, decision-making centers on both internal and external communication behaviors, which are not mutually exclusive. The internal communication process helps direct organizational activities, focusing on maintenance of stability and structure. External communication focuses on bringing about change that establishes a decision path for an organization.[22]

It is imperative that vigilant crisis-management teams proactively anticipate external communication factors, which are often out of the direct control of decision-makers. At the same time, decision-makers must select appropriate internal communication and adapt it to their crisis program as they choose appropriate strategies. Since anticipating crisis focuses on prevention, it helps to reduce uncertainties when crises occur. Anticipating crises, then, constitutes a vigilant response only when the process has managed to scrutinize all the unthinkable potential for technology misuse, failures, and/or distresses. Shrivastava and others refer to this process as identifying the "triggering event"— specific factors identifiable according to place, time, and agents.[17] In preventing terrorism or a major crisis, it is essential to understand that triggering events, though they have low probability of occurrence, still pose threats of great magnitude.

The focus on anticipation shares a concern for detailed insight, which is amplified by current research in risk communication. Renz briefly describes risk communication as communication regarding uncertain physical hazard—as in the case of terrorism.[23] She further argues that risk communication should consider of primary importance of both the various groups who would be involved and the messages created for them. However, one goal of risk communication is proactivity, such that no environmental impact from terrorism catches the public unaware.

The anticipatory model shares this concern for the discovery of details. However, the proposed model shifts the focus from the consequences of technological failure to expectation and prevention of a crisis.

### Rigidity

Rigidity consists of the degree of inflexibility that is built into a particular action or process. Thus, the degree of rigidity that is exercised by a decision-maker could determine how vigilant a crisis response is. This view is consistent with that of the "vigilant interaction theory," which argues that individuals' view of a problem, available options, and consequences will determine the quality of the choices made.[20] Rigidity may exist in the form of a tenacious explanation for an action that becomes irrevocable or public, making the action more difficult to change. Rigidity, in this case, may be advantageous in crisis situations in which decision-makers are called upon to clarify ambiguity and confusion, as well as to maintain and communicate accurate views.[12]

The challenge with rigidity is that it creates a blinder or incapacity that prevents consideration of other alternatives. In some cases, a decision or explanation that is too rigid may seriously intensify a crisis. For instance, it is common for institutional and organizational decision-makers to mistake certain regulatory standards for adequate safeguards against crisis and ensuing liabilities.[12] For example, if the regulation standard suggests that an acceptable level of lead in water is 5% and a report or assessment by a water supply company indicates 4.7%, the organization is more likely to assume it is covered under regulation standards. Thus failure to look at a way to further reduce the lead content or entertain the view that the 4.7% is an indication that something that has not been previously considered may be happening. As long as these regulatory standards are maintained, decision-makers may mistakenly believe they are not liable for accidents or mistakes. However, responsibility in crises should not just be based on adherence to regulatory standards, but also on whether decision-makers were too rigid to consider alternative factors that may have contributed to the crisis.

### Control

Control represents another factor that may influence the vigilant response to a crisis in both a positive and negative manner. Control is viewed as the degree of influence that key decision-makers have at their disposal. The control is often elusive because it has to do with individual perception, especially when the influence is indirect in nature, as is often the case.

Control influences crisis in the sense that it affects how individuals respond to crisis situations given the action taken. For instance, if individuals see themselves as having the ability and authority to do something about a crisis, it is more likely that they will take action. Thus, ability and authority creates empowerment, which could extend to a vigilant response in crisis management. The foundation for this reasoning can be traced to Weick, who argues that when people think they can do more, they pay more attention to their surroundings and issues, which leads to greater ability to control and cope with their environment.[14] When decision-makers are empowered or have greater control, they are able to respond quickly to crisis-triggering events as they unfold. In contrast, individuals with specialized expertise will have a narrow focus that could prevent them from seeing the incident as a crisis-triggering event, so that they miss a chance to prevent a crisis.[12,19]

The anticipation model recognizes the effect of both rigidity and control on the interaction patterns. It stresses that excessive rigidity and inappropriately distributed control can result in one of the following faulty decision-making schemes: (1) failure to recognize positive qualities of alternate decision options, (2) overlooking critical negative aspects of a decision choice, (3) exaggeration of positive aspects of a decision option, and (4) overestimating negative consequences of a decision option. Therefore, crisis decision processes resulting in one or more of these problems will hinder the decision outcome, whereas avoiding these problems fosters vigilant decision-making.[20]

## THE ROLE OF THE MEDIA IN CRISIS

It has been emphasized earlier that key decision-makers during crisis need to keep in mind their audiences and the messages created for them. It should be noted that the delivery and dissemination of those messages can have just as much impact on the ability to prevent or contain a crisis as the messages themselves. The media—the disseminators of important crisis-related information—play a significant role in the success or failure of crisis management. Therefore, a brief review of the role of media in crisis follows.

Attention toward the role of the media in crisis situations has its start during the second decade of the twentieth century when, according to Albrecht, the U.S. government became concerned with protecting the rights of consumers against faulty prescription drugs and from merchants who used fraudulent weights and measures.[12] Likewise, increased concern for the safety of buildings resulted in the establishment of construction standards.

Due to the increasing use of the media to influence public opinion, organizations and managers quickly learned the importance of cooperating with reporters. By the time the Great Depression first emerged, public opinion was becoming a strong force in the United States. Additionally, the press began to create and present events to the public. Eventually, "corporations and governments became very adept at creating a constant flow of incidents that were ideal for selling media."[12] This trend shows the apparent relationship forming between corporate and government entities that enabled them to influence public opinion.

During the latter part of the twentieth century, television technology became more advanced, while radio and print media became fiercer in their reporting, particularly of terrorism and violent crime, in an effort to gain more listeners and readers.[24] As a result of this increased coverage of political violence, media critics argue that the mass media, however unwitting, serve to facilitate the terrorist agenda. While much attention was focused on the role of the media portraying disasters and violent acts to the public, it was not until the 1980s that research began to examine other roles the media played during emergency and disaster situations,[25] such as providing information to help the public cope with disasters.

Media performance during disasters began to receive more attention after the 1980s, especially with increased interest in media operations and performance. The publication of the National Academy of Sciences report *Disasters and the Mass Media* brought to light the many relevant roles the media can play when disaster strikes, particularly educating the public, providing warnings and directions for taking action, as well as disseminating information on the appropriate agencies to contact for assistance.[25]

A major research topic of the last fifteen years has been the way the media disseminate hazard- and disaster-related information.[25] The public often looks to the media as an important source of information regarding the effect of long-term hazards, important disaster threats, and recommended actions in response to certain threats.[26] Tierney and others report that a significant number of studies have examined citizens' willingness to comply with media-broadcast warnings, and claim that television and radio are usually deemed very credible sources of disaster information.[25]

The events immediately following the September 11, 2001, terrorist attacks seemed to bring the public and the news media closer together as news reporting brought comfort to individuals, information that helped them take appropriate courses of action, as well as public spaces in which to engage in discourse about what was happening.[24] According to Nacos, the constant flow of information provided by print, radio, and television made the public feel more involved with the unfolding events.[24] Also, the news media were seen as a valuable resource in assisting crisis managers with communicating important information (e.g., what to do, what not to do). Finally, the dissemination of news provided individuals with public spaces where they could converse with experts and with each other about the terrorist acts, their aftermath, and their implications.[24] Another study suggests that the media play five functional roles as perceived by the public. These five roles—providing information, building solidarity, providing comfort, explaining the significance of an event, and reducing tension—were considered by the respondents to be very important in the event of a crisis, particularly a terrorist attack.[27]

News reports of terrorist attacks and threats can greatly define the events that people actually experience.[28,29] "For many people and in most situations, the mass media are the most salient source of information on hazards and disasters. In large measure, people learn what they know about disasters from the mass media."[25] In fact, public-opinion research reveals that the people who are the least knowledgeable are the most susceptible to media influence.[30] The media are also important sources for crisis managers and policymakers, many of whom have televisions in their offices in order to catch breaking news.[30] Because of the wide reach and immediacy of television, we now expect our policymakers and crisis managers to be on top of emerging events.

The public's understanding of and reaction to a crisis event, particularly one involving terrorist motives, may have a profound effect on an entire community's ability to contain the crisis, cope with its aftermath, and prevent future threats.[26,31] Organizations and agencies who have the responsibility to protect and serve the community need to understand the media's impact on the public's perception of a crisis in order to circumvent any adverse outcomes from news coverage, as well as know how to disseminate mass-media messages that can assist the community during crisis.[30]

Research examining the relationship between the media and the public they serve suggests that the public consists of multiple audiences, and that any message communicated during a crisis must have a clear goal that is understandable to each audience.[32] Otherwise, different audiences may perceive different messages and interpretations from the same action,[30,31] a reality key leaders should expect and anticipate. For example, Seeger, Vennette, Ulmer, and Sellnow have found that gender may be related to the desire for certain types of crisis information.[33] They report that women appeared more interested in reassurances from religious and spiritual leaders, as well as information about closures and cancellations of events. In general, television and other pervasive media outlets tear down the cultural and socioeconomic barriers that otherwise divide people. While television may be an efficient way to send one message to a lot of people, parallel messages and decisions must be developed to address groups with conflicting needs,[30] such as the need to be reassured and comforted versus the need for detailed information about how to act.

Research suggests that in addition to acknowledging multiple audiences, agencies directly responsible for handling the crisis must establish and maintain a good working relationship with the media in order for their messages to be heard and understood by the general community.[32,30] Governments and other agencies are often linked to their community not directly, but through the available media outlets. Thus, the media can serve as a conduit between leaders and the public in the delivery of vital information related to the crisis.[32]

However, agencies should not make the mistake of relying solely on the media to communicate with the public. Albrecht suggests that "waiting for them to make your decisions for you is like waiting for the judge to dismiss a lawsuit against you without showing up to provide reasons or a reasonable defense."[32]

Given that the media serve as a viable outlet through which the community may receive valuable information, a good relationship with the media is extremely important. First, strong ties with the media imply that decision-makers understand the positive contributions news media can make in a crisis situation. According to Tierney and others, the media have been credited with saving many lives and reducing casualties through their effective warnings during natural disasters and their timely and accurate information on various other threats.[25] The media have also made a positive contribution to containing terrorism, as can be seen in the many books on terrorism that are by-products of the news media.[34]

A good relationship also implies maintaining a balance between "protecting the autonomy of the press and managing the flow of information so that the crisis can be resolved in accordance to government policy."[30] Although the press may feel they have a right to be on the scene because of their live broadcast capabilities, spokespersons and crisis leaders must minimize the potential of disclosing damaging information or sending the wrong message to the wrong audience. The potential damage is greatest with television coverage, as politicians have developed a much closer relationship with reporters from television than other media.[30]

Another requirement for a good relationship with the media is that decision-makers know how to utilize the many forms of media communication in order to get the most helpful and appropriate message to the public. In particular, the media are not only a tool, but also a viable partner, along with important officials, in dealing with terrorist threats and containing their negative effects. A major responsibility in communicating via television, radio, and so on, is to ensure that the public fully understands the feasibility and limitations of the choices that can be made in response to a crisis. Terrorists, in their destructive acts, attempt to portray these limitations as signs that government is incompetent or uncaring. However, if the community understands the limits within which crisis managers must operate, then public trust may be maintained.[30]

With regard to the message itself, Albrecht advises that the three or four core messages surrounding the crisis should serve as a guide for how to respond to the event or to any public scrutiny.[32] It is these core messages that will help crisis managers stay on track. Additionally, core messages should be timed to avoid trying the patience of the public or the media. According to Crelinsten, if too much time elapses between the first signs of crisis and public communication about it, reporters, in an effort to find newsworthy information, may seek out dramatic statements or predictions from certain officials.[30] As a result, news coverage of events may be distorted and rumors may be spread by overanxious reporters attempting to produce an eye-catching story. To prevent misinformation and message distortion, Albrecht suggests that imparting information at timed intervals may draw attention away from delicate issues and provide reporters with meaningful material.[32] Information dissemination can take the form of press releases and news conferences that keep reporters supplied with "newsworthy" information.[30]

Along with timing, careful planning of the nature and content of the message may not only minimize message distortion, but also help avoid the exacerbation of the crisis itself.[30] During fast-moving crises, especially during which live television coverage is involved, information received by the camera or microphone can instantaneously feed back to the people directly affected or victimized by the crisis, which can inflame the crisis even more. Live coverage may also feed information to the terrorists themselves, who are watching from far away. Moreover, a crisis experienced locally may have an impact far beyond its actual site when covered by live, nationally syndicated media. Crelinsten suggests that crisis managers and decision-makers anticipate the results of unexpected or unintended information feedback loops and cultivate an awareness of where messages might go, versus where they are intended to go.[30] In light of this potential impact of a local crisis on the national or international community, managers need to adapt their behavior and decision-making to the particular demands of the electronic media.

Research on the effect of media on crisis management has focused heavily on television, perhaps because of the close relationship between policymakers and television newscasters.[30] Jackson argues that television is subject to two impulses—to inform and to entertain. "All too often the two drives are mutually exclusive, the result being either banality or razzmatazz, either stodginess or sensationalism. But now and then they are not incompatible alternatives."[34] Because television can be more presentational than explanatory or discursive,[30] crisis managers and governmental officials can use television to present images of caring, assurance, and calm. More explanatory, complex messages should be left to the print media. Overall, lengthy absences from television by top officials may spark mistrust from the public, provide an empty space to be filled by other (often less reliable) sources, and even trigger a sense of urgency not felt before.

As stated earlier, the media have a large impact on public understanding of a crisis event, as well as public perceptions of policymakers' ability to contain the event. Community members, politicians, and crisis managers look to the media for information and answers to the troubling questions surrounding any crisis event. "Thanks to the way electronic and video technology has continued to improve by leaps and bounds, people intuitively assume that the *way* [a] message comes across is almost as important as the message itself."[32]

## CREATION AND FUNCTION OF CCCs

With a foundation in the anticipatory perspective on crisis management and communication, as well as an understanding of the media's role in crisis management, municipalities can develop CCCs to determine community-specific risks and the best means of response in their community. These assessments would involve audits similar to crisis audits[35] and research into local media outlets.

Standard crisis management in the pre-crisis or preparation stage involves crisis preparation, signal detection, and prevention.[35] CCC members would form a crisis management team[36] and work under the standard belief offered by Pauchant and Mitroff that not all crises can be prevented, but many can be.[37] The CCC members would engage in both annual assessments and immediate responses in their crisis-response efforts.

## Crisis Preparation

Crisis preparation for newly created CCCs is similar to standard procedures for crisis-management teams.[35,38,39] The specific needs of CCCs require early attention to the selection of the CCC team members, completion of a community assessment, identification of spokespersons, and attention to the team communication plan.

The CCC team will be a collection of community and municipal members who have knowledge and expertise, represent the community, and also fulfill specific needs of the team. Ideally CCCs will include individuals with a working knowledge of those elements in the community—industrial, technical, and agricultural—that might become terrorist targets. The CCC team will also need individuals with communication and media expertise, representatives of local government, and at least one individual who can successfully manage the operations of the team. The size of the CCC team will likely fluctuate depending on the size of the community and the number of potential terrorist targets in that general location. According to Coombs and Chandler, crisis team members should possess the ability to make group decisions, function as a team member, enact a crisis plan, and listen.[40] These are also desirable qualities of CCC team members.

Completing a community assessment is the first critical project for the newly completed CCC team. Team members should first attend to the generally recognized terrorist threat targets identified earlier in this chapter. However, members' localized knowledge and expertise will help them consider specific community "sites of interest." These sites could be any local facility, course of production, military or weapons storage place, holding place or any other location that could be used by terrorists or serve as a target. Team members must move beyond the more obvious terrorist targets of national landmarks and nuclear power plants and identify potential sites of interests that may be targeted or used to contribute to an attack elsewhere. For example, the purchase of explosive material or rental of a moving van in one community could be used as a weapon in another location.

A community assessment instrument could eventually be developed with input from the Department of Homeland Security. Such an instrument would guide CCCs through an inventory of widely recognized terrorist targets and then help team members investigate their own communities for local sites of interest. This community assessment phase is critical, fundamental work from which all future efforts will stem. Therefore, adequate time, resources, and human power are essential.

The selection of terror spokespersons will take much less time, but will be a key preparatory task for the CCC team. Appointing a spokesperson who can reach the media quickly with a unified message is critical to crisis response.[41,42] In the event of a terrorist threat, the work of this individual (or individuals) will be crucial. In an organization, the CEO is an obvious choice to serve in this position. Coombs wisely suggests that multiple spokespersons be identified in case one is not available, or if the crisis is prolonged and requires extended availability of an official spokesperson.[35]

For CCC teams, members of the local government would be obvious choices for these positions. An ideal guideline was established by Mayor Rudy Giuliani of New York City after the World Trade Center attack on September 11, 2001. Ideally, the local mayor would be able to serve in this capacity for most communities. Other individuals would be recognizable members of city council, members of industry, or a key leader in the health or public safety sector. In some communities, a clergy member may be a good spokesperson.

Criteria for CCC spokespersons, as with most crisis-management spokespersons, include an ability to work with media. Aside from public speaking skills, these individuals will need to respond to questions with accuracy, tact, and composure. The latter might prove difficult, as spokespersons could be called upon in times of great stress. Therefore, Coombs' suggestion that spokespersons receive media training is wise.[35]

The ability to present a credible, competent appearance is of particular importance for CCC spokespersons. If a CCC spokesperson is called upon, he or she will be addressing a specific geographic community in which all members might be affected. Given the localized nature of their message, there will be fewer listeners who are disinterested or merely interested bystanders. The spokesperson's message will address local events with local impact and consequences. The attention and scrutiny of those receiving the message will be at optimum levels. Therefore, it is important that the spokesperson be credible to the local public and trusted by local media.

The final element of preparation in crisis management typically involves the creation of a crisis-management plan. While we will not detail the elements of standard crisis-management plans here, we do note that the most important steps, with regard to terrorist-related crises, are risk assessment and risk management, each of which are explored below.

## Signal Detection

Signal detection refers to the active process of information gathering. CCC team members will conduct investigations of their community at large and specific areas of concern to determine where risks exist. This segment of crisis preparation will depend on the development of relationships between the CCC membership and areas of risk. For example, in agricultural areas, the CCC will have contact with agriculturalists who might be producing food crops and contractors who supply aerial spraying services. These audits will monitor key individuals in the sites of interest, and changes or possible changes in operation procedures. Whereas standard crisis-preparation practice would suggest that organizations maintain relationships with members of the media, the CCC will establish and maintain similar working relationships with citizens at threatened sites. The goal of these relationships is to monitor local sites at risk for terrorist attack.

CCCs will also monitor broad social, political, or environmental changes that might affect local areas. The CCC can then determine if any changes within or outside the community warrant a concern for their sites of interest. For example, if national alert levels increased based on intelligence that discovered attempts to tamper with water-supply systems, the CCC would alert local water departments to the concern and solidify preparation efforts for public communication in the event of an attack.

The CCC team carries a heavy responsibility in the signal-detection phase by gathering information and maintaining relationships with sites of interest in their community. While the act of gathering information and maintaining networks will be demanding, it is essential to ensure accurate and prompt decision-making. The signal-detection phase also requires decision-making as information is evaluated. Decision-making during a crisis can be difficult and may lead to faulty responses.[21] If, however, CCC teams work efficiently in the signal-detection phase before a crisis hits, they will be able to evaluate thoroughly and critically the level of risk for their community.

Heath suggests two criteria for evaluating such information: likelihood and impact.[43] For CCC team members, the former refers to the potential of any information or signal resulting in an actual crisis event. For example, increased concern over bombings of major transportation bridges and tunnels would rate a low likelihood in sparsely populated areas of the West, while concern about attempts to develop terrorist cells in rural areas would rate high. Impact refers to the extent of damage that could result from a signal turning into an action. Damage can be judged on a number of scales, including loss of life, injuries, economic loss, loss of property, potential to foster community fear and chaos, and estimated time and costs of recovery. CCC teams will need to recruit members with the capacity to make such estimates. Teams will also be able to develop impact scenarios with their contacts in the sites of interest. For example, CCC teams in coastal areas can work with shipping industry representatives and port managers to speculate on the dangers of biological weapons arriving by ship and detonating in ports. CCC teams would focus more attention on terrorist signals that are assigned a higher likelihood. Also, based upon community assessments, CCC teams will be able to prepare impact scenarios prior to any signal detection.

## Prevention

Typical crisis-prevention measures for an organization include issues management, risk management, and relationship building. Issues management,[43,44] which seeks to resolve potential crises in a manner that limits harm to the organization, is of little relevance to terrorist crises. Issues management attempts to limit an issue from reaching its full crisis potential. Terrorist crises are simply not approachable from an issues perspective. If a community faces a terrorist act, the crisis has moved beyond the opportunity, if one ever existed, to address the issue behind the act. In essence, the crisis has already moved from issue to action, and the nature of terrorism suggests that the crisis cannot be reverted back to the issue.

Risk management is more applicable to terrorist threats. Risk-management efforts attempt to limit the risk to the organization,[45] or in this case, the community. CCC teams will devote significant time and planning toward risk avoidance, which is the attempt to lower the likelihood and impact of the terrorist threat. For example, concerns after 9/11 about possible terrorist actions at the annual Oscar awards resulted in significant alterations of the event. This was a risk-aversion measure designed to eliminate the likelihood of attack during the nationally tele-vised program. Arenas pose potential terrorists threats throughout the country. At times of elevated risk, CCCs can work with arena managers and events coordinators to alter the programming or admission proce-dures, as needed, to maintain safety.

The cornerstone of risk management is the relationship between the organization and its stakeholders. For CCCs, the stakeholders include contact people at sites of interest and the general public in the commu-nity. In times of increased terrorist threat, CCCs will have greater success in disseminating information if they have a favorable relationship history with their stakeholders. Coombs and Holladay describe relational history as "the nature of the interaction between the organization and its stake-holders. A favorable relationship history is reflected in good works by the organization, while an unfavorable one is characterized by conflict and failures by the organization to fulfill obligations to stakeholders" (p. 111).[46] Grunig and Repper add that relationship development also benefits signal-detection efforts.[47] For the purposes of CCCs, a strong relational history, especially with the media and public, will prove beneficial when crisis information must be released. Positive relationships with people at sites of interest, the media, and the public will hopefully translate into timely, accurate, and well-received information.

## Information Dissemination and the Media

Much of the standard advice with regard to the media and crisis communication involves establishing and maintaining a good relation-ship with the media; getting the message out quickly to the public through the media; and selecting a credible, media-aware spokes-person.[48,49] While this advice holds value for CCC teams, there are some unique needs with regard to dissemination of terrorist threat information.

An initial question regards who should deliver the message, aside from the CCC spokespersons. CCC teams will need to study the local media to determine which source is the most preferred for critical information. Standard rating systems (e.g. arbitron) will be of some benefit, but additional research will be needed. We recommend that CCC teams do local surveys, or even focus groups, to determine whether there is a preferred source (individual or medium) for terror-alert information. This research might determine that a particular tele-vision or radio announcer would be viewed as more credible or knowledgeable. In the event that CCC teams need to respond quickly, these sources would be of primary importance. Even for noncritical alerts or updates, having preselected sources could be beneficial.

Research can also assess which forms of communication are used by different segments of the community for noncritical terror information. Television, while perhaps the most pervasive form of communication in a crisis, may not be readily accessible or meaningful to all segments of the local population. Moreover, television coverage alone may not encourage citizens to act, or engage in public discourse about a crisis. This function might fall to other forums, such as municipal meetings, local newspapers, senior-citizen publications, pamphlets or flyers distributed at various locations, local cable or radio programming, and so on. These outlets can be useful for conveying terrorist-related information that is less urgent or targeted toward a specific audience. For example, if there is increased concern over terrorists' attempts to purchase or steal handguns and rifles, which media sources or forms would gun owners and sellers be likely to follow? If the concern involves attempts to strike large gatherings, which sources would reach concert attendees or local basketball fans? CCC teams can benefit by predetermining the best media or other form of communication for contacting various elements of the community.

Finally, CCCs can attempt to assess which types of messages would be preferred by the general public. Team members can initially attempt to determine the ideal frequency for updates. For example, the general public may wish only to hear information when the likelihood and impact levels reach a certain point. Local manufacturers or large employers, on the other hand, may desire information with much lower levels of risk.

For terrorist alerts, CCCs can also seek information on which type of risk information the public prefers. Initial questions to ask include the following items:

1. Would the public prefer to hear percentage estimates of the likelihood of terrorist threat in their community?
2. What level of detail should be revealed about terrorist attacks in other communities, or potential attacks in their own community?
3. Should casualty and fatality estimates and possibilities be revealed?
4. Should oral descriptions or visual depictions of terrorist threats or actions be used?
5. Does the public want to know details about the source of the terrorist threat or action?
6. For nonimmediate information, is there a preferred time to receive the information, possibly to avoid children's viewing or listening?
7. Should information be conveyed with a certain level of emotional detachment?

8. When and to what extent should information be conveyed according to audience demographic factors, such as gender, age, or religion, or ethnic identity?
9. What is the public's perception of the anticipated or actual terrorist threat or attack?

Message strategy can also be evaluated by CCCs. Typical crisis-response strategies range from denial to attacking the accuser.[50] These strategies are often used when an organization is struck with a crisis, but many of these strategies could also be used in response to terrorism. For example, the strategies of bolstering, minimization, and corrective action could be used.

Bolstering attempts to reduce the negative by stressing the positive. For example, CCCs could announce that there is an elevated risk of terrorists contaminating water supplies. But, the CCC would then employ a bolstering strategy by explaining how measures have been taken to secure the treatment facilities. Minimization is a strategy that suggests a crisis or threat is not serious. For example, the same CCC team could announce that the threat of water contamination is not a credible threat and that their community is too small to be a likely target for such an attack.

Coombs' research has suggested that when terrorist crises occur, the strategies of ingratiation, mortification, and suffering should be employed. We note that Coombs' definition of terrorism is not focused on matters of homeland security, but involves "intentional actions taken by external actors" (p. 457).[51] He lists product tampering, hostage taking, sabotage, and workplace violence as examples of terrorism. While not specific to homeland security, Coombs' suggestions are still useful to CCCs.

Ingratiation strategies are those that attempt to gain public support and approval. Mortification strategies go a bit further by attempting to "win forgiveness of the publics and to create acceptance of the crisis."[51] Finally, the suffering strategy will play on the sympathy of the public and create a good versus evil (terrorists) dichotomy. These are methods that could be used by CCCs to convey a strong sense of regret for allowing the crisis to happen, while also helping the public keep faith in the entities designed to protect them. For example, a terrorist strike at a large NASCAR function could create havoc and result in significant injuries and deaths. Identification and tributes to the injured and lost combined with blame clearly focused on the responsible terrorist organization would utilize the suffering strategy.

A more assertive strategy would involve corrective action. Corrective action is a crisis response that explains that steps will be taken to fix or prevent future crises. In the event that some attempt at water contamination was made, the CCC could explain in detail how the treatment plant and local government is implementing changes to prevent future contamination attempts. Corrective action strategies were witnessed after 9/11 when airport security measures were improved and additional personnel hired to improve screening procedures.

The strongest strategic response would be to attack the terrorist, a modification of the attack-the-accuser crisis–response strategy.[50] In this case, all blame is focused on the attacker (terrorists), who is portrayed in the darkest light possible. This strategy does not recognize any possible limitations on the part of the community or its government to prepare for terrorists actions. Instead, the focus is entirely on the terrorists and their actions. Immediately following 9/11, some communities feared the possibility of a terrorist renting or stealing a crop duster airplane and spraying toxic chemicals over crops or people. Had a terrorist been caught in such an attempt, the attack strategy would have focused on that person's actions, the unjust nature of the attempt, and the victory of the capture. The response would not have challenged how the terrorist almost succeeded and which flaws would have made that possible for the terrorist to get access to the place and chemicals.

CCC team members have the full range of response strategies from which to choose. Frequently, responses will be comprised of a combination of strategies deemed appropriate given the threat and the audience. For example, a terrorist attack on a dairy farm that attempted to destroy or poison a milk-production facility could be responded to with the attack strategy. All blame would be placed on the terrorists without challenge to the daily producer or FDA.

## CONCLUSION

This chapter advocates the creation of CCCs that are intended to disseminate information to local communities regarding actual or possible terrorist attacks. CCCs would be designed to assess the local community to determine the most likely terrorist threats and the best method of communication for handling such threats.

The creation of CCCs has at its theoretical base the anticipatory model of crisis communication, as well as other existing response strategies (see figure 12.1). This model and its components—anticipation, understanding, and expectation—serve as a guide for the CCC team as

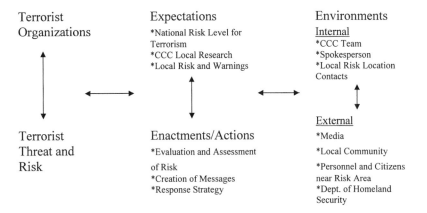

**Figure 12.1**
The uniqueness of this anticipatory model is the interdependency embedded in it. For instance, the anticipation of terror is influenced by both the internal and external environments, which necessitates an understanding of the environment. This leads to the expectations formulated about potential terrorists and terrorist threats/risks. Consequently, a response to the terrorist act or threat is formulated through enactment; finally, whatever actions are taken will influence both the internal and external environments.

it anticipates internal and external communication factors surrounding a crisis in order to select the most appropriate strategies for handling a real or possible terrorist threat. Moreover, the CCC team will conduct research into the local community to determine how key crisis managers and spokespersons can keep in mind the various groups they serve and the messages they create for them.

While a general understanding of terrorist activities and threats to national security are important in keeping our country safe, it is the purpose of this chapter to place emphasis on what local communities can do to handle significant terrorist events. Arguably, it is at the local level that the impact of terrorist activities is most felt, and it is at this level that threats can be most efficiently addressed and prevented. Additionally, the success experienced by one CCC in containing or preventing a terrorist attack may serve as a model for other communities. The application of an anticipatory framework places more power not only in the hands of city authorities and law enforcement, but also with communication practitioners (e.g., public-relations experts). This model implies that practitioners must use a variety of communicative channels to stay connected with the public and to provide them with an accurate picture of the seriousness and pervasiveness of a terrorist attack. For example, in the case of food or water contamination, communication experts need to know how best to use media channels in order to inform the community about affected sources and vulnerable populations.

In addition to coping with a terrorist attack that has already occurred, a CCC team may help a community prevent an attack by learning from past terrorist incidents. For example, a CCC team may learn what actions New York City took before, during, and after 9/11. Decision-makers with knowledge of the worst terrorist attack on U.S. soil may be better able to assess whether such an attack could happen in their own community. Even when a terrorist attack cannot be prevented, an anticipatory framework may provide decision-makers with a more vigilant response that contributes to more effective outcomes.

## NOTES

1. Seikman P. Protecting America's ports. Fortune 2003;148(10):T198C.

2. Bender B. Terror risk seen highest at US ports: tankers in Boston may be vulnerable. The Boston Globe 2003 Jun 21;Sect. A:1,1.

3. Filner B. Making San Diego's port secure. The San Diego Union-Tribune 2003 Aug 22;Sect. B9:2, 6, 7;Sect B7:1,1.

4. Perlstein M. A "top 10" target, N.O. mounts a defense: local security chief provides an update. Times-Picayune 2003 Sep 11;Sect. A:15,1.

5. Runk D. Two found guilty of scouting terrorism targets: "Sleeper cell" had eye on Disneyland. The Record 2003 Jun 4;Sect. A:12,1.

6. Zamora JH. California lists top terror targets. San Francisco Chronicle 2003 Feb 23;Sect. A:1,1.

7. Azar L. 27 sites could be terrorist targets, subcommittee finds. Wyoming Tribune-Eagle 2002 Aug 8;Sect. A:4.

8. Williams S. State cut of funds bigger than most: $8.7 million received to boost anti-terror arsenal. Milwaukee Journal Sentinel 2003 Feb 8;Sect. B:1,1.

9. Barbarisi D. Terrorism in RI: you never know. Providence Journal-Bulletin 2003 May 23;Sect. D:4,1.

10. Zoretich F. Terror threat great, but U.S. more ready, Freeh says. Albuquerque Tribune 2003 Jul 12;Sect A:5.

11. Chalecki EL. A new vigilance: identifying and reducing the risks of environmental terrorism. Global Environ Pol 2002 Feb:2,1:46–64.

12. Olaniran BA, Williams DE. Anticipatory model of crisis management: a vigilant response to technological crises. In: Heath R, editor. Handbook of public relations. Newbury Park, CA: Sage; 2000. p. 581–94.

13. Olaniran BA, Williams DE. Burkian counternature and the vigilant response: an anticipatory model of crisis management and technology. In: Millar DP, Heath RL, editors. Responding to crisis: a rhetorical approach to crisis communication. Mahwah, NJ: Lawrence Erlbaum; 2004. p. 75–94.

14. Weick KE. Enacted sense-making in crisis situations. J Manage Stud 1988;25:305–17.

15. Shrivastava P. Bhopal: anatomy of crisis. Cambridge, MA: Ballinger; 1987.

16. Shrivastava P, Mitroff II. Strategic management of corporate crisis. Columbia J World Bus 1987;22:5–11.

17. Shrivastava P, Mitroff II, Miller D, Miglani A. Understanding industrial crises. J Manage Stud 1988;25:285–303.

18. Smircich L, Stubbart C. Strategic management in an enacted world. Acad Manag Rev 1985;10:724–36.

19. Perrow C. Normal accidents: living with high risk technologies. New York: Basic Books; 1984.

20. Hirokawa RY, Rost K. Effective group decision-making in organizations. Manag Commun Q 1992;5:267–88.

21. Williams DE, Olaniran BA. Exxon's decision-making flaws: the hyper-vigilant response to the Valdez grounding. Public Relations Rev 1994;20: 5–18.

22. Kreps GL. Organizational communication: theory and practice. 2nd ed. New York: Longman; 1990.

23. Renz MA. Communication about environmental risk: an examination of a Minnesota county's communication on incineration. J Appl Commun Res 1992;20:1–18.

24. Nacos BL. Terrorism as breaking news: attack on America. Pol Sci Q 2003;118(1):23.

25. Tierney KJ, Lindell MK, Perry RW. Facing the unexpected: disaster preparedness and response in the United States. Washington, DC: Joseph Henry Press; 2001.

26. Greenberg BS, Hofschire L, Lachlan K. Diffusion, media use and interpersonal communication behaviors. In: Greenberg BS, editor. Communication and terrorism: public and media responses to 9/11. Cresskill, NJ: Hampton Press; 2002. p. 3–16.

27. Perse E, Signorielli N, Courtright J, Samter W, Caplan S, Lambe J, et al. Public perceptions of media functions at the beginning of the war on terrorism. In: Greenberg BS, editor. Communication and terrorism: public and media responses to 9/11. Cresskill, NJ: Hampton Press; 2002. p. 39–52.

28. Shpiro S. Conflict media strategies and the politics of counter-terrorism. Pol 2002;22(2):76–85.

29. Smith D. Media and apocalypse: new coverage of the Yellowstone Forest fires, Exxon Valdez oil spill, and Loma Prieta earthquake. Westport, CT: Greenwood Press; 1992.

30. Crelinsten RD. The impact of television on terrorism and crisis situations: implications for public policy. J Contingencies Crisis Manag 1994;2(2):61–72.

31. Stempel GH III, Hargrove T. Media sources of information and attitudes about terrorism. In: Greenberg BS, editor. Communication and terrorism: public and media responses to 9/11. Cresskill, NJ: Hampton Press; 2002. p. 17–26.

32. Albrecht S. Crisis management for corporate self-defense. New York: American Management Association; 1996.

33. Seeger MW, Vennette S, Ulmer RR, Sellnow, TL. Media use, information seeking, and reported needs in post crisis contexts. In: Greenberg BS, editor. Communication and terrorism: public and media responses to 9/11. Cresskill, NJ: Hampton Press; 2002. p. 53–63.

34. Jackson G. Terrorism and the news media. Terrorism Pol Violence 1990;2(4):521–8.

35. Coombs WT. Ongoing crisis management: planning, managing, and responding. Thousand Oaks, CA: Sage; 1999.

36. Fink S. Crisis management: planning for the inevitable. New York: AMOCOM; 1986.

37. Pauchant TC, Mitroff II. Transforming the crisis-prone organization: preventing individual, organizational, and environmental tragedies. San Francisco: Josey-Bass; 1992.

38. Barton L. Crisis in organizations II. Cincinnati, OH: South-Western; 2001.

39. Lerbinger O. Managing corporate crises: strategies for executives. Boston: Barrington Press; 1986.

40. Coombs WT, Chandler RC. Crisis teams: revisiting their selection and training. In: Barton L, editor. New avenues in risk and crisis management. Las Vegas: UNLV Small Business Development Center; 1996. p. 7–15. (vol 5).

41. Katz AR. Checklist: 10 steps to complete crisis planning. Public Relations J 1987;43:46–7.

42. Murphy P. How "bad" PR decisions get made: a roster of faulty judgement heuristics. Public Relations Rev 1991;17:117–29.

43. Heath RL. Strategic issues management: organizations and public policy challenges. Thousand Oaks, CA: Sage; 1997.

44. Jones BL, Chase WH. Managing public policy issues. Public Relations Rev 1979;5(2):3–23.

45. Smallwood C. Risk and organizational behavior: toward a theoretical framework. In: Barton L, editor. New avenues in risk and crisis management. Las Vegas: UNLV Small Business Development Center; 1995. p. 139–48. (vol 4).

46. Coombs WT, Holladay SJ. Reasoned action in crisis communication: an attribution theory-based approach to crisis management. In: Millar DP, Heath RL, editors. Responding to crisis: a rhetorical approach to crisis communication. Mahwah, NJ: Lawrence Erlbaum; 2004. p. 95–116.

47. Grunig JE, Repper FC. Strategic Management, publics, and issues. In: Grunig JE, editor. Excellence in public relations and communication management. Hillsdale, NJ: Lawrence Erlbaum; 1992. p. 117–57.

48. Slahor S. Media relations during a crisis. Superv 1989;50:9–11.

49. Trahan JV III. Media relations in the eye of the storm. Public Relations Q 1993;38(2):31–3.

50. Benoit W. Image repair discourse and crisis communication. Public Relations Rev 1997;23(2):177–86.

51. Coombs WT. Choosing the right words: the development of guidelines for the selection of the "appropriate" crisis-response strategies. Manag Commun Q 1995;8(4):447–76.

# 13 Integrated Telecommunication Tools for Bioterrorism Response

*Azhar Rafiq and Ronald C. Merrell*

Bioterrorism imperils public health and threatens scarcity with a looming potential for pathology and epidemic havoc on an unprecedented scale. Bioterror events are man-made disasters that, by design, give no warning of onset and demonstrate no predictable pattern of disposition. Biological warfare has been a significant concern for the United States since World War II, and remains a significant threat, especially given the events of the last four years.[1,2] A defenseless civilian population is subjected to the chronic anxiety of possible infections and peril, with little warning or recourse. Bioterrorism entails the introduction of biological pathogens, microorganisms, or specific biologically active substances (i.e. toxins) to harm societies in such a way as to disrupt, overwhelm, or otherwise intimidate a target population. The targeted population is a functional, social, and economic unit with a defined and predictable infrastructure essential to normalcy. The unseen enemy carrying out a terrorist act attempts to assault a group of people by taking advantage of their vulnerabilities and in so doing destabilizes normalcy by rupturing social services and the community network.

The impact of the biological agent may disable or kill large numbers of people immediately, and the event may be over in a few hours. Alternately, it may leave lingering medical, economic, social, or environmental consequences. A large number of victims in a bioterror event could overwhelm and burden the healthcare system and its resources. Previous bioterror events have typically been on a small scale.[3] The entire terror event may unfold at the site of the first case without spreading, or the first victim may be only the first case in an evolving epidemiological disaster. Bioterrorism attacks can thus be classified as either "immediate" or "extended," relative to the event's onset and duration. The immediate events have a sudden onset and result in consequences within hours on the target population. Consequences can be rapidly fatal, eliminating large numbers of people. The extended attack can unfold over time, like a communicable disease, over weeks and months. In either variant effective public health surveillance systems must detect the pathology as a bioterror event by recognizing patterns of signs and symptoms that refer to a possible bioterror agent. Early detection of a covert attack precedes mobilization of resources to contain the inductive biological agent, treat victims, and protect those exposed to the agent. A series of disease-outbreak detection and surveillance systems have been proposed with inclusion of informatics.[4-6] For early detection of population risk, the Center for Disease Control and Prevention (CDC) has proposed the Early Aberration Reporting System, while Tsui and others have proposed a computer-based public health surveillance system (RODS).[7,8] Because the effect of the biological agent may be dispersed in a community, an effective public health surveillance system must have the capacity to detect subtle patterns of disease and distinguish bioterror events from common and natural disease incidents characteristic of the community. According to the report *Combating chemical, biological, radiological and nuclear terrorism: a comprehensive strategy*, prepared by the Center for Strategic and International Studies, the effects of a bioterrorist act may not manifest until after the inductive agent's incubation period.[9]

In bioterrorism, the agent assaults human physiology through some infectious or biologic process. Consequences for the victim may manifest almost immediately, as in the case of toxins, or the biological agent may incubate for days in an asymptomatic or prodromic phase. During this quiescent period the victim could travel considerable distances encompassing the globe. Thus, the disease may affect individuals first exposed or may be transmitted to others during the asymptomatic, prodromal, or active illness phases. Caregivers may be at the greatest risk once exposed to the affected victims. The inoculums may be evanescent or quite durable on fomites, in water supply, or in the atmosphere. The agent usually requires a vehicle for delivery, which may be a food, aerosol, water contaminant, or a vector host animal delivering the agents surreptitiously at sites and times of vulnerability chosen by the terrorist. Thousands of biological agents are capable of causing human infection and thus can be considered potential biological weapons. NATO's *Handbook on Medical Aspects of NBC Defensive Operations* lists thirty-one infectious agents as potential biological warfare agents.[10] A Russian

Table 13.1
"Category A" Biological Agents Classified by the CDC

| Biological Agent | Common Mechanism of Disease | Incubation Period |
|---|---|---|
| Anthrax | Skin contact | 1–6 days |
| Botulism | Foodborne | 12–36 hours |
| Plague | Inhalation | 2–4 days |
| Smallpox | Inhalation | 1–5 days |
| Tularemia | Contaminated food or water | 3–5 days |
| Viral hemorrhagic fever | Physical contact | Immediate effect |

Source: Horn JK. Bacterial agents used for bioterrorism. Surg Infec 2003;4(3):281–7.

panel of experts considers eleven microbial agents from NATO's list to be most likely to be used and concludes that smallpox, plague, anthrax, and botulism are the top candidates.[11] The CDC has established a list of six "category A" agents that constitute the greatest threat to communities in the United States (table 13.1).[12]

The vehicle, the inductive agent, and the population affected, predicts the expected scenario after dispersion of the biological agent. A sparse population has a different mathematics of epidemiology than a dense population. Finally, the scenario of the inductive agent's consequences can unfold in various phases that have unpredictable consequences and realize extensive barriers to incident management (table 13.2). During the early phases, the agent and its consequences may be obscure and lead to public fear and a lack of coordination of actions on the part of official responders.

It is often difficult to decipher a terror event, especially in its early phases. The possibility of an attack, its unknown site of origin, time of induction, and number of victims are cumulative uncertainties that place a burden of unpleasant information upon the public and support

Table 13.2
Phases of a Bioterrorism Event Induction with Possible Mechanisms of Action

| Phases of Induction | Mechanism |
|---|---|
| Site of onset | Unpredictable—dependent on route of application |
| Rate of infection | Delayed—dependent on organism's incubation period |
| Distribution of attack | Widely spread over community infected |
| Casualty management for agent containment | Quarantine and/or medication |

services. These uncertainties make it difficult to control behavior, and may retard economic activity and consume preventive resources. When an attack is suspected or early in its course, information is sparse, hard to confirm, possibly exaggerated by rumor, or extrapolated to grim possibilities. At this early phase of situational identification, the terror event may greatly exceed the actual physical toll of the agent. The terror may lead to severe economic and resource service disruptions, far out of proportion to the actual event. As the event progresses in formation it can be difficult to distribute the action of the healthcare workers effectively without consuming many of the infrastructure resources.

The disadvantage caused by uncertainty regarding the inoculums and their dispersion is not overcome until accurate information is available to identify the agent, its dynamics, and the best course of action to halt its effects. Inaccurate information can result in problems that aid and magnify the perfidy of the terrorist intent. Information, then, is crucial in engaging the public and health responders to take appropriate actions that will limit the effects of the agent and control its spread. Information solutions are as crucial as antibiotics, vaccines, and barrier protection when it comes to a prompt and successful response to the bioterror event.

Bioterror response management often begins within the routine health system, with the medical personnel who treat common infections and ailments in the regional population. Initial detection of an uncommon infection or toxin reaction may elude the primary care physician. When the first case is recognized, it will likely be sent out to the regional healthcare center, where it is more likely to become an index case—if healthcare workers have been empowered by relevant information. In locations where there is a high probability of a bioterror event, it seems prudent that every health worker should have same level of training to detect, contain, and communicate. Required training courses are in development, and with their fully developed form will become part of the routine credentials for all healthcare workers. When these fully trained individuals are properly informed, they become the vanguard of a surveillance and response system for bioterrorism. Their participation also requires an ability to articulate their concerns to responsible local and national parties and in databases constructed for the purpose.

It is assumed that either the healthcare workers in the community or a responder team at the site of the inoculation makes the initial detection of disease outbreak. Bioterror response requires initial communication of accurate information flowing directly from first responders. Prompt action can arrest the spread of the agent, direct effective treatment protocols to exposed victims, and minimize social disruption. The response begins with analysis at or near the site of the event and extends with communication through multiple nodes of authority to a central command and control center located at a geographically distant site. The immediate response implements protocols rehearsed prior to the actual event.

The first response to the event must include surveillance or detection, analysis, and communication of information acquired at the scene. The human disease or toxicity may be one readily recognized by primary responders or may involve pathology totally unfamiliar to them. Lack of recognition may allow critical time to pass, which encourages spread or progress of the disease. Health workers near the scene of the event may also be vulnerable to the agent and quickly become casualties and liabilities to the relief effort, rather than assets to provide information and intervention. The overarching goal is for rapid implementation of expanded services and management of many people, relaying a mass of information and coordinating resources to be applied to the event. Integration of information technology with effective flow of relevant information regarding the consequences and evolution of the unfolding event becomes critical to coordinate a multiagency bioterror response.

Communication confirms ground-zero analysis, gives directives to first responders and other agencies, activates protocols for disaster management, and connects the various nodes in the hierarchy of disaster-event command and control. Effective bidirectional communication also deploys appropriate resources to the right place at the right time. Thus, responders must be equipped with reliable and compatible communication assets that are redundant in case of failure of one modality. The communication equipment must be portable and easily set up. The flow of information should use communication systems equipped with tools that operate independently and complementary to the regional police, fire, and emergency services. The regional services are typically self-contained and configured to transmit incident information directly to the next vertical level of information management, such as command and control centers. Bioterror response entails communication out of the immediate event site and integrates information collection, management, and dissemination with multiple nodes of communication. Continuous onsite surveillance data can be immediately communicated using either wired connections or wireless networks.

Wired communications utilize physical lines to connect two parties in a point-to-point fashion. Wired options include telephone lines for phone linkage or modem dial out for Internet connectivity. During disaster events it is very possible that the Plain Old Telephone System

(POTS) will be not functional, due to cable infrastructure damage, power outages, or lack of access. Phone lines can become overloaded for all landline public phone access (POTS or high-speed fiber-optic lines), as thousands of people try to communicate simultaneously with others beyond the attack site.[13]

It is possible that Internet access by wired systems remain operational and serve as an asset for directing messages outward from the site of incidence and retrieving reference information to evaluate the signs and symptoms from victims. With low-bandwidth Internet-based systems, it is possible to relay relevant patient information for confirmation of diagnosis and treatment, as well as containment protocols from expert physicians in distant locales.[14] Internet connectivity can also provide a portal for continuous real-time relay of patients' physiological parameters, in order to better formulate a treatment plan.[15] However, Internet access can also become limited, in that access routes are difficult to extend to a remote location or mobile units. Additionally, accessibility to a feasible service provider can be a limiting constraint. The degree of access-speed and number of simultaneous users in any specific area is limited to what the service provider considers to be the average and deems to be economically appropriate.

The option of wireless communication is a more feasible alternative. These options include the use of cellular phone, wireless access networks for the Internet, radio, and satellite. Wireless capabilities allow bidirectional communication among geographically dispersed parties with minimal time delay. A comparison of wireless access topologies is outlined in table 13.3 for mobile communications. In general the higher the frequency range of transmission, the greater the information transfer capacity.

Cell phones are functionally similar to radios and have low-power transmitters in them. Many cell phones have two signal strengths: 0.6 watt and 3 watts. In contrast, most CB radios transmit at 4 watts. Therefore, the power consumption of the cell phone, which is normally battery operated, is relatively low. This fact has made handheld cellular phones adaptable to a variety of applications. In order for cell phones to carry out their transmission, they require base stations. Base stations transmit at low power and result in forming a zone of signal capture. Cellular phones within the base station do not transmit very far outside the cell zone. The cellular approach requires a large number of base stations in a city of any size. A typical large city can have hundreds of towers to relay the transmitting signal. Each carrier in each city also runs one central office called the Mobile Telephone Switching Office (MTSO). This office handles all of the phone connections to the

Table 13.3

## Communication Capabilities for Wireless Technology*

| Technology | Frequency | Bandwidth | Power | Users | Cost | Issues |
|---|---|---|---|---|---|---|
| HF (ham) radio | 1–30 MHz | 100–400 bps | + | + | + | antenna ~9 m |
| VHF | 30–200 MHz | 2400–9600 bps | ++ | ++++ | + | <5km to node |
| UHF | 200 MHz–1 GHz | 2400–9600 bps | ++ | ++++ | + | <5km to node |
| Cellular (analog) (1st generation) | 800–900 MHz | 2400–9600 bps | + | ++++ | + | <5 km to node |
| Cellular (digital) (2nd generation) | 1.7–1.8 GHz | 14.4–60 Kbps | ++ | ++++ | ++ | <5 km to node |
| LEO satellite | 1.5–1.7 GHz | 2400–9600 bps | ++ | – | +++ | outside access |
| Geosynchronous satellite | 4.0–24 GHz | 64 Kbps | +++ | – | ++++ | outside antenna dish |
| Wireless Ethernet (3rd generation) | 2.5 GHz | 11–100+ Mbps | + | – | ++ | <30 m to node |

* The plus signs indicate the relative intensity to which that characteristic is applicable for the corresponding communication technology, with a dash (-) referring to minimal application and ++++ indicating most widely applicable.
bps, bytes per second; GHz, giga hertz; HF, high frequency; Kbps, kilo bytes per second; km, kilo meters; LEO, low earth orbit; m, meters; Mbps, mega bytes per second; MHz, mega hertz; UHF, ultra high frequency; VHF, very high frequency.

normal land-based phone system and controls all of the base stations in the region. More advanced digital cellular phones can function in a web-based interface for information management.

As evidenced in the tragic events of September 11, 2001, in New York, situations of panic can easily overload cellular phone communication system infrastructures, causing them to be inoperable. In New York, tremendous demand to simultaneously relay a very large volume of calls caused signals to be dropped and the system to fail. Current emergency-response telecommunication systems fail to support the information needs required for a response to bioterror, or any other disaster-management situation.

The possible remaining options for effective communication are radio or satellite. The advantages of using these modalities are many. Remote locations can be reached economically and with great ease, and information can be broadcast simultaneously to numerous parties. Amateur radio communications provide the greatest operational flexibility with a wide range of available frequencies for two-way radio-frequency (RF) communications. A range of frequencies is available. At the low end are medium frequencies at 18 to 20 megahertz. Very high frequency and ultra high frequency bands peak at 200 megahertz to 1 gigahertz. Extremely high frequency segments range upward from there.[16] Studies with a radio link in the low range at a frequency of 9.675 megahertz have proven that it is feasible to transmit medically relevant data in text format in real time to distant consultants.[17] RF communication is flexible in that repeaters, or automatic relay stations, can increase signal transmission range from remote locations. However, damage to radio towers, base stations, or repeaters can disable RF communication.[18]

In contrast to RF communication, satellite linkage provides a mechanism for global communication when other wired or wireless resources are unavailable. To manage portability and minimal power requirements, handheld terminals relaying the signals with low earth orbit (LEO) satellites provide an effective communication alternative.[19] LEO satellites are much closer to earth than geostationary satellites and are not stationary. Geostationary satellites occupy fixed positions in the sky, since they orbit synchronously with the earth's rotation and are used mainly for commercial communications. Because of the shorter distance to the LEO satellite, earth-based transmitters and receivers can be smaller, with lower power requirements. In order to access the LEO systems, the satellite phone must be used outside. The additional advantage with LEO connectivity is that the satellite phone can operate in almost any geographic location and communicate with any other phone in the world. With the transmission rate at almost half that of an ISDN (128 kilo bits per second) access line, the LEO transmission can support basic videoconferencing, image transfer and text, as well as voice transmission. The limitation of handheld satellite units is that they provide only one channel for telephone calls or e-mails sent and received. Satellite technology with the Very Small Aperture Terminal (VSAT) configuration, which requires antenna 1.2 to 2.4 meters long or a transportable equivalent, can simultaneously handle multiple telephone connections and Internet access.[20]

The third-generation telecommunication platforms offer another solution and are most feasible in a hybrid configuration. Using wireless Ethernet connections to a computer or telephone with a transmission rate of 2.5 gigahertz, it is possible to transfer 11 to 100 megabits per second. Transmissions must occur, however, less than 10 meters from the transmitting node, which could be a barrier in a situation of emergency case management. However, if an emergency vehicle functions as the node and communicates to Internet by satellite, a hybrid solution is possible that provides an option for large bandwidth access while maintaining mobility.

With intact communication resources, the vertical information-relay hierarchy dictates that first responders transmit the immediate, on-site survey to the regional command and control center. This information, including disease incidence, size and character of outbreak, and a survey of victims, is then disseminated down the chain of public health agencies to better unify tracking of the disease outbreak across a wider base of communities. The CDC has proposed the protocol illustrated in figure 13.1 for dissemination of information regarding the disease outbreak and public health alerts, starting with the parties that initially detect the disease pattern. In order to encourage effective information exchange, the CDC has implemented the Health Alert Network (HAN), which integrates information and communication protocols linking local, state, and federal agencies involved in public health management. HAN is designed to be a medium for electronic transmission of information and data, integrating a National Electronic Disease Surveillance System (NEDSS) and the Epidemic Information Exchange (Epi-X). NEDSS is designed to support electronic collection and transmission of disease data, facilitating the rapid detection and response to outbreaks.

Command and control is considered as the most important activity in bioresponse.[21] In coordinating the response to a disaster event, command and control is responsible for controlling the spread of the disease, monitoring the disease progression, and coordinating the allocation of resources to manage the situation.[22] In order to generate a coordinated and sustained management of the disaster event, command and control requires the following four essential elements:

1. Information about the event to conduct complete situational analysis of impact and consequences.

2. Adequate communication infrastructure to relay accurate, bidirectional information to and from the responders at site of incidence.

3. Access to a complete reference data warehouse at the center in order to perform proper data analyses, statistical predictions, and to link field responders to expert consultants for real-time interaction.

4. Appropriate telecommunication tools and protocols to coordinate participation of various agencies, allocate resources, and relay updated information to first responders.

## Situational Analysis

The first responder team surveying a potential bioterror event will be required to assess the situation and gather clinical assessments of patients, physical assessments of the event site, and early sampling to

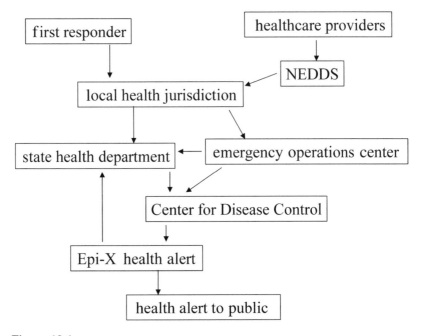

**Figure 13.1**
The CDC's proposed Health Alert Network (HAN) shows the flow of information from healthcare providers and/or first responders to the medical community and the public. NEDSS and Epi-X are existing CDC communications networks designed to promote information sharing.

characterize the biological agent. This capability to acquire preliminary raw data from the disaster site requires ideal tools and extensive training to recognize the potential biological terror. First responders may be able to analyze the data set using interactive databases and information sources distributed to the responder from resources archived in electronic databases within tools such as Personal Digital Assistants (PDA) or tablet PCs. The data set is transmitted immediately to the command and control center in order to validate the actions of the first responders and initiate the coordinated effort.

This initial analysis is a matter of clarifying the suspicion and then seeking more definitive answers. For example, the first responder may observe skin lesions and suspect smallpox or anthrax. The first responder's training should equip him or her to collect pertinent data, protect him or herself, consult interactive databases or information sources, and seek advice from more expert individuals. The first responder should also be able to contact the next echelon of emergency response to report their concerns. Thus, a primary information and telecommunication needs of these responders is to access appropriate information resources, in this case, to compare visual data on skin changes and patient symptoms. These information resources could be web-based or PDA software that has been created for bioterror incidents.

These mobilized workers responding to a potential bioterror event should have electronic diagnostic tools, such as video and audio dictation, to warehouse the data in digital format and relay remotely for telemedicine consultation with authorities, who might render a diagnosis before the victim contaminates others. They are also charged with analysis of the environment to provide clues to the mode of inoculation and probable routes of spread. The responder should also have the training and tools to take samples for subsequent biological analysis, and the ability to contain the situation to some degree. Important decisions are made at this encounter and telecommunications should be seamless to the next echelons of response.

## Communication Infrastructure

The command and control structure must have a reliable communications infrastructure. Reliance upon HF radio in chaotic situations is nostalgic and denies the potential of wireless broadband. The infrastructure should also not rely wholly on regional telecommunications such as cell phones. Cell and HF radio are portable and can serve as part of a backup for emergency situations. However, the amount of data that can potentially be collected in a bioterror situation is enormous and requires the faster rate of data transmission associated with LEO satellite infrastructure or a repeater to relay back to a base station with better equipment. The telecommunications topology should be carefully considered, put into position for deployment well ahead of time, periodically used in training exercises, tested frequently, and maintained in the event of emergency by appropriate technical staff members, as well as the command and control center.

## Reference Data Warehouse

The center should have the ability to do complex mathematical modeling and trend analysis, and to distribute evidence-based practice protocols to respond to prediction modeling of unfolding consequences.

The information technology (IT) team should allow evolution of the database received from the field and make that interactive with other databases to determine the nature of the crisis in question. The IT should allow rapid preparation of instructional software for the field workers to guide their work with additional documentation supplementing any voice command relayed from command and control.

## Telecommunication Tools

The tools should include ways to empower the various agencies with proper instruction for ongoing analysis, treatment, and containment. Since many bioterror events will involve simultaneous sites, the coordination of multidirectional information exchange and instruction is essential for the command and control center to manage the unfolding bioterror event. With these tools in place, managers of bioterror response can take solace in at least some modicum of order and timeliness. The managers, responders at various levels, and the public can be kept in an information continuum. Generally free of rumor and frightful supposition, the public and responders thus thwart a major weapon of bioterror. There are a number of studies that applied the principles mentioned above to test situations. The following two examples are offered.

### The Isolated Health Worker in the Field

Health workers are trained to be information managers in variable environments with dense information support to aid in case management. The transposition of such a medical person to a site without information support is not necessarily consistent with the best medical practice. A similar situation prevails should terrorism or a natural disaster deprive a medical worker of dependable access to decision support information. In this study a group of medical personnel traveled to Kenya to conduct patient-care surveys and assist in clinical-care programs. The area lacked all communications and had no source of electrical power. A team of programmers with Medical Informatics and Technology Application Consortium (MITAC) at Virginia Commonwealth University (VCU) developed a system of information support which provided solar power, LEO satellite connectivity to Internet, telemedicine consultation with physicians at VCU, and an electronic medical record (EMR) for patient data archiving. Consequently, field medical workers in Kenya were able to accumulate medical data into a database that was reconciled for all investigators on a regular basis and was consolidated into a backup server at VCU daily. MITAC, in conjunction with students at VCU's school of medicine, validated this working model of information support during evaluation of 2,700 patients in four remote villages in Kenya. This exercise included the integration of personal digital assistance (PDA) devices with an integrated EMR (figure 13.2). Satellite telephone technology added a layer of communications between the ambulant healthcare workers in the field with the consulting physician at VCU. The exercise confirmed the ability to integrate technology for transmission of relevant patient data to a remote host site and conduct relevant medical consultations to guide patient care when needed.

With satellite-based Internet connection, the ambulant medical personnel could download all messages in the morning and respond off-line if there was no urgency. In urgent situations, real-time consultation was possible at 64 kilobits per second, Internet protocol speed. Each worker had a PDA with drug information and quick reference for general diagnostics. The PDA's were synchronized at night to combine all patient data, which then was available as if each worker had in fact seen all patients. This evolving database served as a multiplier for each health worker, who relied very little on anecdote even for unfamiliar medical tasks and conditions. The manager of the project reviewed the data back in the United States and provided insight and directions to the Kenya team based upon the flow of data, which he could review at least twice daily and as needed.

Over a three-week period, more than 400 children were included in this project, and data for the study evolved to the final outcome by incremental inclusion and updates. The workers' satisfaction with the technology indicated strong user-friendly qualities. Utilization of the software and consultation was almost total. The cost was some $0.28 per patient. It was clear that even in an area where there is no information infrastructure—or even a power grid—considerable headway could be made toward sustaining an electronic and information continuum for patient management.

*Attack on a Sporting Event*

It is frightful to think of the possibility of introducing a potent biological agent into a densely gathered and highly vulnerable population such as the attendees at a large sporting event. At a recent sporting event in California, a situational awareness exercise was conducted for dealing with potential mass-casualty events. Particulate monitor sensors were placed at various points around the stadium as though keeping

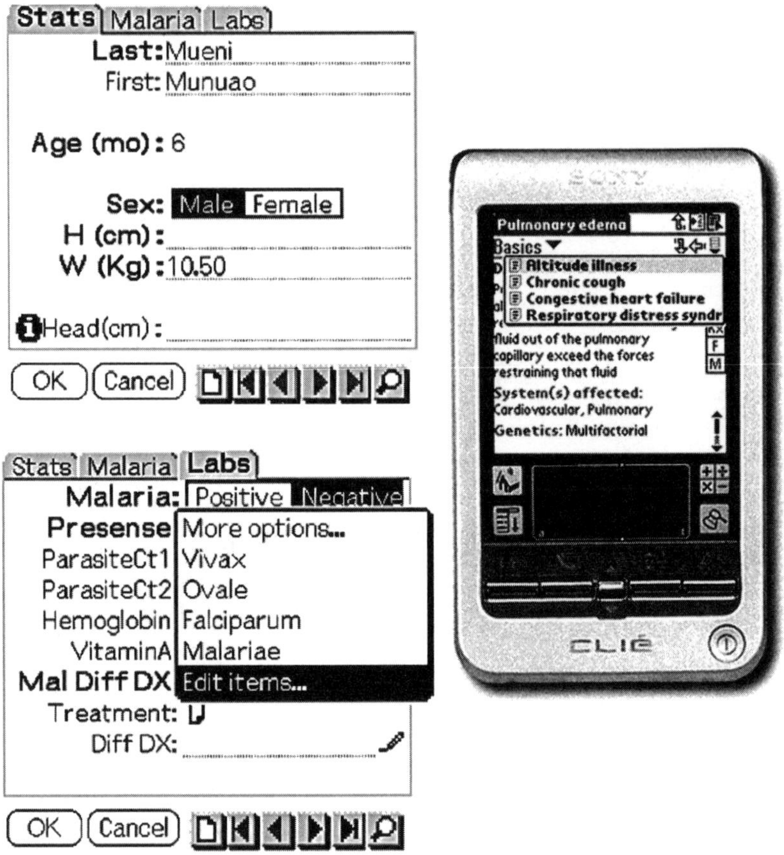

**Figure 13.2**
**Personal Digital Assistant (PDA) with Palm Operating System and Screen Images of the Electronic Medical Record (EMR) Integrated for Patient Data Collection**

vigilant watch for some agent such as the DNA of anthrax. The biosensors were in radio relay to a web server in real time outside the stadium (figure 13.3). A JAVA servlet application received and decoded the data for insertion into a relational database. The data stream was monitored by personnel in the stadium periphery who were alerted that a sensor was engaged. Data streams from the sensor were transmitted by cell phone to a remote management center in Richmond, Virginia (figure 13.4). In the exercise, the cell phone was to fail, and software had been installed to automatically switch the critical information to an Iridium satellite phone with LEO satellite linkage. The cellular phone frequency

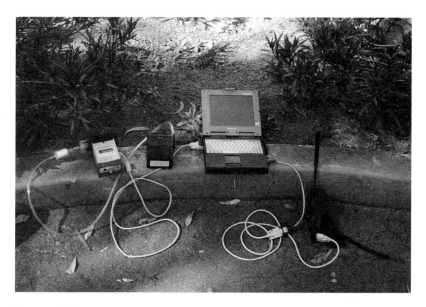

**Figure 13.3**
**Integrated Air Particulate Monitoring System Inclusive of MIE Particulate Monitor, Laptop, and Iridium Satellite Handheld Phone**

channels operated at 824 to 894 megahertz with full-duplex communication and a transmission rate of 19,200 bits per second (bps). In contrast, the data rate for the Iridium satellite connection was limited to approximately 2,400 bps but was sufficient for the text data stream. The exercise was successful in that data flow was continuous despite loss of cell phone linkage. In addition, the data were transmitted in short bursts of packets and demonstrably less vulnerable to interruption due to potential Internet problems.

## CONCLUSIONS

Considering recent advances in technologies, there is no reason to compromise an effective bioterror response with poor telecommunication and information management. With effective planning and training, telecommunication assets can be ubiquitous, pervasive, redundant, and robust. The terrorist party expects to inflict chaos upon a frightened and defenseless population. However, this expectation can be thwarted, curtailed, and perhaps prevented when responsible and responsive surveillance systems are in place that detect disease occurrence, help

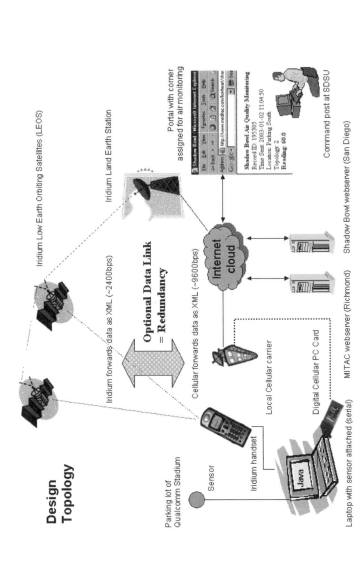

**Design Topology**

Iridium Low Earth Orbiting Satellites (LEOS)

Iridium Land Earth Station

Portal with corner assigned for air monitoring

Iridium forwards data as XML (~2400bps)

**Optional Data Link = Redundancy**

Cellular forwards data as XML (~9600bps)

Internet cloud

Parking lot of Qualcomm Stadium

Local Cellular carrier

Sensor

Iridium handset

Digital Cellular PC Card

Command post at SDSU

Laptop with sensor attached (serial)

MITAC webserver (Richmond)

Shadow Bowl webserver (San Diego)

Shadow Bowl Air Quality Monitoring
Record ID 195305
Time Sent 2003-01-02 11:04:50
Location: Parking South
Topology 2
Reading: 60.0

**Figure 13.4**

**Schematic of Network Architecture Used in Relay of Data Acquired from Particulate Monitor and Relayed over Redundant Wireless Communication Systems to Remote Command Centers and Backend Servers**

*Source:* Courtesy of VCU/MITAC, 2003.

contain further dissemination, and communicate relevant event-significant data. The defense against bioterror is largely an information-management phenomenon that requires health workers and public-safety officials to be included in surveillance of incidents based on prior event scenarios and to arrive with detailed information for detection and initial response. When the public is instructed in a controlled situation, rich with reliable information, panic is prevented, which results in greater safety through more capable management. New technologies in evolution will continue to greatly simplify disaster communications and enhance information management in both the acquisition and transmission modalities.

## NOTES

1. Zilinskas RA. Confronting biological threats to international security: a biological hazards early warning program. Ann NY Acad Sci 1992;666:146–76.

2. Zilinskas RA. Terrorism and biological weapons: inevitable alliance? Perspect Biol Med 1990;34:44–72.

3. Tucker JB. Historical trends related to bioterrorism: an empirical analysis. Emerging Inf Dis 1999;5(4):1–5.

4. Gesteland PH, Gardner RM, Tsui FC, Espino JU, Rolfs RT, James BC, et al. Automated syndromic surveillance for the 2002 Winter Olympics. J Am Med Inform Assoc 2003;10:547–54.

5. Kohane IS. The contributions of biomedical informatics to the fight against bioterrorism. J Am Med Inform Assoc 2002;9:116–9.

6. Teich JM, Wagner MM, Mackenzie CF, Schafer KO. The informatics response in disaster, terrorism, and war. J Am Med Inform Assoc 2002;9: 97–104.

7. Hutwagner L, Thompson W, Seeman GM, Treadwell T. The bioterrorism preparedness and response Early Aberration Reporting System (EARS). J Urban Health 2003;80:i89–i96.

8. Tsui FC, Espino JU, Dato VM, Gesteland PH, Hutman J, Wagner MM. Technical description of RODS: a real-time public health surveillance system. J Am Med Inform Assoc 2003;10:399–408.

9. Bacastow TM. Using information technology to combat terrorism. Washington, DC: Center for Strategic and International Studies; 2001.

10. Departments of the Army, Navy, and Air Force. NATO handbook on the medical aspects of NBC defensive operations. Washington, DC: Departments of the Army, Navy, and Air Force; 1996.

11. Vorobjev AA. Criterion rating as a measure of portable use of bioagents as biological weapons. Washington, DC: National Academy of Sciences; 1994.

12. Horn JK. Bacterial agents used for bioterrorism. Surg Infec 2003;4(3):281–7.

13. Zimmermann H. Communications for decision-making in disaster management. Geneva: ITU-T Workshop on Telecommunications for Disaster Relief; 2003.

14. Lee S, Broderick TJ, Haynes J, Bagwell C, Doarn CR, Merrell RC. The role of low-bandwidth telemedicine in surgical prescreening. J Pediatr Surg 2003;38:1281–3.

15. Harnett BM, Satava R, Angood P, Merriam NR, Doarn CR, Merrell RC. The benefits of integrating Internet technology with standard communications for telemedicine in extreme environments. Aviat Space Environ Med 2001; 72:1132–7.

16. Hutchinson C. The ARRL handbook for radio amateurs. Newington, CT: The National Association for Amateur Radio; 2001.

17. Praba-Egge AD, Hummel RS, Stewart N, Doarn CR, Merrell RC. Remote telemedicine services by high frequency radio link. J Clin Engr 2003;38:55–61.

18. Wood M. Disaster communications Part I—global. 1996. Available from: www.relifweb.int/library/dc1/dcc1.html. Accessed November 14, 2003.

19. Whalen DJ. Communication satellites: making the global village possible. 1997. Available from: www.hq.nasa.gov/office/pao/History/satcomhistory.html. Accessed November 14, 2003.

20. Bell C. The role of satellite communications in disaster management. Johannesburg: African Aid, Disaster Management and Relief; 2003.

21. Marine corps Doctrinal Publications—MDCP 6 Command and Control. 1996. Available from: www.doctrine.usmc.mil/mcdp/html/mcdp6.htm. Accessed November 26, 2003.

22. Rosen J, Grigg E, Lanier J, McGrath S, Lillibridge S, Sargent D, et al. The future of command and control for disaster response. IEEE Engr in Med and Biol 2002;21(5):56–68.

# 14 Thinking the Unthinkable: How Industry Is Reinventing and Communicating Disaster Recovery in a Post-9/11 World

*John Rhoads*

In the weeks and months following September 11, 2001, a steady stream of commentary flowed from the desks of journalists claiming that every aspect of the American psyche had been changed forever. But is that true? In some cases it has only taken the business community two short years to dull the details of 9/11. In meetings one can already hear businessmen and women complaining of the "panacea of excuses" that September 11 has afforded the business community for nonperformance. Comments like this illuminate a troubling trend: Planning for large-scale disasters like September 11 has returned to the back seat in lieu of day-to-day business concerns that seem to demand immediate attention.

If the Department of Homeland Security is to be believed and another terrorist attack is almost certain, this trend is frightening. To forget the near collapse of our business infrastructure in the aftermath of 9/11 would amount to gross negligence on the part of business leaders. Though time blurs the details of the events, it must not dull our sense of urgency. Instead, leaders must shift their view of business continuity from the vacuum of "disaster recovery" to a legitimate extension of risk-management philosophy. Accordingly, in the next few pages we will examine opportunities for growth in the area of business continuity. In this examination, it is vital to begin by addressing problems with the traditional business approach. Next, it is important to supplement this discussion by looking at some alternative disaster-recovery models that are better suited to meet modern business needs. Finally, we should focus our attention on some emerging issues in business-continuity planning.

## ASSESSING THE THREAT: PROBLEMS WITH THE TRADITIONAL APPROACH

After the terrorist attacks on the World Trade Center (WTC) and Pentagon, business leaders began to play the "what if" game. Leaders were forced to question the level of their preparedness for a large-scale disaster. Until this point, only passing thoughts had been devoted to crisis preparedness. And the "business-continuity plan" (if there even was one) was really a simple, small-scale disaster-recovery plan aimed at mitigating loss and restoring functionality after a crisis. Invariably it was the dusty old Federal Emergency Management Agency (FEMA) manual that someone at the home office developed with little or no input from the real world. And in keeping with its value as a relic, it sat untouched on a remote shelf and was only consulted during the clean up after a disaster.

In a post-9/11 world, however, some businesses are taking the lead in developing workable plans to address real threats. Communicators are central to this mission. These companies are shifting from a disaster-recovery strategy that relegates itself to being the "tornado team" to a more holistic, multidisciplinary approach. In these businesses, overall business continuity is emerging as a core value and competency. This approach is designed to assure that regardless of the changes in the business and political environment, the organization has developed a culture that can anticipate and respond in a manner that protects the interests of employees, shareholders and the general public. Gary Sikich explains that in the traditional model, most emergency responses employ a piecemeal approach consisting of risk management, legal tactics, and operations procedures.[1] Worse yet, many responses are so slapdash that most of these parties are never even consulted (p. 45). The result is a disjointed plan, likely to create chaos and confusion, and even exacerbate problems when crises occur. In table 14.1, Grimaldi outlines some hurdles that many continuity planners encounter in the development of a viable plan.[2] As evidenced by his explanation, communication is the key to developing a plan that speaks directly to the needs of stakeholders, with a message and in a manner that they understand. The facts are lucid; to develop a viable and dynamic approach to business continuity, regular communication with all stakeholders before, during, and after the crisis is foundational.

In order to see how central (and overlooked) the role of the communicator has become to business continuity, consider the following

**Table 14.1**
**Common Flaws in Continuity Plans**

| Problem with Traditional Approach | Explanation |
|---|---|
| One size fits all | The business-continuity plan is not task-specific to the organization. Off-the-shelf plans do not contain the necessary level of specificity. A clear task analysis is crucial. This requires open dialogue amongst all stakeholders. |
| Deficiencies in testing | Tests, if conducted at all, are on a small scale and unlikely to represent real-world conditions. In a sterile test environment, the response protocol is already well-communicated and unlikely to create the same level of unexpected challenges as a real crisis. |
| Inadequate maintenance | Plans have not been updated since their original draft and are no longer able to respond to real-world concerns. Ongoing stakeholder communication can help avoid this obstacle. |
| Lack of involvement of senior management | Because these plans require the use of human and capital resources, senior management must support these efforts. Whoever champions these efforts must reside at the senior levels of the organization and be empowered to make decisions regarding both. |
| No enterprise-wide solution | The diversity of business objectives creates tension with the organization in trying to establish the goals of the plan. Objectives have not been shared among the internal stakeholders. |
| No management contingency plans | Often, plans do not anticipate the unavailability of a manager during a crisis. For example, the media contact (which is generally a member of senior management) may be directly affected by the crisis. |
| No immediate threat | Other business objectives compete for scarce resources, and the nonimmediate nature of the plan causes the project to be prone to delays. |

questions that a business can use to audit its current business-continuity plan needs:

- Communication continuity: Who are the people in my organization designated to respond in a crisis? What if that person is one of the affected parties? Does everyone know what s/he can or cannot say to the media?
- Personnel communications: Do I know how to communicate to my employees when they are not at work? What is their preferred method of communication?
- Shareholder communication: How do I communicate to my shareholders that I have a plan to respond? What is the best way to update shareholders about my ongoing success or challenges during and after the crisis?

- Vendor communications: Have I identified my crucial vendors (those that are critical to my mission as an organization)? What if they are affected by the crisis? Do they have a recovery plan? Are there alternate vendors available?
- Media relations: Does the media know who to direct their questions and inquiries to? Do my employees know who to refer the media to? Do all of my media contacts have the same information?

## A NEW BUSINESS-CONTINUITY MODEL: $P^2R^2$

The traditional model used by most organizations has served the business community well. However, prior to 9/11, the model proposed by FEMA was focused mostly on short-term natural disasters, with some consideration given to man-made and technological emergencies. The strength of this plan was its focus on preparations that help mitigate losses from a crisis. However, no plan could have conceived of a disaster on the scale of 9/11. Today, for a plan to be viable, it must anticipate large-scale disasters affecting entire geographies, as well as a limited crisis in a contained area. But rather than a wholesale rejection of this well-conceived model, $P^2R^2$ represents the natural evolution of the FEMA plan.

The main difference between $P^2R^2$ and the FEMA model is that $P^2R^2$ begins with a prevention phase that precedes FEMA's mitigation step (outlined in figure 14.1). The prevention phase focuses on creating a culture of risk awareness, rather than focusing on the mitigation of loss. A risk-aware culture is one that avoids some activities altogether, based on an ongoing risk-benefit analysis. This approach focuses on the early identification and coordination of all stakeholders. The plan then asks those stakeholders to conduct a detailed evaluation of the frequency and severity of risk. This analysis results in (1) rejection of the activity because of undue risk, or (2) acceptance of the activity with a full understanding of the risks involved. Regardless of the choice, the business benefits from a detailed examination of the inherent and latent risks associated with its activities. Additionally this approach supplements FEMA's mitigation step. The analysis conducted in the prevention phase of $P^2R^2$ helps assure that plans to mitigate loss are viable and address the real concerns that stakeholders have expressed during the prevention phase.

Given the size and geographic diversity of modern business, no plan can anticipate the broad range of possible disaster situations. However, 9/11 caused some organizations to modify their approach to the traditional

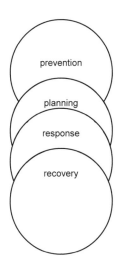

**Figure 14.1**
**P²R²: A New Four-Part Disaster Preparedness Model**

FEMA four-part model. Many organizations began to consider that a crucial step in managing risk was to adopt a robust risk review process. In the P²R² model, as opposed to the traditional FEMA model, each potential disaster situation and its corresponding recovery are addressed in four steps, with each subsequent step building on the foundation of risk awareness.

As table 14.2 demonstrates, the primary difference from the FEMA plan concerns the first step. Rather than a focus on mitigation of risk, the focus in P²R² is on elimination of risk, while mitigation is done during the planning phase. A more detailed analysis of each phase of the P²R² model follows below.

### Step One: Prevention

As with any good risk-management strategy, one of the most effective ways to shield the assets of the company from undue exposure is to simply avoid situations that would expose the organization to unnecessary risk. The challenge of this strategy lies in a thorough identification and understanding of risk.

While risk can never be completely prevented, the organizational focus in this first step should be to identify and eliminate undue risk. For example, a facility in a flood-prone area may avoid some exposure to undue risk by placing administrative offices on a higher level of the building in order to prevent damage to crucial business and administrative

Table 14.2
Comparison of FEMA and P²R² Models

| FEMA | P²R² | Differences |
|------|------|-------------|
| Mitigation reducing the effect of a given loss. | Prevention avoiding activities with unnecessary risk. | FEMA planning focuses on strategies to mitigate loss in the event of a crisis; P²R² prevention focuses on cost/benefit analysis of risk and elimination of activities which present undue risk. |
| Preparedness preparing and implementing strategies to cope with losses and mitigate damage for all risk. | Planning preparing strategies to cope with losses and mitigation of damages of accepted risk. | P²R² narrows the scope of planning to only those risks that have been deemed acceptable by stakeholders. |
| Response organizational reaction during the crisis. | Response organizational reaction during the crisis. | No difference. |
| Recovery restoration of normal business processes. | Restoration restoration of normal business process evaluation of plans effectiveness. | In addition to operational recovery the P²R² plan invites ongoing review and risk assessment to refine the Business-continuity plan. |

records. Likewise, when selecting sites for future businesses locations, leaders should consider the risks associated with locations in target-rich areas. This idea is not revolutionary; companies routinely look at risk factors in assessing whether or not to engage in an activity. It is standard fare for businesses to research statistics like crime and natural disasters before selecting work sites. Yet until September 11, 2001, no one considered the prestige of a building as a factor in its risk profile. It follows then that the real advantage of the new model is its focus on a systematic evaluation of risk before any business activity even begins. Before any measures can be taken, however, the most crucial portion of prevention is an objective review of business functions by all stakeholders. This process best insures that the inherent and latent threats have been identified and prioritized in terms of frequency and severity.

### Risk-Awareness Culture

One of the biggest challenges facing leaders in the prevention phase is building a culture equipped to identify and assess risk. Pepper explains that no matter how hard executives of a company may try, they cannot unilaterally define the "culture" that has been attributed to their organization by stakeholders.[3] He contends that culture develops through negotiation. During multiple interactions, a company's observable behavior produces what stakeholders identify as its culture. In other words, a corporation's culture is not simply the message that a company chooses to embrace; it is the totality of its discourse and behavior. Culture is measured as much by the reaction of the company, as the action of the company. The corporation's reputation emanates from its behavior and action. Reputation is not dictated—it is negotiated among all of its stakeholders[4] (see Conrad,[5] Pepper,[3] Gray, and Ballmer[6]).

This is particularly true in a crisis situation. Stakeholders are more likely to filter out bad or negative news about an organization if the organization has already established a good reputation or image. One of the goals for crisis communicators is to encourage customers to see failure as an anomaly and to draw on the reservoir of goodwill for the company, presuming that it has been established. Creating a risk-management culture is central to this objective.

Too often, when companies speak of risk management, they mean insurance. But risk-management philosophy is at the core of business. Simple math can reveal the direct effects of a poor risk-management philosophy—higher number of accidents and more severe consequences. Yet there are also numerous indirect effects of poor risk management, such as employee turnover, and shareholder impact, are often overlooked. To address both the direct and indirect effects of poor risk management, many organizations are moving to the model illustrated in figure 14.2.

This model dispels the notion that risk management is merely a safety and insurance program. Instead, the model mandates a close, ongoing analysis of potential risks, followed by a decision to decline business that represents undue risk or to accept the business risk that can be effectively managed. However, that risk must be continuously managed and monitored to ensure that accepted risk never becomes risk that should be avoided. The culture relies on properly motivated and empowered teammates and an openness by the organization to receive feedback on perceived risks. Heath explains that people will often endure untold risks if they feel that the company has fully disclosed risks and been open to the concerns of the stakeholders.[7] Additionally, this approach adds value to the continuity-planning process by opening up avenues of communication with stakeholders. In some cases, the stakeholder may be in a better position than management to spot emerging risk issues.

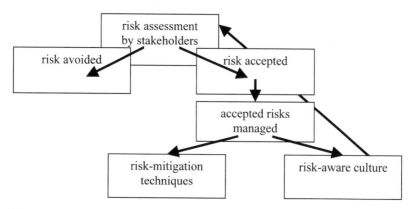

**Figure 14.2**
**This Model Mandates a Close, Ongoing Analysis of Potential Risks**

Even if the company has committed itself to developing a risk-aware culture, identifying the stakeholders needed to accomplish this task is not always simple. Of course, there are highly visible stakeholders within business continuity, but others are not so obvious. For example, many organizations would readily identify employees as stakeholders in a crisis situation but would completely ignore external stakeholders, like environmental impact groups. This issue becomes particularly troublesome for environmentally sensitive businesses, like chemical companies, that operate in target-rich areas where external stakeholders, including local homeowners and activist groups, will demand a seat at the table when assessing risk. Management at such businesses should carefully consider early dialogue with these external stakeholders, who can often have a significant impact on the organization. Companies that ignore the concerns and expectations of these stakeholders, especially in potential crisis situations, do so at their own peril. Researchers have examined and established that the performance of a company over time is tied in part to its social commitment to its external stakeholders.[8,9]

The rules of the prevention phase are the same whether the organization is dealing with a disaster of its own making or something as significant and unpredictable as 9/11: (1) identify stakeholders early, (2) build a culture of open and ongoing dialogue in advance, (3) let the stakeholders tell you their expectations and values, and (4) tell them yours.

One proactive measure is to make a firm commitment to the social concerns of external stakeholders through early and ongoing dialogue on emerging risk issues. Hooghiemstra points to the success of Shell Oil Company's "profits and principles" program.[10] With the *Exxon Valdez* crisis still fresh in the minds of many, Shell published their 1998 commitment in a pamphlet entitled *Profits and Principles: Does There Have to Be a Choice?* Shell emphasized for its stakeholders that it was part of the Shell reputation to be concerned about social responsibility—that it understood and accepted the charge to act responsibly while conducting a potentially dangerous business. Based on this stance it seems clear that for Shell, economic success and good corporate citizenship are not mutually exclusive. The focus of Shell's campaign was to assure its external stakeholders of its reputation for profitability and social responsibility. The program focused first on Shell's business performance, demonstrating that it is consistent with social responsibility and profitability. Second, the company examined whether its culture is consistent with these values. Finally, the campaign focused on how Shell is perceived by its stakeholders with regard to profitability and social responsibility. The importance of the final point cannot be overstated. External stakeholders will engage in risk-benefit analysis with the organization and even endure exposure to high levels of risk—provided that they have been afforded a place at the table to discuss their concerns, and that these concerns have been factored into final decisions. In light of the growing terrorism threat, it also makes good business sense for a company to communicate with its external stakeholders about measures taken to assess and address this threat before a crisis occurs.

Sauerhaft also points out the importance of communicating openness to input from all stakeholders.[11] Often, if a socially responsible organization fails to communicate the fact, stakeholders perceive it to be apathetic to social concerns. When it comes to social responsibility, whether it's true is not always the most important fact in persuading stakeholders of an organization's social conscience. Perception is reality (p. 3). Additionally, Crable and Vibbert contend that there is an added benefit to corporate social responsibility. Organizations that actively choose to be responsible will be less likely to receive a regulatory response (p. 6).[12] The message is clear: if the organization is open to input from all stakeholders, then let it say so—and loudly.

### Step Two: Planning

Armed with a clear understanding of which risks are (and are not) avoidable, the next step in preparing for any disaster is to create and implement a plan to minimize its impact. Always preparing for the worst-case scenario, plans must, with minimal interruption, (1) shield the company's personnel and assets, and (2) restore operational capacity following a crisis. Planning specifically denotes measures implemented prior to an impending crisis. These measures are not meant to fully anticipate all needs during a crisis but merely to lessen the severity of its impact. Again, an effective communication strategy is crucial in assessing the scale of the potential impact. Whether preparing for a hurricane, a chemical spill, or a terrorist attack, ongoing dialogue will produce a more well-rounded plan.

At a minimum, effective operational planning should include the following internal stakeholders:[13]

- A team leader chosen from senior management, or someone with enough support to call upon the capital and human resources of the organization before a crisis is imminent
- A finance director with authority to make capital expenditures
- A legal representative who can provide counsel regarding the company's civil and criminal legal liabilities
- A risk manager with a strong command of loss-control strategies (safety, insurance, etc.)
- A communication specialist, preferably with pre-existing relations between external stakeholders (media, interest groups, industry groups) as well as employees
- A human resources representative who can make decisions regarding the welfare of employees
- A security specialist devoted to risk mitigation and avoidance

Podolak points out that these team members should understand that their roles are "pre through post" crisis.[13] As such, each member should also serve as the internal stakeholders in the prevention phase of the model.

Once the team has been assembled and has shared its objectives, its members must begin to focus on operational contingency planning. At the same time, communicators must work to develop a plan that supplements the team's agreed-upon goals. Again, it is important to reiterate that the value of both plans is greatly diminished if the first phase of $P^2R^2$ has not been completed. Organizations can manage their internal or external reputation to protect fiscal performance and foster growth. However, no plan to manage perceptions can ever be effective until there has been an accurate assessment of existing perceptions from stakeholders. This process is foundational. Too often external or internal stakeholders are identified, yet organizations fail to acknowledge their needs, or even their existence. After identifying stakeholders during the prevention phase, however, the organization can do a better job of communicating in a consistent manner.[14,15]

The central goal of communicators during this phase is to develop a plan to effectively manage the multiple stakeholder perceptions of the organization. Jane Jordan writes that the ultimate goal is to build and reinforce confidence.[16] A step as simple as a well-communicated matrix listing communication responsibilities is a great start. As with most plans, this matrix should be listed by job title and not the name of the responsible party to avoid confusion. Additionally, a primer on the basics of communication is an effective place to start. Jordan explains that one of the biggest mistakes is to assume that people know what to do or say in the event of a crisis. Thus, the communication plan is as crucial as the operational plan.

To develop an effective crisis communication plan, Gilman and Davis suggest the following steps:

- Get support from senior management
- Continue ongoing dialog with employees, media, and shareholders
- Create and maintain an updated contact database (media, political, employee, stakeholder)
- Predesignate appropriate reporting channels during a crisis
- Compile a resource directory (online and hardcopy)
- Test (planned and unplanned)
- Appoint, equip, and authorize a crisis team, including a communication officer
- If applicable, make sure a company spokesperson is available during the plan formation
- Prepare company website response
- Be prepared with dark sites and standby statements
- Set up a communications triage philosophy to assess and address the most pressing inquiries first. (p. 40)[17]

## Step Three: Response

Since most companies' approaches to continuity grew out of a disaster-recovery program, response to a crisis is probably the most studied facet of business continuity. The "what do we do if" game has been played out in boardrooms for years. As a result, businesses are more experienced at completing this element of planning. During this phase, the main goal of communicators should be to reinforce that the safety and security of employees and the public is the top priority; all other messages should fall beneath this goal.

It is impossible to overstate the value of communication during this step. Often organizations make the mistake of creating the appropriate response without ever communicating its action and availability. For example, if senior management went to the trouble of creating a program that offers psychological counseling to teammates but never communicated its availability in a way that was meaningful or even noticeable to employees, efforts have been wasted. The real challenge for the communicator during this phase is to bolster confidence that the organization has a plan to respond to the crisis, and that the plan is consistent with organizational values and prior messages. Consistency is key in terms of message content and frequency.

It is axiomatic that one can never over-communicate in a crisis situation, but it is highly important that the communication is well coordinated. Crisis communication must speak in the same voice as the stated goals of the organization. Even companies with mature disaster-recovery plans often overlook this element during the chaos. Another note with regard to the communication plan is that there should always be a way to alert and coordinate with offsite and backup communicators. As was the case with many companies during 9/11, the person in the home office with the responsibility to spearhead communication efforts may be unavailable due to the disaster. Whether the backup is a third-party public-relations firm or an offsite member of the management team, the backup communication must figure into the plan.

During the response phase, a primary function of the communicator is to deal with seemingly contradictory messages in a way that bolsters the credibility of the organization. A response plan that does not coordinate all communication channels is likely to end up fighting contradictory messages within their own organization.[18] Worse yet, the organization that ignores the matter of communication completely is likely to allow their position to be framed for them through their own silence. Heath explains the importance of developing a plan that identifies all stakeholders and communicates to each one with consistency and integrity (p. 123, 228).[7] The organization will be judged on the perception of their response to the crisis—even if that crisis was not a result of their negligence. The choice is simple. The organization can either actively communicate its response or roll the dice and hope that the media and other external sources communicate the desired message.

To see an example of a consistent response, one need not look further than Johnson and Johnson's response to the Tylenol scare of the

1980s. Upon discovery of the tainted capsules, their quick and highly visible response to forego profits and discontinue distribution of their product communicated volumes about their values as a provider of healthcare products. Johnson and Johnson understood that the real disaster results when stakeholders' expectations are violated by a company's response to a crisis, leaving them open to feelings of uncertainty, isolation, and even outrage.

Another consideration for communicators is ongoing education about assumed risks. For example, during a crisis, an organization may need to remind stakeholders of previous dialogue about risk and benefits and reinforce its commitment to interactive dialogue that continually reassess the risks involved (p. 341).[7] However this step should be followed by a joint commitment to monitor the ongoing risk and update future plans accordingly. In the event of a crisis, how the organization is currently responding is also crucial to preparing for a future crisis.

Interestingly, there are some companies that actively choose silence during this phase. This strategy is usually ill advised. Organizations that choose to maintain silence are likely to allow their detractors to fill the void for stakeholders. For example, on September 11, 2001, when New York City Mayor Rudolph Giuliani hit the streets within minutes of the first attack, the response from even his detractors was positive. In contrast to this, the seeming absence of President Bush created significant opportunities for criticism. While the president probably had ample reason to believe he was a target of the attack (and the choice to remain out of communication may have been the right one), the perception was radically different. His silence amounted to a temporary relinquishment of his ability to control the message. However, a plan of communication with stakeholders, in this case the entire American public, which spoke in general terms about the need to not disclose his location and that he and his staff were closely monitoring the situation, would have communicated a message of control and thus reduced criticism.

Additionally, communicators must understand that *during* a crisis is not the ideal time to begin building a relationship with stakeholders. Businesses and their selected communicators must be able to draw from a reservoir of goodwill formed with stakeholders long before the crisis. Any ambiguity or mixed message is unlikely to be construed in favor of the company in question. As Steve Miller, CEO of Waste Management put it: "[E]very front [in] business is more difficult if you lack a solid reputation" (p. 36).[4] Accordingly, Texaco stands as one of the most egregious examples of this disharmony between internal and external reputation. Vershoor pointed to Texaco's 1996 Annual Statement that extols Texaco's treatment of employees according to the "values" and "vision" of a responsible employer and corporate citizen.[19] Yet it was during this same period that Texaco lost a headline-grabbing racial-discrimination lawsuit. This corporate-identity crisis prevented Texaco from being able to draw off of a reservoir of goodwill during a disastrous $176 million lawsuit (p. 1511).[20] It is easy to understand why a violation of expectations would produce disharmony. The scenario is framed in a syllogism that goes something like this: "A company says it believes in X, and a company that believes in X, should do Y, but this company did not do Y (or, worse yet, it did Z)." In a crisis situation, stakeholders are likely to view the company through the lens of its previous communication practices and expect consistency with prior messages. Any company that waits for a disaster to engage in communication invites criticism and loses the opportunity to frame its response to the relevant issues. Any communication from such a company is likely to be received dubiously.

Again, each phase relates back to the adequate assessment of stakeholder expectations. Often, dissatisfaction results from an expectation that the company should behave in a specific way that it has not behaved.[20] Research indicates that once someone feels that his or her expectations of company behavior are violated, a feeling of powerlessness results. These feelings culminate in frustration, helplessness and negativity.[21,22] Employees, for example, will point to the hypocrisy or apathy within an organization, especially if they feel that organization's treatment of a crisis is not consistent with its previously stated values.[23]

The Internet is the perfect venue for addressing the company's ongoing efforts for dealing with a crisis. While it can be used extensively during the planning phase, it is an invaluable resource to assure that information is widely available. Likewise, if an intranet is established by the company as the preferred means of communication, it provides a single communication outlet that can be monitored for message consistency. The financial services firm of Morgan Stanley Dean Witter (MSDW) provides one example of effective intranet use. On September 11, 2001, the company lost 13 employees, 24 floors of working space, and suffered displacement of 3,500 employees. MSDW turned to its intranet site to create a virtual community for those affected. The company used the website to create webcasts and to inform employees of hotlines and resources that were available, as well as to reinforce policies and procedures aimed at quickly restoring business.[24] One could guess that the only reason for the success of this strategy is that communication via the web was part of the company culture prior to September 11, 2001.

Crisis-response teams are another effective means of communicating during crisis. Similar to the planning team, these teams generally represent a broad cross section of all stakeholders. However, the central goal of this team is to meet the immediate needs of stakeholders during and immediately following a crisis. For this team, it is also a good idea to provide access to a trusted nonmanagement team member who can alert the team to misinformation that may be prevalent within nonmanagement layers of the organization. For example, executives from MSDW cite the success of their "rumor team," during the aftermath of the 9/11 tragedy. The role of this group was simply to talk to the employees to gather the gossip so that rumors could be addressed on the company's website.[23]

## Step Four: Restoration

The ability to return business to a normally functioning operation is the ultimate goal of any plan. Business partners and customers count on the company's ability to minimize future risks and reestablish normal business relationships. However, if the previous steps of prevention, planning, and response are not appropriately addressed, no company can restore services in the most efficient and safe manner.

Often, the failure of the restoration portion of a plan is simply the failure to consider that restoration may be a matter of months or years, rather than days or weeks. Madeline Bowden, an executive with Solomon Smith Barney admitted that prior to 9/11 their plan was focused on momentary interruption in the business model.[25] In fact many organizations make similar unwarranted assumptions about restoration in their business-continuity plan. First, they assume that the interruption will subside and normal business will resume in the same affected location. No one ever dreamed that a business continuity plan for a company located in the WTC should have to anticipate the complete annihilation of the facility. Until 9/11, business-continuity plans were focused on a temporary solution until the main office could be brought back online. Second, plans did not anticipate that an entire geographic region would be affected. The attacks on the WTC and Pentagon and the subsequent halt of all activity in New York City and Washington, DC, left many companies handcuffed. Previously, companies simply assumed that if their New York offices were temporarily unavailable, they would handle immediate needs out of other metropolitan areas. No one ever felt the need to ask: "What happens if *all* communication and transportation is unavailable?"

*Emerging Concerns*

In addition to deeper operational concerns, there are new concerns. The real disaster no longer ends with the restoration of business services. In fact, the lingering effects on personnel can leave a lasting impact on businesses for years to come. The fiscal and psychological impact of 9/11 created ripples that will not be fully felt for years. There are strong business examples of disasters that still affect local populations and employees decades after the actual incident. For example, nearly twenty years after the Union Carbide disaster, which killed hundreds in Bhopal, India, DuPont (which now owns Union Carbide) is still dealing with the long-term fiscal and cultural results of the crisis.[1] Rebuilding the physical production facilities was the easiest task. Complicating the issue is the fact that as organizations become more global in scope, their cultural makeup is likely to mirror this change. It is crucial to understand that differing cultures may have widely differing views on how to deal with crisis or its geopolitical causes and effects. For example, in the days following the 9/11 terrorist attacks, many employers became concerned about the ongoing safety and welfare of Arab-American employees and felt the need to implement measures to protect those employees from race-based violence.

Another emerging issue that employers are currently coping with in the wake of 9/11 is the increase in post-traumatic stress disorder (PTSD) claims. In most states, PTSD claims would be compensable under a workers' compensation scheme. However, the lingering effects and the very nature of PTSD might result in claims remaining latent before incurring large losses. Since many large and small companies maintain a level of self-insurance, not only do PTSD claims affect their staffing resources but also their bottom line. Even for employers with progressive programs that address the psychological impact of disasters, the sheer size of the population affected by 9/11 is unprecedented.

Communication of resources also remains a challenge during the restoration phase. How does management inform employees that grief counseling is available and convince employees to avail themselves of this resource? Again, communication is key. Organizations could spend thousands, even tens of thousands of dollars, making these resources available, but unless the availability is communicated to employees in a meaningful way, the offer is likely to go unnoticed. In service industries, including many affected by 9/11, employees are the company's only assets. Recovery of the business is entirely dependent on the recovery of its personnel. To illustrate this point, Madeline Bowden, a vice president with Solomon Smith Barney, one of the larger tenants in the WTC, explains that a lack of crisis counseling would have communicated a lack of care. However, prior to 9/11, the company had gone to great lengths to send the message that they valued their employees. So inactivity would have created an inconsistent message from which they would never have recovered.[25]

Organizational solvency also creates threats to stakeholders. As insurers were downgraded, and in some cases disappeared altogether, many companies were left wondering who would honor claims arising from the crisis. Fortunately, the federal government stepped in to bridge the gap, but what about a future crises? The federal government cannot continue to honor claims arising from future attacks, so organizations must communicate the measures they have taken to assure solvency in the event of an attack. Has the organization moved its operations base to a less target-rich area? Procured terrorism coverage from a reputable insurer? Have plans been made to communicate the stability of the organization to its employees and shareholders?

## CONCLUSION

Long-term answers to continuity issues are required because long-term business viability is at stake. The events of 9/11, along with recent statements by the Department of Homeland Security about the inevitability of future attacks, make the excuse of unforseeability much less available to business leaders. This creates additional challenges that should drive leaders to adopt the role of a responsible business steward in business-continuity planning. Leaders can no longer claim ignorance as an excuse for failing to plan for large-scale disasters. Business-continuity planning must begin well before a disaster, and communication that is early and often can only solidify these efforts. The only way to determine a plan's viability is to use regular ongoing communication to assess how well it addresses stakeholder expectations.

With regard to stakeholders, organizations must begin to view interaction as "transaction." In other words, groups within the public will look to the company's behavior (past and present) to help define its overall message. So business continuity also means continuity of message. If a company says that it values its employees and public safety as much as its profits, it must not forget that message during a crisis. Inconsistency here will result in long-term damage. When it comes to emergency responses, stakeholders believe in the old adage: "People [and companies] are like teabags; put them in hot water to find out what they're made of."

## NOTES

1. Sikich GW. Crisis management planning for corporate America—post 9/11. Continuity Insights 2003 Jun/Jul;1:45–8.

2. Grimaldi RJ. Why do business continuity plans fail? Risk Manag 2002 May;49:34–9.

3. Pepper GL. Communicating in organizations: a cultural approach. New York: McGraw-Hill; 1995.

4. Nakra P. Corporate reputation management: CRM with a strategic twist. Public Relations Q 2000; Summer:35–42.

5. Conrad C. Strategic organizational communication: cultures, situations and adaptation. New York: Holt, Rhinehart and Winston; 1985.

6. Gray ER, Balmer JT. Managing the corporate image and corporate reputation. Long Range Plan 1998;31:695–702.

7. Heath RL. Management of corporate communications: from interpersonal contacts to external affairs. Hillsdale, NJ: Lawrence Erlbaum; 1994.

8. Waddock S, Graves S. The quality of management and the quality of stakeholders relations: are they synonymous? Bus Soc 1997;36:250–79.

9. Preston L, O'Bannon D. The corporate social-financial relationship: a typology and analysis. Bus Soc 1997;36:419–34.

10. Hooghiemstra R. Corporate communications and impression management: new perspectives on why companies engage in social reporting. J Bus Ethics 2000;27:55–68.

11. Sauerhaft S. Atkins C. Image wars: protecting your company when there's no place to hide. New York: John Wiley & Sons; 1989.

12. Crable RE. Vibbert SL. Managing issues and influencing public policy. Public Relations Rev 1985;11:3–16.

13. Podolak A. Creating crisis management teams. Risk Manag 2002 Sep;49:54–7.

14. Vendelo MT. Narrating corporate reputation: becoming legitimate through storytelling. Int Stud Manag Organ 1998;28:120–37.

15. Dutton JE, Dukerich JM. Keeping an eye on the mirror: image and identity in organizational adaptation. Acad Manag J 1991;34:517–54.

16. Jordan J. Building confidence in a crisis. Continuity Insights 2003 Jun/Jul;1:22–4.

17. Davis SC, Gilman AD. Communications coordination. Risk Manag 2002 Aug;49:39–42.

18. National Research Council. Improving risk communication. Washington DC: National Academy Press; 1989.

19. Texaco. Annual report to shareholders. Texaco, Houston, TX; 1996.

20. Verschoor CC. A study of the link between a corporation's financial performance and its commitment to ethics. J Bus Ethics 1998;17:1509–16.

21. Ashforth BE. The experience of powerlessness in organizations. Organ Behav Hum Decis Process 1989;43(2):207–42.

22. Beetham D. The legitimation of power. Atlantic Highlands, NJ: Humanities Press International; 1991.

23. Heath RL. Strategic issues management: organizations and public policy changes. Thousand Oaks, CA: Sage; 1997.

24. Ferris GL. Response and recovery at Morgan Stanley. Risk Manag 2002 Dec;49:24–7.

25. Dealing with disaster: lessons learned one year later. Risk Manag 2002 Dec;49:12–7.

# 15 Toward a Paradigm of Managing Communication and Terrorism

## H. Dan O'Hair, Robert L. Heath, and Jennifer A. H. Becker

As is suggested in the first chapter of this volume, communication and terrorism are inextricably linked. The chapters following that introduction make similar connections, explaining how terrorism can be more effectively managed through communication processes and the formations of meaning of one sort or another. This chapter recommends specific options for addressing terrorism threats and moves our thinking to elevated levels for viewing terrorism from a communication perspective.

Today, crisis situations in general, and terrorist threats in particular, require an unparalleled focus on communication issues involving heretofore complacent, ignored, or neglected audiences. These audiences include the following: the general public, from whom we need information about their knowledge, beliefs, and behaviors regarding the anticipation and outbreak of a threat; governmental officials, who are not only decision-makers but sources of communication that the public must trust; and health professionals, who must become media savvy in order to perform their roles in a more effective manner.[1]

One way of framing the communication issues relevant to terrorism is to begin with an examination of the rationale of society. Distinguished anthropologist Mary Douglas suggests that among the many rationale for the organization of society, two are vital: the assignment of blame for unfortunate events and the organization by specialty to reduce risk. Thus, one can argue that the rationale of society is a collective management of risk. One can easily account for many professions based on what they contribute to the reduction of risk for the collective good. One such profession would be early responders, including fire and police personnel. Intelligence agencies and risk assessors and planners would add to the list. Teachers, medical personnel, researchers, engineers, trainers, and so forth—the list is long. Does it also include clergy who help invoke spiritual management of risk to account for the mysteries of life? Communication scholars and professionals could be added to the list. Preparing for, averting, mitigating, and following up in myriad ways after the work of terrorism is one crucial aspect of this risk management. It requires the allocation of social capital and material equity.[2]

Crisis planning, training, and response are vital aspects of collective risk management. One of the more troubling aspects of crisis preparedness is the lack of planning among organizations and communities. A sense of optimism can push crisis preparation too far to one end of the continuum. Optimistic bias occurs when people feel that they are less susceptible to risk than others and leads people to believe that they are more likely to experience positive consequences from events than negative. A serious result of this effect is that people underestimate their level of risk.[3] Corporate spokespersons reported in a survey that they were unprepared for a bioterrorism threat and that few of their represented organizations had plans in place. Many of these survey respondents perceive a large distance between their organizations and the potential of a threat on the magnitude of the anthrax crisis. These same people were probably experiencing optimistic bias.[3]

There is no shortage of suggestions for how terrorism can be controlled. Political, scientific, social, and layperson opinions abound. Depending on the perspective, a long continuum of options is available to individuals, professionals, and communities in preparing for terrorist attacks. Reid suggests that terrorism is best controlled through the following actions: weakening or eliminating the individual terrorist; controlling, "hardening," or eliminating routes of terrorist attack; decreasing terrorist funding and sponsorship; and/or making the terrorist's goal too expensive to pursue.[4] From our perspective, it is the latter of these strategies in which communication can play the most salient role.

Any philosophy of communication tailored to discussions of terrorism needs to revisit the timeless concern of processes and meaning. By what processes does communication occur? And to the development of what meaning that informs and guides collective action? These questions need careful analysis.

The analysis reconsiders the rationale of the democratic process instantiated in the First Amendment to the U.S. Constitution. People are encouraged to engage in debate and persuasion to examine issues for forming policy. Terrorism can be a corrupting factor in this scheme, it would seem, when it opts for coercion instead of more orderly debate. Aside from the element of criminal behavior, terrorists' penchant for coercion seems to predispose persons against them. It alters and distorts the tradition of public debate and collective resolution of concerns.

Pessimism and fear push to the center of consciousness from both sides when terrorism becomes part of the social equation. It can replace enlightened decision-making. The design and implementation of community support services and policy debates require careful attention if they are to mitigate the damaging presence of dysfunctional approaches of social influence. Communication scholarship has a strong tradition of addressing such challenges.

In this chapter we offer a number of perspectives organized into four sections: policy initiatives, community preparedness and response, communicating with the public, and interagency cooperation. The perspectives we offer ask that a different approach or new twists on old approaches be considered as we plan for potential terrorist activities. While we do not profess to know all the answers to managing communication and terrorism, we hope to enjoin collective thinking about these issues as part of a process of confronting terrorism potentialities.

## COMMUNICATION POLICY INITIATIVES

Policies toward terrorism response and preparedness are developed and refined through communication processes. Likewise, policy is administered and implemented by means of communication. In this section, we explore issues related to policy and the prevailing assumption among policymakers (and those who implement it) that acts of terrorism must be addressed in-kind. A direct, reactive strategy to terrorism does not usually help to curb future terrorist acts, especially in the long term. This are what Perlman calls first-order change.[5] This strategy attempts to focus on the obvious superficial problems and symptoms presented by terrorism; it does not address the sources of the issues. First-order change strategies also have the tendency to distract policymakers and implementers from pursuing other, more meaningful responses to the sources of terrorism.

Retribution or vengeance is first-order responses. The mindset leading to such reactions can be fueled by punimania, or an overwhelming urge to punish, which may or may not be justified, when punishment (1) does not address or resolve the root causes of the problem, (2) generates more suffering for innocent people in widening circles over time and space, and (3) has the probability of making things worse, even for the punisher. There are many examples of this, but an obvious one is the escalation of violence between the Israelis and Palestinians.[5] Strategies of communication pursuing first-order change focus on narrow courses of action with a restricted range of options. Tendencies toward groupthink are more likely.

Second-order change focuses on the deep structure of the system. Second-order change strategies are likely not as popular among distressed groups who have experienced terrorism, yet they have greater potential for long-lasting results. Second-order strategies tackle the root causes driving terrorists. They question the motives, lifestyle, values, and even the plight of those identifying themselves as terrorists or those who live with and support them—a systems perspective so to speak. Perlman suggests that this unconventional thinking can lead to alterations in how the systems in which terrorists live and connive can be fundamentally changed for the good. Various communications policies should include criteria that illuminate and encourage dialectical thinking, devil's advocacy, constructive controversy, and concurrence seeking.[6,7] In this way, multiple viewpoints are offered, considered, and debated, and tunnel vision is arrested.

Another means of addressing terrorism on a policy level stresses de-escalation in the tensions experienced by parties involved in the context of terrorism. One such approach is that proposed by Osgood, which he terms GRIT, or graduated and reciprocated initiatives in tension reduction.[5] Although commonly applied at the international relations level, GRIT would be appropriate in a number of contexts. The idea is to begin a symmetrical and reciprocated process of moves and countermoves that demonstrate good faith in scaling back the aggressive stances usually employed in terrorism contexts. As parties gain a semblance of confidence and trust in their counterparts, tension is reduced allowing greater opportunities for reasoning and negotiation. Similar to second-order change, the goal is to engage processes of understanding by uncovering the deep issues that create hostile feelings among potential terrorists. Variations on this theme can be observed in contexts such as the progress being realized in the protracted conflict between Northern Ireland and Great Britain, or with hostage-taking contexts.

Highly specific communication policy recommendations are difficult to advance due to the contextual nature of terrorism and the unique circumstances evolving from the multiple parties in any one terrorism situation. What we have laid out are some general guidelines that sketch a path toward considering multiple viewpoints in planning for terrorism and a plea for a longer-term perspective for dealing with deep causes, which precipitate terrorism in the first place.

## COMMUNITY PREPAREDNESS AND RESPONSE

When we speak of community, we do so in two ways. In a geographic sense, we think of communities as composites of individuals who work, live, and play in close geographic proximity in "local communities." However, geographic convenience does not itself create a sense of community. The "bowling alone" syndrome testifies to the penchant for members of local communities to wrap themselves in their families and refrain from civic engagement. Another way of thinking about communities is from a perceptual sense where proximity may or may not influence how a community is constituted. We know about communities of scholars and communities of practice; even spiritual groups and softball leagues think of themselves as communities. Key to both concepts of community is how they are fashioned and sustained through communication. In this section we discuss ideas for facilitating community and communities in light of terrorist threats.

We are intrigued with a concept of *communication capital* advanced by Camara. Communication capital refers to an individual's ability to draw upon information and emotional resources in order to come to grips with crisis situations. Communication capital includes drawing on different kinds of experiences, observations, media systems, emotions, expert opinions, and other resources to inform researchers how individuals respond to situations, including critical and life-altering events.[8] It stands to reason that people who build up their communication capital through readily available and reliable information sources will be better able to weather crises than those with less capital. Much was written about the spike in communication activities just after the airliners crashed into the World Trade Center on 9/11. Many people crowded around television sets; others reached out to friends and loved ones through land-based and cellular phones; still others turned to the Internet as a trusted medium for information and connection with others. Classrooms and boardrooms became communities of grief, horror, fear, and eventually consolation, sympathy, and healing. All the while these people began building their communication capital reserve by engaging in these communities.

*Social capital* is a related concept, whose central thesis is that social networks are valuable. Social capital grows from the communicative relationships that people form through sharing information, ideas, feelings, and favors. Eventually people begin to trust one another. Similar to the premise underlying the movie *Pay It Forward*, social capital relies on the goodwill of others who are willing to perform self-less acts for the betterment of others. Inherent in this notion is the idea of reciprocity. One good deed creates opportunities for other good deeds to follow. Reciprocity is not so much based on obligation but on the belief that helping behavior, civic engagement, public service and so forth are the right things to do, and that setting examples will raise the bar of participation even further. Social capital works best through intertwined interpersonal relationships that develop into social networks, which in turn grow into communities. Many benefits accrue to those with social capital, such that people with strong networks recover from illness more quickly compared to those who are isolated or alone. Happier marital couples experience fewer infectious illnesses and longer life expectancy.[9] Beyond the personal benefits, however, social capital is essential for strengthening communities. It is through social capital, networks, and communities that threats of terrorism fade. Hanging together and forming common bonds are formidable obstacles to terrorist attack. Strong communities with a store of social capital are best positioned to prevent terrorism in the first place and to respond most effectively in the event of terrorist acts.

In a similar fashion, *communication infrastructure theory* is a story-telling system that consists of stories, narratives, and conversations among ordinary people. Much like social capital, these narratives serve to build an infrastructure or reservoir of civic-mindedness that serves urban centers in their quest to respond to events crisis. It is fueled by people telling stories to one another, media producing or recounting stories, and organizations facilitating communication and civic engagement.[10]

As with other infrastructures, communication infrastructures are usually invisible until something happens to impair their functioning. For example, when electrical failures or transportation shutdowns occur inhibiting our everyday media connections, acute awareness of the communication system as a precondition to attain everyday goals quickly emerges. After 9/11, we observed a turning point at which a usually invisible community-based communication infrastructure became visible.[10]

Story telling is more than an idle activity, reasons Walter R. Fisher; it is the rationale of human communication: homo narrans—humans as story tellers. Narrative theory reasons that humans order their cognitive and communicative experience as a story. Their form and content drive the way people think, act, and communicate. Accordingly, terrorism is a unique narrative that interrupts other narratives. Terrorists seek to alter the normal or traditional narratives. Communication analysis can, therefore, usefully advise on how narratives can accommodate to the presence of terrorism. The altered narrative, then, re-informs that rationale for the collective management of risk. Such stories can create a sense of resilience.[11]

*Resilience* is a community-building idea we find particularly compelling. Resilience is a notion promulgated by Grotberg that refers to the thoughts, feelings, and even the spirit of individuals toward their community and its members.[12] It is perceived as an ideal state in which communities and its members possess an optimistic, pliable, and hardy perspective toward both normal and crisis conditions. Resilient communities are those that enjoy strong relationships within and outside the family, understand the need for vibrant community services (such as education, health, social, welfare), and are energetic in developing a community climate that is compassionate, empathic, respectful, and communicative. Research has discovered that resilient communities possess four common characteristics.[12]

Collective self-esteem: The community takes pride in its image and the values that it stands for. Community values can include physical appearance, a caring climate for its members, and even cultural or social experiences. Members of the community enjoy its reputation.

Cultural identity: Situated as one of the more essential factors, cultural identity with the community is strong even in the face of change, turmoil, or crisis. New problems or emergency issues become part of the context of the community and are handled by applying traditional cultural values.

Social humor: Part of resilience is the ability to put things into perspective. A resilient community cannot take itself too seriously. It must be able to joke about itself in order to demonstrate the importance of humor in its lives. Humor brings people together even more closely and helps to take the edge off more serious challenges, fashioning a more creative climate for enjoying life.

Collective honesty: Resilience would be meaningless without a community insisting that its members, organizations, and institutions pursue a sense of honesty throughout its reaches. Resilient communities remain mindful of the prominence of integrity in its leaders and officials and go to great lengths in rooting out corruption, dishonesty, and fraud.

How do resilient communities overcome threats or even acts of terrorism? Through resilient acts that construct strategies to discourage terrorism. According to Grotberg, "Resilient people can deal with acts of terror. They become stronger as they refuse to succumb to the tragedies perpetrated by terrorists. Their resilience is enhanced as they recognize the support of the community, and indeed, the nation, in overcoming the destructive aspects of terrorism. Terrorists have good reason to fear resilient people. Resilience triumphs over terror."[12]

Resilient, socially networked communities where stores of communication capital reside offer greater comfort and security than disconnected communities. How can members of communities move toward these goals if they are so inclined? A number of government materials are available for helping states and communities in joining together to create systems of preparedness (www.ojp.usdoj.gov). Another means of creating awareness for community building is to enlist the support of friends and neighbors to carry out a survey such as the Social Capital Community Benchmark Survey[13] below:

How many of your neighbors' first names do you know?

How often do you attend parades or festivals?

Do you volunteer at your kids' school? Or help out senior citizens?

Do you trust your local police?

Do you know who your U.S. senators are?

Do you attend religious services? Or go to the theater?

Do you sign petitions? Or attend neighborhood meetings?

Do you think the people running your community care about you?

Can you make a difference?

How often do you visit with friends or family?

Answers to the survey questions serve two purposes. First, when people answer questions about the social capital in their community, it creates self-awareness about their own personal needs for generating more social capital. Secondly, by summing or aggregating responses from many people in the community, a profile emerges from the mindset of community members toward their local network and communication infrastructure. Publicizing these results in the local paper and publishing them on the website of the local municipality will help communicate the needs of the community to building stronger bonds internally.

A final community-building activity is becoming involved in the Public Conversations Project (www.publicconversations.org). While the model for engaging people in local, community dialogue is designed for controversial topics where conflict exists, this model can be successfully employed as a means to bring people together to communicate about what is important to them. Through this process, people get to know one another, build social capital, and join in building a stronger community.

## COMMUNICATING WITH THE PUBLIC

When we speak of communicating with the public about terrorist threats or acts, a process of risk communication begins to unfold. Risk communication is a process that involves getting information about potential or actual crises into the hands of individuals who can act on it in a timely, responsible, and effective manner. It is a multifaceted process that focuses on the exchange of information pertaining to risk, and can be conveyed through media or channels including websites, public meetings, group discussions, press releases or conferences, public service announcements, hot lines, as well as online and print publications.[14]

Risk assessment must be a two-way street. Organizations and agencies entrusted with preventing and responding to terrorism must have a better understanding of what the public perceives and understands as well as a greater sensitivity to the public's likely behavior during a crisis. In order to make this happen, much greater cooperation and communication among the media, decision-makers, scientific community, and the public is imperative.[15]

Toward this end, processes and outcomes of risk assessment become a vital part of the collective management of risk. Such outcomes can include:

- Information gathering about risk (intelligence and surveillance)
- Coordination of intelligence and surveillance
- Dissemination of intelligence and surveillance
- Perspective building to establish norms and roles for terrorism-specific risk management
- Risk-management infrastructures for emergency/first response, community preparedness, and social support and restoration
- Crisis planning and response

In crisis situations, critical players must be able to assess a more representative picture of public knowledge and behavior than media reports or calls from frightened citizens.[16] "Relevant research agencies (universities, think tanks, or government) should establish the capacity to move quickly to the scene of a disaster and study immediate responses while they are occurring."[15] During times of crisis, understanding public opinion is critical, and allows crisis managers and public officials to determine what the public knows and believes, who they trust, and what actions they are likely to take. The time has come for a more responsive means of determining public knowledge and beliefs during a crisis. One way of responding to this challenge is through short-duration surveys. These measures truncate the time-consuming process of public-opinion surveys and have proven to be just as reliable and valid as traditional surveys. During the anthrax crisis of 2001, these surveys informed health authorities about (1) levels of public confidence in official messages, (2) precautions people were taking, (3) knowledge about treatment, and (4) attitudes toward vaccinations.[16] Generating public information of this nature is an essential step toward constructing the type of interactive communication process so necessary during crises.

Risk communication involves sources and targets at multiple levels. The individual level is often a target for risk-assessment messages (employees, public), groups and organizations (social groups, places of employment) play symmetrical roles in risk messages serving as both source and target, and the institutional level (government, scientific community) most often serves as a source of information dissemination. Although multiple levels exist where risk communication is directed, it is an inherently cross-level process where interaction among levels occurs both naturally and strategically.[17] For example, CDC's new emergency communication system consists of five audience-centered communication teams: media, federal partners, clinicians, public, and public-health partners, along with two media-communication teams (hotlines and website).[18]

### Benefits and Challenges

The benefits of risk communication include providing contexts and opportunities for assisting decision-makers with critical information, building trust among various stakeholders, and providing a forum for dialogue among various stakeholders involved in the process of risk management.[14]

Shortcomings of the risk communication process involve conflict and disorganization among stakeholders, inadequate planning and preparation processes, and lack of resources.[14] Moreover, risk communicators serve multiple audiences who are often dissatisfied with the communication process. Government officials, scientists, and members of the risk-management community feel that the public responds irrationally to risk information and has difficulties understanding and assimilating risk information. On the other hand, the lay public often distrusts risk messages and sometimes questions the authority or legitimacy of the message source.[14]

Agencies and organizations intent on communicating risk messages face large obstacles in getting serviceable and practical information in the hands of the public. They are particularly challenged in assembling a knowledge base on critical audience and message characteristics, including: (1) message effectiveness and competence, (2) suitability of the message source, (3) ethical and moral issues, and (4) the context of risk communication (where, how, and when information is presented).[14] Public trust in risk communication is a critical issue as well. Trust is diminished when there is a lack of agreement among experts, coordination among risk-management organizations, sensitivity to the communication needs of the audience, access or disclosure, and public participation in risk-management plans.[19]

Logic and best practices suggest a synergy between risks, crises, and issues. Issues can increase risks and result from risk perceptions and policy recommendations. Crises occur when risks manifest themselves. Poor crisis response can lead to increased risk and the emergence of issues. For these reasons, an issues-management approach can provide planning, increased standards of corporate responsibility, issue monitoring, and communication responses.[20]

## Local Mindset

A critical communication challenge is building a preparation mindset among members of the public through calculated, evolving, and cooperative activities using such venues as school programs, public education, public participation in planning processes, and educating and training citizen's groups.[14] During the anthrax crisis, the CDC placed field communicators at the source and released information locally by the scientists working the case. Information about local communication and activities was then communicated up to the national office, creating a reversal of previous communications procedures. Even the national media wanted information from the local source of the crisis.[21] Make no mistake—this phenomenon is real. At the local level, health officials (local health offices, and doctors or hospitals) are perceived to be the most trusted spokespersons during a bioterrorist event. If the crisis was at the national level, then CDC spokespersons were viewed as most trusted by this survey.[22]

## Processing Information

Targets of risk communication do not process information in a vacuum. How they perceive and evaluate risk information is influenced by their judgments of how others interpret and respond to these same messages. These significant others could be valued social groups, family members, trusted official sources, or occupational groups.[17] It is also important to remember that during crises, individuals experience difficulty in processing information. The urgency, uncertainty, and anxiety of the situation create cognitive distractions that hamper normal decision-making efforts. Humans have a tendency to expect the worst, which in turn affects their trust in normally respected sources of information. In order to respond effectively, messages must be crafted to maximize clarity, accuracy, and truthfulness.[23] In addition, context must be taken into consideration in messages. Context includes audience beliefs, competing messages, and earlier messages absorbed by receivers.[24]

Covello and colleagues have summarized some of the more significant issues to be considered in crafting messages for the public.[14] During crisis situations, receivers of messages are likely experiencing stress, which produces psychological and emotional distractions (termed the "mental noise model"). In order to compete with these distractions messages must be clear, concise, and memorable. A second factor to consider in crisis situations is the tendency that negative information is given greater weight than positive information (termed the "negative dominance model"). Message strategists must weigh the various pieces of information they feel are important to the audience and balance the negative and positive so that receivers do not over emphasize the negative aspects of the entire message. A third consideration is the issue of trust. Audiences must be able to trust the message and the messenger. In a "trust-determination model" trust has to be developed over time. When delivering messages, it helps to have third-party endorsement by credible people. Trust can also be enhanced when messages include care and empathy, dedication and commitment, competence and expertise, and honesty and openness. Aside from identifying the relevance of individual communicators in this risk-assessment and response model, the real challenge is to create and support a communication infrastructure that serves the collective needs of individuals. Ideas, opinions, protocols, and responses survive not because of the authority or credibility of individual sources, but because they serve the needs of the entire infrastructure.[20]

O'Hair and colleagues argue that messages are most likely responded to based on two processes: interpretation and evaluation.[25] During interpretation, receivers ask about the relevance of the message. Does the message really affect them? Is the message culturally appropriate? Are other messages competing for their attention? Evaluation suggests a process of weighing and interpreting the message. Do they understand the message as intended? Do they feel the message will help them? Did the message arrive on time? Do they trust the message and the messenger? Did the message cause the receivers to act in ways intended by the messenger? These questions can be used in developing an "audience profile" that will guide the crafting of messages.

## Involving the Media

The public has a tendency to want information from a variety of sources following a crisis, regardless of quality and reliability, and they want it from local governmental and nongovernmental sources and from federal sources.[26] The media play an almost omnipotent role in making this happen. Unfortunately, journalists may be some of the more poorly prepared players in a terrorism event. Research has shown that many journalists lack medical understanding for delivering accurate news and that they are more fearful and stressed during crises than the public.[26] We therefore need to improve media coverage by educating reporters, informing them quickly, involving them fully, and being forthright and honest. This would help to reduce sensationalistic reporting, superficial coverage of critical events and information, subjectivity, and low ethical and professional standards.[27] As a result, the general public and governmental officials will place greater faith in the media's role in communication and terrorism.

## Ethical and Professional Challenges

Communicating risk messages to the public carries with it some ethical responsibilities. Ethical risk communication can be judged by five values: (1) voice, or the extent to which targets participate in the communication process; (2) self-determination, or the level at which targets can determine their own actions; (3) honesty, or the extent to which the message exhibits conventional standards of honesty; (4) pluralism, or the level at which the message portrays multiple points of view; and (5) equality, or the level at which the message reaches and affects all members in the intended target audience.[17] Officials constructing risk-communication strategies should apply these standards to their messages. After all, the more a group perceives that it is being communicated to in an ethical, considered manner, the more likely it will be to trust the messages they are being asked to act on.

There are additional issues that will challenge those sending messages to the public.[28] First, how do officials (or even the media) decide when to withhold information from the public? Is it ethical to do so at all? If so, what are the parameters in making such a decision? How will this affect trust in the future? Another issue involves a long-term goal of making terrorism routine. Is it appropriate and ethical to help people integrate the threat of terrorism into their normalcy? Should we ask people to make the threat of terrorism part of the fabric of who they are? How about the importance of acknowledging uncertainty? Should risk messages ask the public to accept the fact that they cannot know with any level of certainty that terrorism is a threat for them? Finally, is it appropriate to over-reassure the public with messages? Or is it the responsibility of officials to be perfectly honest with the public and allow them to deal with their fear and uncertainty as reasonable decision-making human beings?

In sum, communicating with the public may be the most important issue for managing terrorism. Many of the chapters in the volume repeat the chorus for clear, effective, and honest communication in the context of terrorism threats, although many take very different approaches. Where government officials fall short is in investing adequate resources for an effective communication system. Until that challenge is met, the public will continue to remain skeptical about what it is told.

The events of previous terrorist crises sounded an alarm for greater preparedness among the various stakeholders who must respond in those emergency times. The time is long past for training public health officials, governors, city officials, and respected community leaders about the principles and practices of emergency risk communication.[29] These measures should include training in media relations and management, better interagency cooperation, and a greater sensitivity to literacy and cultural issues as they relate to communicating with the public.[30]

Terrorist attacks are different from natural disasters. They inflict more stress and psychological trauma and as such require a different preparation and response plan from mental-health organizations who are depended upon during emergency situations.[31] Although risk communication is a primary objective during crises, evidence suggests that many organizations are poorly prepared to provide this service. The 2001 anthrax attacks are a case in point. Furthermore, a survey of state mental-health departments revealed that few have a risk-communication plan in place or strategies for working with the media in the event of an attack.[31]

## INTERAGENCY COMMUNICATION

A wide range of agencies and organizations are affected by and concerned about terrorism. Such agencies include, but are not limited to, first responders (e.g., police, fire, hazardous materials, and other emergency rescue teams); healthcare organizations; public and environmental health officials; leaders and officials in communications, energy, transportation, and tourism; and federal, state, and local government leaders.

These agencies are well served to develop, revisit, and refine terrorism preparedness and response programs that facilitate effective communication and action.[32] Officials must consider not only how terrorist attacks may affect their own agencies, but other agencies with whom they are interdependent. The effects of terrorism often are amplified when considered in aggregate. For example, if an act of terrorism damages emergency-response systems and communication systems, people at a rescue site are doubly in peril.

Thus, interagency communication is prerequisite to the coordination of activity in preparation for and in response to terrorism. In order to reduce the potential for terrorism and to mitigate its effects, agencies must communicate effectively and responsively. Above all, they should be committed to working together as an integrated and unified team, to prepare for terrorism and to restore normality following an act of terrorism.[33] Many studies on interagency collaboration point to leadership as a key element in bringing disparate units together. It is imperative that leaders among these agencies develop a sense of shared values and trust as they work together for essential common goals.[34,35]

Preparedness for terrorism has been the province of several different U.S. government agencies, but historically their efforts have been deficient and disjointed.[36] Four months before the 9/11 attacks, President Bush named the Federal Emergency Management Agency (FEMA) as the chief agency in charge of coordinating federal, state, and local responses to terrorism. Although other federal agencies offer similar services, the president said, "To maximize their effectiveness, these efforts need to be seamlessly integrated, harmonious, and comprehensive."[37]

However, great strides are still needed to achieve "seamless" integration through interagency communication. For example, the FBI, CIA, and other intelligence agencies held information about al Qaeda prior to 9/11; however, the agencies did not effectively communicate to pool their intelligence and prevent the attacks.[38] Offering additional examples,

Alter reports that there are "no fewer than 11 different databases [that] are used by border-security agencies, none of which is compatible with the others; that agencies needing to communicate use different frequencies; that the nuclear-response teams (Department of Energy) and radiological-weapons response teams (Health and Human Services) are totally uncoordinated."[39]

It was not until after 9/11 that the president called for a new Office of Homeland Security and charged it with unifying homeland defense activity. The tremendous shift of responsibility from FEMA to the Office of Homeland Security in itself posed challenges. Some argue that Homeland Security Director Tom Ridge, who lacks power over personnel and budgets, was poorly positioned to effectively coordinate agencies under his command.[39]

Issues of power and politics also complicate interagency communication. Turf wars resulting from entrenched positions along historical or partisan lines impede effective coordination among agencies.[37] For example, when the military's four major regional commanders requested that FBI and Treasury Department agents join their staffs to improve coordination between military and civilian agencies, some administration officials balked.[39] Although the move would reduce bureaucratic delays for commanders (some of them ten time zones away from Washington), Washington officials worried that giving up agents would inflate the commanders' power and that the heads of the FBI and Treasury Department would "ultimately undercut the defense secretary's authority."[40]

### Elements of Effective Interagency Communication

A key element of effective communication is responsiveness to changing and emerging needs, conditions, and technologies. Agencies must perceive that sufficient preparation and response to terrorism never ends, but rather remains an ongoing challenge. They must remain open to new ideas and tools that augment their capacities and be flexible to changes. Indeed, the best preparedness and response plans include multiple contingency plans to facilitate prudent action in extraordinary times.[32] Agencies must recognize that even the best-laid plans demand modification in light of changed constraints and objectives. As such, plans should be reviewed periodically in light of environmental changes. For example, prior to September 11, 2001, few plans accounted for a commercial airliner flying into a building; the 9/11 attacks necessitated review and modification of plans.

## Technology

Technology can play a key role in enhancing responsiveness. FEMA encourages first responders to use an instant-messaging service to locate and talk to each other in case of a terrorist attack or other emergency situation. The technology is believed to be secure from hackers. Such technology may have cleared up confusion that hindered rescue efforts following the 9/11 attacks.[41]

While technology can enhance interagency communication, it can also be a source of crisis itself. Federal government agencies vary considerably in preventative measures they have taken to prevent cyberattack.[42] Moreover, although more than fifty federal agencies are responsible for protecting critical information cyberstructures, their efforts and policies are largely uncoordinated and even in conflict.

## Developing a Program

When developing preparedness and response programs, there are several key considerations. One first step is to develop a broad statement that describes the overall direction, policy, and message of the program.[43] A global message serves to orient collaborators who are internal and external to the agency. Moreover, agencies should take inventory of their resources, and design strategies for effective deployment of them.[43] In doing so, they should assess strengths and weaknesses in their organizational capacity to detect and respond to crises and to communicate with other collaborating agencies.[32] When programs are developed, they should be communicated in writing with clarity, precision, and concision, then disseminated to key parties.

## Testing Preparedness

How can agencies test their preparedness? The best check is to practice.[32,33] Actual enactment of response plans is the best way to anticipate strengths and weaknesses between individual agency and interagency action. Practice sessions, particularly when repeated under increasingly distressing circumstances, can underscore the need to update certain aspects of response plans. For example, in May 2003, an extensive exercise was enacted in response to a simulated terrorist attack in Seattle.[44] The exercise, which involved dozens of federal, state, and local agencies, was successful overall, although some failings were pinpointed to communication problems. Agencies seeking to improve their response to terrorism also can look toward other disaster recovery efforts for pointers. For example, the Homeland Security department has studied NASA's response to the *Columbia* disaster.[45]

NASA has been applauded for its smooth coordination of more than 130 federal, state, and local agencies that worked together to retrieve debris.

## CONCLUSION

Themes recur. One such theme is the battle between reaction and proaction. Without doubt, the attack on the World Trade Center and the Pentagon caught the nation in most aspects, if not all, in a reactionary mode. One valuable theme in this book is the advantage to be created by proaction. Proaction can strike at the root of terrorism and have infrastructures in place in the event that attacks occur.

The soundness of crisis preparation and response suggests that a crisis is both a potential and probable event that can affect business as usual. The timing of the event and its magnitude are often unpredictable, but preparation and prevention are not.

Policy often necessarily results from problem recognition and recovery. One aspiration of the authors of this book is the development of theoretical and best-practices guidelines that can assist in proactive preparation and response. Once embarrassment and outrage have served their usefulness, proaction can occur. Such efforts do not and should not occur in a vacuum. Generations of scholarship and best practices can be brought to bear to solve problems and create protocols. This book is intended to do so, in the spirit that risk management is a collective challenge and a rationale for society and professions. Communication scholars and professionals believe that by understanding the communication aspects of social problems, solutions based on communication can be offered for the betterment of society.

## NOTES

1. Koplan J. Communication during public health emergencies. J Health Commun 2003;8:144–5.

2. Douglas M. Risk and blame: essays on cultural theory. London: Routlegde Press; 1992.

3. Salmon C, Park H, Wrigley B. Optimistic bias and perceptions of bioterrorism in Michigan corporate spokespersons. Fall 2001 J Health Commun 2003;8:130–43.

4. Reid WH. Controlling political terrorism: practicality, not psychology. In: Stout CE, editor. The psychology of terrorism: a public understanding. Westport CT: Praeger Publishers; 2002. p. 1–8. (vol 1).

5. Perlman D. Intersubjective dimensions of terrorism and its transcendence. In: Stout CE, editor. The psychology of terrorism: a public understanding. Westport, CT: Praeger Publishers; 2002. p. 17–47. (vol 1).

6. O'Hair D, Friedrich G, Dixon L. Strategic communication in business and the professions. 5th ed. Boston: Houghton Mifflin; 2005.

7. Deutsch M, Coleman PT. The handbook of conflict resolution: theory and practice. San Francisco: Jossey-Bass; 2000.

8. Camara SK, Street T. Crisis uncertainty: a nation living in fear after the attack on America—war on terrorism. Iowa J Commun 2002;35(1):163–85.

9. Baker W. Achieving success through social capital. San Francisco: Jossey-Bass; 2000.

10. Kim Y, Ball-Rokeach S, Cohen E, Jung J. Communication infrastructure and civic actions in crisis. In: Greenberg B, editor. Communication terrorism: public and media responses to 9/11. Cresskill, NJ: Hampton Press; 2002. p. 289–304. Star, S. Bowker, G. How to infrastructure. In: Lievrouw LA Livingstone SM, editors. Handbook of new media: social shaping and consequences of ICTs. Thousand Oaks, CA: Sage; 2002; p. 151–162. Hirschbury P, Dillman D, Ball-Rokeach S. Media system dependency theory: Responses to Mt. St. Helens. In: Ball-Rokeach S, Cantor M, editors. Media, audience, and social structure. Beverly Hills: Sage; 1986. p. 117–26.

11. Fisher WR. Human communication as narration: toward a philosophy of reason, value, and action. Columbia, SC: University of South Carolina Press; 1987.

12. Grotberg EH. From terror to triumph: the path to resilience. In: Stout CE, editor. The psychology of terrorism: a public understanding. Westport, CT: Praeger Publishers; 2002. p. 185–208. (vol 1).

13. Social Capital Community Benchmark Survey. Available from: www.cfsv. org/communitysurvey.

14. Covello V, Peters R, Wojtecki J, Hyde R. Risk communication, the West Nile virus epidemic, and bioterrorism: responding to the communication challenges posed by the intentional or unintentional release of a pathogen in an urban setting. J Urban Health 2001;78:382–91.

15. Burke T. Regulating risk: the challenges ahead. In: Burke T, Tran N, Roemer J, Henry C, editors. Regulating risk: the science and politics of risk. Washington, DC: International Life Sciences Institute; 1993. p. 87–101.

16. Blendon R, Benson J, Desroches C, Weldon K. Using opinion surveys to track the public's response to a bioterrorist attack. J Health Commun 2003;8:83–92.

17. Rimal R, Flora J. Moving toward as framework for the study of risk communication: theoretical and ethical considerations. In: Burleson B, editor. Communication yearbook. Beverly Hills: Sage; 1995. p. 320–42. (vol 18).

18. Prue C, Lackey C, Swenarski L, Gantt J. Communication monitoring: shaping CDC's emergency risk communication efforts. J Health Commun 2003;8:35–49.

19. Shore D. Communicating in times of uncertainty: the need for trust. J Health Commun 2003;8:13–4.

20. Heath RL. Strategic issues management: organizations and public policy challenges. Thousand Oaks, CA: Sage Publications; 1997.

21. Robinson S, Newstetter W. Uncertain science and certain deadlines: CDC responses to the media during the anthrax attacks of 2001. J Health Commun 2003;8:17–34.

22. Pollard W. Public perceptions of information sources concerning bioterrorism before and after anthrax attacks: an analysis of national survey data. J Health Commun;8:93–103.

23. Rudd R, Comings J, Hyde J. Leave no one behind: improving health and risk communication through attention to literacy. J Health Commun 2003;8:104–15.

24. Vanderford M. Communication lessons learned in the emergency operations center during CDC's response: a commentary. J Health Commun 2003;8:11–2.

25. O'Hair D, O'Rourke J, O'Hair M. Business communication: a framework for success. Cincinnati: South-Western; 2001.

26. DiGiovanni C, Reynolds B, Harwell R, Stonecipher E, Burkle F. Community reaction to bioterrorism: prospective study of simulated outbreak. Emerg Infect Dis 2003;9:708–12.

27. Rowen F. Public participation and risk communication. Int J Emerg Ment Health 2003;4:253–8.

28. Sandman P. Bioterrorism risk communication policy. J Health Commun 2003;8:146–7.

29. Courtney J, Cole G, Reynolds B. How the CDC is meeting the training demands of emergency risk communication. J Health Commun 2003;8:128–9.

30. Payne J, Schulte S. Mass media, public health, and achieving health literacy. J Health Commun 2003;8:124–5.

31. Hall M, Norwood A, Fullerton C, Ursano R. Preparing for bioterrorism at the state level: report of an informal survey. Am J Orthopsychiatry 2002;72:486–91.

32. Kuhr S, Hauer JM. Intergovernmental preparedness and response to potential catastrophic biological terrorism. J Public Health Manag Prac 2000;6(4):50–6.

33. Hillier T. Bomb attacks in city centers. FBI Law Enforcement Bull 1994;63(9):13–7.

34. Einbinder SD, Robertson PJ, Garcia A, Vuckovic G, Patti RJ. Interorganizational collaboration in social service organizations: a study of the prerequisites to success. J Child Poverty 2000;6(2):119–40.

35. Foster MK, Meinhard AG. A regression model explaining predisposition to collaborate. Nonprofit Volunt Sect Q 2002;31:549–64.

36. Zuckerman MB. With the urgency of war. U.S. News World Rep 2002;132(21):64–5.

37. McCutcheon C. Members welcome Bush's plan for strengthening counterterrorism and urges [sic] more concrete action. CQ Wkly 2001; 59(19):1098.

38. Johnston D. Report of 9/11 panel cites lapses by C.I.A. and F.B.I. The New York Times 2003 Jul 25;Sect A:1 (col. 5).

39. Alter J. Better late than never. Newsweek 2002;139(24):33.

40. Schmitt E. 4 commanders seek staff role for the F.B.I. The New York Times 2001 Nov 20;Sect A:1 (col. 5).

41. FEMA's instant messaging service. Fire Eng 2003;156(7):48.

42. Mecham M. Cyber uncoordinated. Aviat Week Space Technol 2002; 157(5):17.

43. Fabian N. Post September 11: some reflections on the role of environmental health in terrorism response. J Environ Health 2002;64(9): 78–80.

44. Kershaw S. Terror scenes follow script of no more 9/11's. The New York Times 2003 May 13;Sect. A:21 (col. 1).

45. Covault C. Homeland legacy. Aviat Week Space Technol 2003;158(19): 33–4.

# Appendix:
# Resource Centers

## EMERGENCY CONTACTS

Centers for Disease Control and Prevention (CDC) emergency response
line: (770) 488-7100
National Domestic Preparedness Office (for civilian use): (202) 324-9025
National Response Center (for chemical-biological hazards and terrorist
events): 1-800-424-8802, (202) 267-2675
United States Department of Defense, United States Army Soldier and
Biological Chemical Command, Domestic Preparedness Office: (410)
436-3382
USAMRIID emergency response line: (888) 872-7443

## FEDERAL AGENCIES:
## EMERGENCY OPERATIONS CENTERS

Alaska Volcanic Observatory: (907) 786-7497
Aviation Weather Center, Storm Prediction Center: (816) 58-3427
Canada Government Emergency Operations Coordination Center: (613)
991-7000
Department of Defense (DTRA)/Department of Energy: (703) 325-2102,
(703) 325-2102, (505) 845-4667
Department of State Operations Center: (202) 647-1512
FBI Operations Center (Washington, DC): (202) 324-6700
FEMA Alternate Operations Center (FAOC): (912) 225-4756, 1-800-792-6196
FEMA Disaster Finance Center (Berryville, VA): (540) 542-7300

FEMA Disaster Information Systems Clearing House: (540) 542-2189
FEMA Hyattsville National Processing Service Center: (301) 209-4000
FEMA MERS Operations Center (MOC) (Denver, CO): (303) 235-4847, 1-800-311-7021
FEMA MERS Operations Center (MOC) (Maynard, MA): (978) 461-5501, 1-800-213-8965
FEMA MERS Operations Center (MOC) (Thomasville, GA).
FEMA MERS Operations Center (MOC) (TX): (940) 898-5280, 1-800-260-5110
FEMA MERS Operations Center (MOC) (WA): (425) 487-4449, 1-800-395-6042
FEMA Operations Center (FOC): (202) 898-6100, (540) 665-6100, 1-800-634-7084
FEMA Mount Weather Operator: (202) 566-1600
FEMA National Emergency Training Center: (301) 447-1000
FEMA National Interagency Emergency Operations Center (NIEOC): (202) 646-2470
FEMA National Processing Service Center (Denton, TX): (940) 891-8500
FEMA National Teleregistration Center (Denton, TX): (940) 591-7100
FEMA National Teleregistration Center (Mt. Weather, Berryville, VA): (540) 542-7109
FEMA Virginia National Processing Service Center (Mt. Weather, Berryville, VA): (540) 542-7717
Joint Nuclear Accident Coordinating Center (JNACC)
National Centers for Environmental Predictions (Kansas City, MO)
National Coordinating Center for Telecommunications (NCS): (703) 607-4900
National Hurricane Center: (305) 229-4470
National Interagency Coordination Center (Boise, ID): (208) 387-5400
National Interagency Fire Center (Boise, ID): (208) 387-5512
National Interagency Fire Desk (Washington, DC): (202) 205-1450
National Response Center: 1-800-424-8802
National Weather Service, general/severe weather information, local and extended forecast (recording), river-stage forecasts (recording), Washington, DC weather information: (703) 260-0209, (703) 260-0307, (703) 260-0305, (703) 260-0105
Nuclear Regulatory Commission Operations Center (301) 816-5100
Office of the Secretary of Defense Crisis Coordination Center: (703) 769-9320
Tsunami Warning Center (Alaska): (907) 745-5235
Tsunami Warning Center (Hawaii): (808) 689-6655
Typhoon Warning Center (Guam): (671) 344-4224

U.S. Marshals Service (Washington, DC): (202) 307-9100; 1-800-336-0102

USGS National Earthquake Information Center, 24-hour recorded message: (303) 273-8500, (303) 273-8516

White House Situation Room: (202) 456-9431

## UNITED STATES DEPARTMENT OF DEFENSE MILITARY COMMANDS

Director of Military Support (DOMS) (for after-duty hours, use Army Operations Center): (703) 697-3203

Fifth U.S. Army (Fort Sam Houston, TX): (210) 221-2955

First U.S. Army (Fort Gillem, GA): (404) 469-3280, (404) 469-3288

National Airborne Operations Center (NAOC): (402) 422-1891

National Military Command Center (NMCC): (703) 697-6340

U.S. Air Force Operations Center: (703) 695-7220

U.S. Army Forces Command (FORSCOM): (404) 464-5222

U.S. Army National Guard Command Center: (703) 607-9350

U.S. Army Operations Center: (703) 697-0218

U.S. Atlantic Command (USACOM): (757) 322-6000; DSN 262-6000

U.S. Coast Guard Command Post: (202) 267-2100

U.S. Marine Corps Operations Center: (703) 695-7366

U.S. Navy Operations Center: (703) 695-0231

U.S. Pacific Command (USPACOM): (808) 477-7227

U.S. Transportation Command (TRANSCOM) mobility control center (MCC): (618) 256-8105

## FEDERAL EMERGENCY MANAGEMENT AGENCY (FEMA) REGIONAL OPERATIONS CENTERS

| Region | Office Number | Fax Number | Stu-III Number |
|--------|---------------|------------|----------------|
| I | (978) 461-5400 | (978) 461-5415 | (978) 461-2947 |
| II | (212) 225-7258 | (212) 225-7252 | (212) 225-7033 |
| III | (215) 931-5757 | (215) 931-5590 | (215) 931-5757 |
| IV | (770) 220-5600 | (770) 220-5435 | (770) 220-5283 |
| V | (312) 408-5304 | (312) 408-5302 | (312) 408-5462/5560 |
| VI | (940) 898-5433 | (940) 898-5231 | (940) 898-5375 |
| VII | (816) 283-7600 | (816) 283-7601 | (816) 283-7605 |
| VIII | (303) 235-4779 | (303) 235-4777 | (303) 235-4787/4946 |
| IX | (415) 923-7091 | (415) 923-7050 | (415) 923-7004 |
| X | (425) 487-4660 | (425) 487-4471 | (425) 487-4633 |

## STATE EMERGENCY MANAGEMENT OFFICES

Director, Alabama Emergency Management Agency
5898 County Road 41
P.O. Drawer 2160
Clanton, AL 35046-2160
Ph: (205) 280-2285
Fax: (205) 280-2444
URL: www.aema.state.al.us/

Director, Alaska Division of Emergency Services
P.O. Box 5750
Fort Richardson, AK 99505-5750
Ph: (907) 428-7039
Fax: (907) 428-7009
URL: www.ak-prepared.com

Director, Arizona Division of Emergency Services
5636 East McDowell Road.
Phoenix, AZ 85008
Ph: (602) 231-6245
Fax: (602) 231-6356
URL: www.state.az.us/es/

Director, Arkansas Department of Emergency Management
P.O. Box 758
Conway, AR 72033
Fax: (501) 730-9754
URL: www.adem.state.ar.us/

Director, California Office of Emergency Services
2800 Meadowview Rd.
Sacramento, CA 95832
Ph: (916) 262-1816
Fax: (916) 262-1677
URL: www.oes.ca.gov/

Director, Colorado Office of Emergency Management
Division of Local Government
Department of Local Affairs
15075 South Golden Rd.
Golden, CO 80401-3979
Ph: (303) 273-1622

Fax: (303) 273-1795
URL: www.dola.state.co.us/oem/oemindex.htm

Director, Connecticut Office of Emergency Management
Department of Public Safety
360 Broad Street St.
Hartford, CT 06105
Ph: (203) 566-4343
Fax: (203) 247-0664
URL: www.mil.state.ct.us/OEM.htm

Director, Delaware Emergency Management Agency
165 Brick Store Landing Rd.
Smyrna, DE 19977
Ph: (302) 659-3362
Fax: (302) 659-6855
E-mail: jmulhern@state.de.us
URL: www.state.de.us/dema/hW1min62x.htm

Director, District of Columbia Emergency Management Agency
2000 14th Street, NW, 8th Floor
Washington, DC 20009
Ph: (202) 727-6161
Fax: (202) 673-2290
URL: www.dcema.dc.gov

Director, State of Florida Division of Emergency Management
2555 Shumard Oak Blvd.
Tallahassee, FL 32399
Ph: (904) 413-9969
Fax: (904) 488-1016
E-mail: Joe.Myers@dca.state.fl.us
URL: www.floridadisaster.org

Director, Georgia Emergency Management Agency
P.O. Box 18055
Atlanta, GA 30316-0055
Ph: (404) 624-7000
Fax: (404) 635-7205
URL: www.State.Ga.US/GEMA/

Vice Director, Hawaii State Civil Defense
3949 Diamond Head Rd.

Honolulu, HI 96816-4495
Ph: (808) 734-2161
Fax: (808) 733-4287
E-Mail: gburnett@scd.state.hi.us
URL: scd.state.hi.us

State Director, Idaho Bureau of Disaster Services
4040 Guard Street, Bldg. 600
Boise, ID 83705-5004
Ph: (208) 334-3460
Fax: (208) 334-2322
E-mail: jcline@bds.state.id.us
URL: www.state.id.us/bds/bds.html

Director, Illinois Emergency Management Agency
110 East Adams St.
Springfield, IL 62701
Ph: (217) 782-2700
Fax: (217) 785-6043
URL: www.state.il.us/iema

Director, Indiana Emergency Management Agency and Department of
Fire and Building Services
302 West Washington Street, Room E-208
Indianapolis, IN 46204-2760
Ph: (317) 232-3980
Fax: (317) 232-3895
URL: www.ai.org/sema/hW1min62x.html

Administrator, Iowa Division of Emergency Management
Department of Public Defense
Des Moines, IA 50319
Ph: (515) 281-3231
Fax: (515) 281-7539
E-mail: dsanders@max.state.ia.us
URL: www.state.ia.us/government/dpd/emd/hW1min62x.htm

Deputy Director, Kansas Division of Emergency Preparedness
2800 S.W. Topeka Blvd.
Topeka, KS 66611-1287
Ph: (913) 274-1401
Fax: (913) 274-1426
E-mail: genek@agtop.wpo.state.ks.us
URL: www.ink.org/public/kdem/

Executive Director, State of Kentucky Office of Disaster and
Emergency Services
EOC Building
Boone National Guard Center
Frankfort, KY 40601-6168
Ph: (502) 564-8682
Fax: (502) 564-8614
E-mail: rpadgett@kydes.dma.state.ky.us
URL: webserve.dma.state.ky.us

Assistant Director, Louisiana Office of Emergency Preparedness
P.O. Box 44217
Baton Rouge, LA 70804
Ph: (225) 342-1583
Fax: (225) 342-5471
URL: www.loep.state.la.us

Director, Maine Emergency Management Agency
State Office Building, Station 72
Augusta, ME 04333
Ph: (207) 287-4080
Fax: (207) 287-4079
E-mail: john.w.libby@state.me.us
URL: www.state.me.us/mema/memahome.htm

Director, Maryland Emergency Management Agency
Camp Fretterd Military Reservation
5401 Rue Saint Lo Dr.
Reistertown, MD 21136
Ph: (410) 517-3600
Fax: (410) 517-3610
Toll-free: (877) 636-2872
E-mail: dmcmillion@mema.state.md.us
URL: www.mema.state.md.us/

Director, Massachusetts Emergency Management Agency
400 Worcester Rd.
P.O. Box 1496
Framingham, MA 01701-0317
Ph: (508) 820-2010
Fax: (508) 727-4764

E-mail: drodham_EPS@state.ma.us
URL: www.magnet.state.ma.us/mema/homepage.htm

Deputy State Director, Michigan Division of Emergency Management
4000 Collins Rd.
P.O. Box 30636
Lansing, MI 48909-8136
Ph: (517) 336-6198
Fax: (517) 333-4987
URL: www.msp.state.mi.us/division/emd/emdweb1.htm

Director, Minnesota Division of Emergency Management
Department of Public Safety
Suite 2231
444 Cedar St.
St. Paul, MN 55101-6223
Ph: (612) 296-0450
Fax: (612) 296-0459
URL: www.dps.state.mn.us/emermgt/

Director, Mississippi Emergency Management Agency
1410 Riverside Dr.
P.O. Box 4501, Fondren Station
Jackson, MS 39296-4501
Ph: (601) 352-9100
Toll-free: 1-800-442-6362
Fax: (601) 352-8314
URL: www.mema.state.ms.us or www.memaorg.com

Director, State of Missouri Emergency Management Agency
P.O. Box 116
2302 Militia Dr.
Jefferson City, MO 65102
Ph: (573) 526-9146
Fax: (573) 634-7966
E-mail: mosema@mail.state.mo.us
URL: www.sema.state.mo.us/semapage.htm

Administrator, Montana Division of Disaster and Emergency Services
1100 North Main
P.O. Box 4789
Helena, MT 59604-4789
Ph: (406) 444-6911

Fax: (406) 444-6965
URL: www.state.mt.us/dma/des/index.shtml

Assistant Director, Nebraska State Civil Defense Agency
National Guard Center
1300 Military Rd.
Lincoln, NE 68508-1090
Ph: (402) 471-7410
Fax: (402) 471-7433
E-mail: krogman@nrcdec.nrc.state.ne.us
URL: www.nol.org/home/nmd/nema.htm

Chief, Nevada Division of Emergency Management
Capitol Complex
2525 South Carson St.
Carson City, NV 89701
Ph: (702) 687-4240
Fax: (702) 687-6788
E-mail: bowen@sierra.net
URL: www.state.nv.us/dmv_ps/emermgt.htm

Director, New Hampshire Governor's Office of Emergency Management
State Office Park South
107 Pleasant Street
Concord, NH 03301
Ph: (603) 271-2231
Fax: (603) 225-7341
URL: none

Deputy State Director, New Jersey Office of Emergency Management
P.O. Box 7068, Old River Rd.
West Trenton, NJ 08628-0068
Ph: (609) 538-6050
Fax: (609) 538-0345
URL: www.state.nj.us/lps/njsp/outfit-p.html

Director, New Mexico Division of Emergency Management
Department of Public Safety
P.O. Box 1628
13 Bataan Blvd.
Santa Fe, NM 87504-1628
Ph: (505) 476-9600

Fax: (505) 476-9650
URL: www.dps.nm.org/emc.htm

Director, New York State Emergency Management Office
22 Security Building, State Campus
Albany, NY 12226-5000
Ph: (518) 457-9996
Fax: (518) 457-9995
URL: www.nysemo.state.ny.us/

Director, North Carolina Division of Emergency Management
116 West Jones St.
Raleigh, NC 27603
Ph: (919) 733-3718
Fax: (919) 733-5406
URL: www.dem.dcc.state.nc.us/

Director, North Dakota Division of Emergency Management
P.O. Box 5511
Bismarck, ND 58506-5511
Ph: (701) 328-8100
Fax: (701) 328-8181
E-mail: dfriez@state.nd.us
URL: www.state.nd.us/dem

Deputy Director, Ohio Emergency Management Agency
2825 W. Dublin Granville Rd.
Columbus, OH 43235-2206
Ph: (614) 889-7150
Fax: (614) 889-7183
URL: www.state.oh.us/odps/division/ema/

Director, Oklahoma Department of Civil Emergency Management
P.O. Box 53365
Oklahoma City, OK 73152
Ph: (405) 521-2481
Fax: (405) 521-4053
URL: www.onenet.net/~odcem/

Director, Oregon Division of Emergency Management
595 Cottage Street, NE
Salem, OR 97310

Ph: (503) 378-2911 ext. 225
Fax: (503) 588-1378
URL: www.osp.state.or.us/oem/oem.htm

Director, Pennsylvania Emergency Management Agency
2605 Interstate Dr.
Harrisburg, PA 17110-9364
Ph: (717) 651-2001
Fax: (717) 651-7800
URL: www.pema.state.pa.us/

Director, Rhode Island Emergency Management Agency
645 New London Ave.
Cranston, RI 02920-3003
Ph: (401) 946-9996
Fax: (401) 941-1891
URL: www.state.ri.us/riema/riemaaa.html

Director, South Carolina Emergency Preparedness Division
Office of the Adjutant General
1100 Fish Hatchery Rd.
West Columbia, SC 29172
Ph: (803) 737-8500
Fax: (803) 737-8570
E-mail: mckinney@strider.epd.state.sc.us
URL: www.state.sc.us/epd/

Director, South Dakota Division of Emergency Management
500 East Capitol
Pierre, SD 57501-5070
Ph: (605) 773-3233
Fax: (605) 773-3580
E-mail: garyw@dem.state.sd.us
URL: www.state.sd.us/state/executive/military/sddem.htm

Director, Tennessee Emergency Management Agency
3041 Sidco Drive
P.O. Box 41502
Nashville, TN 37204-1502
Ph: (615) 741-6528
Fax: (615) 242-9635
URL: www.tnema.org

State Coordinator, Texas Division of Emergency Management
Department of Public Safety
P.O. Box 4087, North Austin
Austin, TX 78733-0225
Ph: (512) 465-2443
Fax: (512) 424-2444
URL: www.txdps.state.tx.us/dem/

Director, Utah Division of Comprehensive Emergency Management
State Office Building, Room 1110
Salt Lake City, UT 84114
Ph: (801) 538-3400
URL: www.cem.ps.state.ut.us/

Director, Vermont Division of Emergency Management
Waterbury State Complex
103 South Main Street
Waterbury, VT 05671-2101
Ph: (802) 244-8721
Fax: (802) 244-8655
URL: www.dps.state.vt.us/

Director, Puerto Rico Civil Defense Agency
Office of the Governor
P.O. Box 5127
San Juan, PR 00906
Ph: (809) 724-0124
Fax: (809) 725-4244
URL: None

Deputy Director, Virgin Islands Office of Civil Defense and
Emergency Services
102 Estate Atmon
St. Croix, VI 00820
Ph: (809) 773-2244
Fax: (809) 774-1491
URL: None

State Coordinator, Virginia Department of Emergency Management
10501 Trade Ct.
Richmond, VA 23236-3713
Ph: (804) 897-6502

Fax: (804) 897-6506
URL: www.vdem.state.va.us

Director, Washington State Emergency Management Division
Building 20, M/S: TA-20
Camp Murray, WA 98430-5122
Ph: (253) 512-7000
Fax: (253) 512-7200
URL: www.wa.gov/wsem/

State Director, West Virginia Office of Emergency Services
Main Capitol Building, Room EB-80
Charleston, WV 25305-0360
Ph: (304) 558-5380
Fax: (304) 344-4538
URL: www.state.wv.us/wvoes

Administrator, Wisconsin Division of Emergency
Government
2400 Wright St.
P.O. Box 7865
Madison, WI 53707
Ph: (608) 242-3232
Fax: (608) 242-3247
URL: badger.state.wi.us/agencies/dma/wem/hW1min62x.htm

Coordinator, Wyoming Emergency Management Agency
5500 Bishop Blvd.
Cheyenne, WY 82009
Ph: (307) 777-4920
Fax: (307) 635-6017
E-mail: wema@wy-iso.army.mil
URL: wema.state.wy.us

Manager, American Samoa Territorial Emergency Management
Coordination
Department of Public Safety
P.O. Box 1086
Pago Pago, AS 96799
Ph: (011) (684) 633-2331
Fax: (684) 633-2300
URL: None

Director, Guam Division of Civil Defense Emergency Services Office
P.O. Box 2877
Agana, GU 96910
Ph: (011) (671) 477-9841
Fax: (671) 477-3727
URL: ns.gov.gu/

Civil Defense Coordinator, Mariana Islands Office of Civil Defense
Capitol Hill
Saipan, Mariana Islands 96950
Ph: (011) (670) 322-9529
Fax: (670) 322-2545
URL: None

Civil Defense Coordinator, Republic of the Marshall Islands
P.O. Box 15
Majuro, Republic of the Marshall Islands 96960
Ph: (011) (692) 730-3232
Fax: (692) 625-3649
URL: None

Special Assistant to the President of Micronesia Disaster Coordination
Office of the President
P.O. Box 490
Kolonia, Pohnpei, Micronesia 96941
Ph: (011) (691) 320-2822
Fax: (691) 320-2785
URL: None

Palau NEMO Coordinator
Office of the President
P.O. Box 100
Koror, Republic of Palau 96940
Ph: (011) (680) 488-2422
Fax: (680) 488-3312
URL: None

## WORLD HEALTH ORGANIZATION WORLDWIDE WEB ADDRESSES

Control of tropical diseases: www.who.ch/ctd/

Dealing with a cholera emergency—essential information: www.who.ch/chd/pub/cholera/cholemer.htm

Emerging and other communicable diseases surveillance and control (EMC): www.who.ch/emc/

Guidelines for cholera control: www.who.ch/chd/pub/cholera/cholguid.htm

Pan American Health Organization (PAHO): www.paho.org/PAHO disasters preparedness and mitigation in the Americas: www.paho.org/spanish/ped/pedhome.htm

Weekly Epidemiological Record, World Health Organization (WHO-WER) www.who.ch/wer/wer_home.htm

WHO global program for vaccines: www.who.ch/gpv/

## UNITED NATIONS' WORLDWIDE WEB ADDRESSES

Detailed collection of economic data and socio-economic indicators published by the World Bank. Standardized data presented for numerous individual countries (161 in the 1994 edition) make this an ideal reference for international comparisons: www.ciesin.org/IC/wbank/wtables.html

Global Information and Early Warning System on Food and Agriculture (FAO-GIEWS): www.fao.org/giews

OCHA emergency information by country or region: www.reliefweb.int/dha_ol/contlist.html

References to refugee, human rights, and related literature: www.unhcr.ch/refworld/refbib/biblio/reflit.htm

UNAIDS: www.unaids.org

United Nations Children Fund (UNICEF): www.unicef.org/

United Nations Development Programme (UNDP): www.undp.org

United Nations International Decade for Natural Disaster Reduction (IDNDR): www.idndr.org

United Nations Office for the Coordination of Humanitarian Affairs—OCHA online humanitarian report, 1997: www.reliefweb.int/dha_ol/pub/humrep97/index.html

UNRISD War Torn Societies Project: www.unicc.org/unrisd/wsp/

UN Subcommittee on Nutrition (UN-SCN): www.unsystem.org/accscn

World Bank: www.worldbank.org

World Food Programme (WFP): www.wfp.org/

## INTERNATIONAL ORGANIZATIONS' WORLDWIDE WEB ADDRESSES

Gemini: www.oneworld.org/gemini

International Organization for Migration (IOM): www.iom.ch/

Maps, facts and figures, reports, news releases, and publications on the countries (over fifty) in which the ICRC is currently active: www.icrc.org

Regional Disaster Information Centre (Latin American-Caribbean) (CRID): www.disaster.info.desastres.net/crid
Reporting on Red Cross/Red Crescent action as it happens: www.ifrc.org/

## EMERGENCY REFERENCE SITES

AlertNet: www.alertnet.org/alertnet.nsf/?OpenDatabase
American College of Emergency Physicians (ACEP): www.acep.org
Asian Disaster Preparedness Center, AIT (ADPC): www.adpc.ait.ac.th
ATSDR's Hazardous Substance Release and Health Effects Database; Agency for Toxic Substances and Disease Registry: atsdr1.atsdr.cdc.gov:8080/hazdat.html
British Columbia Earthquake Response Plan: hoshi.cic.sfu.ca/~pep/eqplanaa.html
Brown University Humanitarianism and War Project: www.brown.edu/Departments/Watson_Institute/H_W/H_W_ms.shtml
Centers for Disease Control and Prevention, Atlanta: www.cdc.gov
Complex Emergencies Response and Transition Initiative: www.tulane.edu/~CERTI/certi.html
CRED, Catholic University of Louvain: www.md.ucl.ac.be/entites/esp/epid/misson/
Databases on emergency statistics and bibliographic references (CRED): www.md.ucl.ac.be/entites/esp/epid/mission
Emerging infectious diseases: www.cdc.gov/ncidod/EID/eidtext.htm
Famine Early Warning System (FEWS): www.fews.org
Federal Emergency Management Agency, USA: www.fema.gov/EMI/edu/higher.htm
General information on tsunamis, their effects, and population response mechanism: swww.geophys.washington.edu/tsunami/intro.html
Global Disaster Information Network: members.nova.org/~lroeder/info.htm
Hazardnet is a new informational service for natural and technological hazards. Good links from this site on a variety of hazard information: hoshi.cic.sfu.ca/~hazard/
Humanity Development Library: www.oneworld.org/globalproject/humcdrom
International Emergency and Refugee Health Program (CDC): www.cdc.gov/nceh/programs/internat/ierh/ierh.htm
Links to a variety of hazard mitigation information: www.fema.gov/
Medicine and global survival (M&GS): www.healthnet.org/MGS/
Morbidity and Mortality Weekly Report, CDC, Atlanta: www.cdc.gov/epo/mmwr/mmwr_wk.html
National Disaster Medical System, Health and Human Services: www.oeps_ndms.dhhs.gov

National Library of Medicine, Natural Hazards Center: Research and applications, information center–Colorado: www.nlm.nih.gov/databases/freemedl.html

An online information service addressing emerging diseases: www.outbreak.org/cgi-unreg/dynaserve.exe/index.html

Oxford University Refugee Studies Programme: www.qeh.ox.ac.uk/rsp/

UCLA Center for Public Health and Disaster Relief: www.ph.ucla.edu/cphdr/

University of Buffalo, National Center for Earthquake Engineering Research: nceer.eng.buffalo.edu

University of Colorado Natural Hazards Center: www.Colorado.EDU/hazards/

University of Hawaii Center of Excellence in Disaster Management and Humanitarian Assistance: website.tamc.amedd.army.mil/

University of Pittsburgh Global Disaster Health Network: www.pitt.edu/%7Eghdnet/GHDNet/

University of Wisconsin Disaster Management Center: www.engr.wisc.edu/dmc/

U.S. Centers for Disease Control and Prevention (CDC): www.cdc.gov

U.S. Committee on Refugees: www.refugees.org

Volunteers in Technical Assistance (VITA): www.vita.org

WorldAid: www.worldaid.org

## NONGOVERNMENT ORGANIZATIONS' WORLDWIDE WEB ADDRESSES

Adventist Development and Relief Agency (ADRA): www.adra.org

African Research and Medical Foundation (AMREF): www.amref.org/

Association of Medical Doctors of Asia: www.amda.or.jp/econtents/news/apro.html

CARE: www.care.org

Christian Aid: www.christian-aid.org.uk/main.htm

Church World Service (CWS): www.ncccusa.org/CWS/emre/

Doctors without Borders USA: www.dwb.org/index.htm

Food for the Hungry: www.fh.org/wcn/index.html

InterAction: www.interaction.org/

International Medical Corps: www.imc-la.com/

Lutheran World Relief: www.lwr.org

Médecins Sans Frontières (MSF): www.msf.org

Norwegian Refugee Council: web.sol.no/nrc-no/

Oxfam: www.oneworld.org/oxfam/

Refugees International: www.refintl.org/

Save the Children UK (SCF): www.oneworld.org/scf/
Save the Children USA: www.savethechildren.org/
World Vision USA: www.wvi.xc.org/

## INTERNATIONAL GOVERNMENT ORGANIZATIONS' WORLDWIDE WEB ADDRESSES

Central Intelligence Agency: www.odci.gov/cia
European Community Humanitarian Office (ECHO): europa.eu.int/en/comm/echo/echo.html
Intergovernmental Conference on Emergency Telecommunications: www.itu.int/newsroom/projects/ICET/
North Atlantic Treaty Organization: www.nato.int
OFDA: www.info.usaid.gov/hum_response/
U.K. Department for International Development (DID): www.oneworld.org:80/oda/index.html
U.S. Agency for International Development (USAID): www.info.usaid.gov

## NEWS AGENCIES' WORLDWIDE WEB ADDRESSES

*The Economist*: www.economist.com
*The Guardian*: www.guardian.co.uk/
*MSNBC*: www.msnbc.com
*Nando Times*: www.nando.net
*New York Times*: www.nytimes.com
*One World*: www.oneworld.org
*PanAfrican*: www.africanews.org/PANA/news
*The Times*: www.the-times.co.uk
*USA Today*: www.usatoday.com/usafront.htm
*Voice of America*: gopher.voa.gov

## JOURNALS' WORLDWIDE WEB ADDRESSES

*Annals of Emergency Medicine*: www.acep.org/annals
*British Medical Journal*: www.bmj.com/bmj/
*Journal of Infectious Diseases*: www.journals.uchicago.edu/JID/
*Journal of the American Medical Association (JAMA)*: www.ama.assn.org/public/journals/jama
*The Lancet*: www.thelancet.com/
*The Medical News*: www.themedicalnews.com
*New England Journal of Medicine (NEJM)*: www.nejm.org

# INFORMATION ABOUT BIOLOGICAL AGENTS

Cordesman AH. *Defending America Redefining the conceptual borders of homeland defense: Biotechnology and biological weapons.* Center for Strategic and International Studies, 1800 K Street NW, Washington, DC 20006, (202) 775-3270. Available from: www.csis.org, listed under Homeland Defense.

Cordesman AH. *Defending America Redefining the conceptual borders of homeland defense: The risks and effects of indirect, covert, terrorist, and extremist attacks with weapons of mass destruction—Challenges for defense and response.* Center for Strategic and International Studies, 1800 K Street NW, Washington, DC 20006. Telephone: (202) 775-3270.

U.S. Department of Defense, U.S. Army Soldier and Biological Chemical Command, Domestic Preparedness Office. *Improving local and state agency response to terrorist incidents involving biological weapons.* Prepared in response to the Nunn-Lugar-Domenici domestic preparedness program. 2000 Aug 1. Telephone: (410) 436-3382.

# INFORMATION ABOUT CHEMICAL AND HAZARDOUS AGENTS

Agency for Toxic Substances and Disease Registry, Hazardous Substance Release/Health Effects Database: atsdr1.atsdr.cdc.gov:8080/hazdat.html

Biological agent information papers, USAMRIID: www.nbc-med.org/BioAgents.html

CBDCOM website homepage: www.apgea.army.mil

CBIAC homepage: www.cbiac.apgea.army.mil

Centers for Disease Control and Prevention: www.cdc.gov

Chemicals in the environment: OPPT chemical fact sheets: www.epa.gov/chemfact/

Cordesman, AH. *Defending America Redefining the conceptual borders of homeland defense: The risks and effects of indirect, covert, terrorist, and extremist attacks with weapons of mass destruction—Challenges for defense and response.* Center for Strategic and International Studies, 1800 K Street NW, Washington, DC 20006. Telephone: (202) 775-3270.

Decontamination: 206.39.77.2/dmcr/NBC/chemicas/Decontam.htm

Disaster Management Central resource: 206.39.77.2/DMCR/dmrhome.html

Disaster preparedness, decontamination, and chemical warfare: www.infotrieve.com/healthworld/preview

Emergency Response and Research Institute: www.emergency.com

ERDEC safety office material safety data sheets: www.cbdcom.apgea.army.mil

Fire science information: www.firesci.com

Hazardous materials operations page: www.emergency.com/hzmtpage.htm

HAZMAT information: www.emergency.com

NBC Medical Defense Library: 206.39.77.2/DMCR/dmrhome.html

Northwest Fisheries Science Center: material safety data sheet searches: research.nwfsc.noaa.gov/msds.html

Nuclear, biological, and chemical medical website with field manual 8-285: www.nbc-med.org

Organization for the Prohibition of Chemical Weapons (OPCW) in The Hague, the Netherlands. OPWC is responsible for implementing the Chemical Weapons Convention (CWC). *Decontamination of chemical warfare agents: An introduction to methods and chemicals for decontamination*: www.opcw.nl/chemhaz/decon.htm

U.S. Department of Defense, U.S. Army Soldier and Biological Chemical Command, Domestic Preparedness Office, Chemical Team. *Guidelines for responding to a chemical weapons incident*. Prepared in response to the Nunn-Lugar-Domenici domestic preparedness program. 2001, Mar. Telephone (410) 436-3382.

U.S. Department of Health and Human Services, Public Health Service, Agency for Toxic Substance and Disease Registry; recommendations from their website entitled *Unidentified chemical pre-hospital management*. "Medical management guidelines for acute chemical exposures": aepo-xdv-www.epo.cdc.gov/wonder/prevguid

U.S. Department of Transportation, Transport Canada, and the Secretariat of Transport and Communication Mexico. *2000 Emergency response guidebook: A guidebook for first responders during the initial phase of a dangerous goods/ hazardous materials incident*. 2000 Jan. Telephone: (202) 366-4900.

USAD Health and Human Services homepage: www.os.dhhs.gov/

USAMRICD open literature publications and books, 1981–1996: chemdef. apgea.army.mil/instbilb.htm

## INFORMATION ON RADIOLOGICAL AND NUCLEAR CRISIS

U.S. Department of Defense, Military Medical Operations Office, Armed Forces Radiobiology Research Institute. *Medical management of radiological casualties handbook*, 1st ed. Bethesda, MD 20889-5603. 1999 Dec. Available from: www.afrri.usuhs.mil.

# Bibliography

## GENERAL

Advisory Panel to Assess Domestic Response Capabilities for Terrorism Involving Weapons of Mass Destruction. Toward a national strategy for combating terrorism. Second annual report to the President and the Congress. Governor Gilmore III. Cover letter. 2000 Dec 15. p. 4–5.

Commission to Assess the Organization of the Federal Government to Combat the Proliferation of Weapons of Mass Destruction. Combating proliferation of weapons of mass destruction, pursuant to public law 293. 104th Congress. 1999 July 14. p. 10.

Cordesman A, Senior fellow for strategic assessment. Defending America redefining the conceptual borders of homeland defense. Homeland defense: federal policy and programs to deal with the threat of attacks with weapons of mass destruction. Rough draft for comment, Center for Strategic and International Studies. 1800 K Street NW, Washington, DC 20006. 2000 July 18. p. vi.

Countering the changing threat of international terrorism, June 8, 2003. Accessed October 3, 2003.

Federal Emergency Management Agency, U.S. Fire Administration. Fire department response to biological threat at B'nai B'rith headquarters Washington, DC. Technical report series, report 114 of the Major Fires Investigation Project. Investigated by Jeff Stern. 1997 Apr 24. p. 3.

Hoffman B. Terrorism and WMD: some preliminary hypotheses. The Nonproliferation Review 1997 May:45–53.

Kansas City Department of Health. Bioterrorism: threats and events. Kansas City, MO; Rev. December 4, 2000.

Ledlow G, Johnson J, Cwiek M. Bioterrorism and business: think globally, act locally. In: Delener N, Chao C-N, editors. Beyond Boundaries: Challenges of Leadership, Innovation, Integration, and Technology. Global Business and Technology Association International Conference. 2002 July. p. 683–93. ISBN: 0-9657171-4-3.

National Bioterrorism Forum, Association of Medical Surgeons of the Uniformed Services. Louisville, KY: 2002 Nov 12.

Report of the Council on Scientific Affairs. Medical preparedness for terrorism and other disasters. Resolution 411, A-00; Recommendation 2, CSA Rep. 2, A-00. Michael A. Williams, MD, chair, at the Medic WMD 2000 Conference, executive summary. 2000 Apr 3–6. p. i.

U.S. Commission on National Security/21st Century. Road map for national security: imperative for change. The phase III report of the U.S. Commission on National Security/21st Century. 2001 Feb 15.

U.S. Department of Defense, Office of the Inspector General. Audit report: management of national guard weapons of mass destruction—civil support teams. Report number D-2001-043. 2001 Jan 31. p. i.

U.S. Department of Justice and the Federal Emergency Management Agency. Emergency response to terrorism self study. FEMA/USFA/NFA-ER: SS. June 1999. Available from: www.usfa.fema.gov. E-mail: usfapubs@fema.gov; fax: (301) 447-1213.

U.S. General Accounting Office. Combating terrorism: observations on the Nunn-Lugar-Domenici domestic preparedness program. Testimony before the Subcommittee on National Security, International Affairs and Criminal Justice, Committee on Government Reform and Oversight, House of Representatives. Statement of Richard Davis, director, National Security Analysis, National Security and International Affairs Division. 1998 Oct 2.

U.S. General Accounting Office, Critical Infrastructure Protection. Comprehensive strategy can draw on year 2000 experiences. GAO/AIMD-00-1. 1999 Oct. p. 4.

U.S. General Accounting Office. Combating terrorism: issues in managing counterterrorist programs. Testimony before the Subcommittee on Oversight, Investigations, and Emergency Management, Committee on Transportation and Infrastructure, House of Representatives. Statement of Norman J. Rabkin, director of National Security Preparedness Issues branch, National Security and International Affairs Division. 2000 Apr 6. p. 1–2.

U.S. General Accounting Office. Combating terrorism: linking threats to strategies and resources. Testimony before the Subcommittee on National Security, Veterans Affairs, and International Relations, Committee on Government Reform, House of Representatives. Statement of Norman J. Rabkin, director of National Security Preparedness Issues branch, National Security and International Affairs Division. GAO/T-NSIAD-00-218. 2000 July 26. p. 2.

U.S. General Accounting Office. Combating terrorism: federal response teams provide varied capabilities; opportunities remain to improve coordination. Report to Congressional requesters. GAO-01-14. 2000 Sep. p. 4.

## RISK ASSESSMENT

Advisory Panel to Assess Domestic Response Capabilities for Terrorism Involving Weapons of Mass Destruction. First annual report to the president and the Congress: assessing the threat. 1999 Dec 15.

Cordesman AH. Defending America redefining the conceptual borders of homeland defense: the risks and effects of indirect, covert, terrorist, and extremist attacks with weapons of mass destruction—challenges for defense and response. Washington, DC: Center for Strategic and International Studies; 2001 Feb 14.

Federal Emergency Management Agency. Guide for all-hazard emergency operations planning: state and local guide (101), chapter 6, attachment G: terrorism. 2001 Apr. p. 6-G-8 and tab E.

Hopmeier, M. Countering the changing threat of international terrorism. Report of the National Commisson on Terrorism, pursuant to public law 277, 105th Congress. 2000 June 8. Available from: www.counteringthechangingthreatofinternationalterrorism.htm. Accessed November 12, 2003.

Kortepeter MG, Cieslak TJ, Eitzen, EM. Bioterrorism. Journal of Environmental Health 2001;63(6):21–4.

Ledlow G, Johnson J, Cwiek M. Bioterrorism and business: think globally, act locally. In: Delener N, Chao C-N, editors. Beyond boundaries: challenges of leadership, innovation, integration, and technology. Global Business and Technology Association International Conference. 2002 July. p. 683–93. ISBN: 0-9657171-4-3.

U.S. Commission on National Security/21st Century. New world coming: American security in the 21st century—major themes and implications. The phase I report on the emerging global security environment for the first quarter of the 21st century. 1999 Sep 15.

U.S. Department of Defense, Office of the Secretary of Defense. Proliferation: threat and response. 2001 Jan. Available from: www.defenselink.mil.

U.S. Department of Defense, Office of the Undersecretary of Defense for Acquisition, Technology and Logistics. Protecting the homeland: report of the Defense Science Board. Summer 2000 study, executive summary, vol. 1. Washington, DC; 2001 Feb.

U.S. Department of State, Office of the Secretary of State. Patterns of global terrorism 2000. Released by the Office of the Coordinator of Counterterrorism. 2001 Apr. Available from: www.fbi.gov. Accessed October 6, 2003.

U.S. General Accounting Office. Combating terrorism: need for comprehensive threat and risk assessments of chemical and biological attacks. Report to Congressional requesters. GAO/NSIAD-99-163. 1999 Sep.

U.S. General Accounting Office. Combating terrorism: observations on the threat of chemical and biological terrorism. Testimony before the Subcommittee on National Security, Veterans Affairs, and International Relations; Committee on Government Reform; House of Representatives. Statement of Henry L. Hinton Jr, assistant comptroller general, National Security and International Affairs Division. GAO/T-NSIAD-00-50. 1999 Oct 20.

U.S. General Accounting Office. Combating terrorism: issues in managing counterterrorist programs. Testimony before the Subcommittee on Oversight, Investigations, and Emergency Management; Committee on Transportation and Infrastructure; House of Representatives. Statement of Norman J. Rabkin, director of National Security Preparedness Issues branch, National Security and International Affairs Division. 2000 Apr 6.

Zeller S. Protection money. Government Executive 2003 June. p. 38.

## SCREENING AND IDENTIFICATION

bioterrorism.slu.edu/. Accessed October 10, 2003.

Disaster exercise manual. Emergency: guidelines on exercising emergency operations plans for local government. Emergency Management Division, Department of Michigan State Police. EMD PUB-702. Publication 09-99.

Jones RW, Kowalk MA, Miller PP (editor), Tarrant R. Critical incident protocol: a public and private partnership. Michigan State University, School of Criminal Justice, Global Security Institute, University Outreach Office, Tarrant and Associates, Inc.; 2000. Supported by Grant 98-LF-CX-0007, U.S. Department of Justice.

Keith GS. Pre-incident planning for industrial and commercial facilities fire protection handbook. 18th ed. Quincy, MA: National Fire Protection Association; 1997.

National Association of County and City Health Officials. The role of local public health agencies and the Health Alert Network program in a national surveillance system. Ph: (202) 783-5550. 2000 Apr.

NBC News Today Show. Newscast of 7:00–8:00 a.m. 2003 Dec 26.

Site emergency planning workbook. Emergency Management Division, Department of Michigan State Police. EMD PUB-602. Publication 5-95; 1995.

U.S. Department of Defense, U.S. Army, U.S. Army Soldier and Biological Chemical Command. Domestic preparedness: compendium of weapons of mass destruction courses sponsored by the federal government. Appendix A. Performance Objectives Matrix, Aberdeen Proving Ground, MD; 2000 Jan. Domestic Preparedness Hotline: 1-800-368-6498.

U.S. Department of Justice, Office of Justice Programs, National Institute of Justice. A guide for explosion and bombing scene investigation. Technical working group for bombing scene investigation, NCJ 181869. Available from: www.ojp.usdoj.gov/nij/pubs-sum/181869.htm. Accessed June 2000.

U.S. Department of Transportation. IAFF training for radiation emergencies: first responder operations. Student text unit 2: recognition, identification, detection; and student text unit 4: introduction to radioactive materials; 1999 June.

U.S. General Accounting Office. Combating terrorism: analysis of federal counterterrorist exercises. Briefing report to Congressional committees. GAO/NSIAD-99-157BR. 1999 June.

Wagoner WD. Comprehensive plan/hazard mitigation interface; integration of emergency management into the community planning. Planning Department Team, Livingston County Department of Planning. Winter, 1998–1999.

www.business-marketing.com/store/article12.html. Accessed October 24, 2003.

www.fema.gov/ppt/reg-x/congress.ppt. Accessed December 20, 2003.

www.house.gov/rothman/pdf/terrorism_grants.pdf    and    fpc.state.gov/documents/organization/7931.pdf. Accessed December 20, 2003.

www.hshsl.umaryland.edu/resources/terrorism.html. Accessed December 20, 2003.

www.iaem.com/terrorism_preparedness_and_res.shtml. Accessed December 20, 2003.

www.ilpi.com/terrorism/training.html. Accessed December 20, 2003.

www.msp.state.mi.us/division/emd/emdwebl.htm. Michigan State Police Emergency Management Division contains publications on emergency management. 2003 Oct 24.

www.sbcfire.com/dp/. Accessed December 20, 2003.

seem.findlay.edu/terrorism/. Accessed December 20, 2003.

www.vdem.state.va.us/prepare/terrorismtoolkit/terrguide/ and www.vdem.state.va.us/library/famdis.cfm. Accessed December 20, 2003.

## PREVENTION, DETERRENCE, AND PLANNING

Central Intelligence Agency. Chemical/biological/radiological incident handbook. 1998 Oct. Available from: www.cia.gov/HW1min62x.html. Accessed October 20, 2003.

English JF, Cundiff MY, Malone JD, Pfeiffer JA (APIC bioterrorism task force) and Bell M, Steele L, Miller JM (CDC hospital infections program bioterrorism working group). Bioterrorism readiness plan: a template for healthcare facilities. Association for Professionals in Infection Control and Epidemiology (APIC); 1999 Apr 13.

Federal Bioterrorism Forum, held by the U.S. Department of Defense, Centers for Disease Control and Prevention, Federal Emergency Management Agency, Food and Drug Administration, Department of Health and Human Services, and the Public Health Service. AMSUS Conference, Louisville, Kentucky. 2002 Nov 12. Authors Gerald Ledlow and Mark Cwiek were invited as expert guests representing community preparedness and community interests.

Federal Emergency Management Agency. Guide for all-hazard emergency operations planning. State and local guide (SLG) 101; 1996 Sep.

Federal Emergency Management Agency. Urban search and rescue response system: task force equipment cache list. A component of the Federal Response Plan under Emergency Support Function 9. 1999 Mar 30.

Speier AH, Nordboe D (editor). Psychological issues for children and adolescents. This publication was produced under an interagency agreement between the Federal Emergency Management Agency and the Center for Mental Health Services, Substance Abuse and Mental Health Services Administration. This publication was previously published under the title Manual for Child Health Workers in Major Disasters. The first edition, printed in 1981, was written by Norman L. Farberow and Norma S. Gordon. The second edition revises and updates the first edition. Portland Ridley served as the CMHS publications and editorial coordinator. Additional copies are available at no charge from National Mental Health Services Knowledge Exchange Network, P.O. Box 42490, Washington, DC 20015. Toll-free number: 1-800-789-2647. Available from: www.mentalhealth.org/.

U.S. Department of Defense, U.S. Army, U.S. Army Center for Health Promotion and Preventive Medicine. Biological warfare agents as potable water threats. Medical issues information paper no. IP-31-017. 1998 Mar 24.

U.S. Department of Defense, U.S. Army, U.S. Army Soldier and Biological Chemical Command. Domestic preparedness. Aberdeen Proving Ground, MD; 1999 Mar. Domestic Preparedness Hotline: 1-800-368-6498.

U.S. Department of Defense, U.S. Army, U.S. Army Soldier and Biological Chemical Command. Domestic preparedness: compendium of weapons of mass destruction courses sponsored by the federal government. Aberdeen Proving Ground, MD; 2000 Jan. Domestic Preparedness Hotline: 1-800-368-6498.

U.S. Department of Defense, U.S. Army, U.S. Army Soldier and Biological Chemical Command, Health and Safety Functional Working Group, Chemical Weapons Improved Response Program. An alternative health care facility: concept of operations for the off-site triage, treatment, and transportation center (OST$^3$C). Mass Casualty Care Strategy for a Chemical Terrorism Incident, Aberdeen Proving Ground, Maryland 21010. 2001 Mar.

U.S. Department of Health and Human Services, Centers for Disease Control and Prevention (CDC). Biological and chemical terrorism: strategic plan for preparedness and response. Morbidity and Mortality Weekly Report 49(RR-4). Recommendations and Reports; 2000 Apr 21.

U.S. Department of Justice, Federal Emergency Management Agency. Emergency response to terrorism self study. FEMA/USFA/NFA-ERT:SS; 1999 June. Available from: www.usfa.fema.gov. E-mail: usfapubs@fema.gov; fax: (301) 447-1213.

U.S. Department of State, Bureau of Diplomatic Security. Countering terrorism: security suggestions for U.S. business representatives abroad. Publication 10619; Rev. 1999 June.

U.S. Department of Transportation. IAFF training for radiation emergencies: first responder operations. Student text unit 2: Recognition, identification, detection; student text unit 4: introduction to radioactive materials; and unit 7: personal protective equipment. 1999 June.

U.S. Department of the Treasury, Bureau of Alcohol, Tobacco, and Firearms. Bomb threats and physical security planning. ATF P 7550.2. 1987 July.

U.S. Environmental Protection Agency, Office of Solid Waste and Emergency Response. LEPCs and deliberate releases: addressing terrorist activities in the local emergency plan. Factsheet, EPA 550-F-01-005. 2001 May. Available from: www.epa.gov/ceppo/. Hotline: 1-800-424-9346.

U.S. General Accounting Office. Combating terrorism: observations on the Nunn-Lugar-Domenici domestic preparedness program. Testimony before the Subcommittee on National Security, International Affairs and Criminal Justice, Committee on Government Reform and Oversight, House of Representatives. Statement of Richard Davis, director, National Security Analysis, National Security and International Affairs Division. 1998 Oct 2.

## TRAINING AND APPLICATION

American College of Emergency Physicians, American College of Surgeons. Equipment for ambulances. Available from: www.acep.org/policy/PO400164. htm and www.acep.org/policy/PO400192.htm. Accessed October 4, 2000.

American Hospital Association. Hospital preparedness for mass casualties. Final report, summary of an invitational forum, supported by the U.S. Department of Health and Human Services, Office of Emergency Preparedness. 2000 Mar 8–9.

Central Intelligence Agency. Chemical/biological/radiological incident handbook. 1998 Oct. Available from: www.cia.gov/HW1min62x.html. Accessed October 20, 2003.

Federal Emergency Management Agency. An orientation to hazardous materials for medical personnel: a self-study guide. IS 346. 1998 Apr.

U.S. Department of Defense, U.S. Army, U.S. Army Soldier and Biological Chemical Command. Domestic preparedness. Aberdeen Proving Ground, MD; 1999 Mar. Domestic Preparedness Hotline: 1-800-368-6498.

U.S. Department of Defense, U.S. Army, U.S. Army Soldier and Biological Chemical Command. Guidelines for incident commander's use of firefighter protective ensemble (ffpe) with self-contained breathing apparatus (SCBA) for rescue operations during a terrorism chemical agent incident. Aberdeen Proving Ground, MD; 1999 Aug. Domestic Preparedness Hotline: 1-800-368-6498.

U.S. Department of Defense, U.S. Army, U.S. Army Soldier and Biological Chemical Command. Guidelines for mass casualty decontamination during a terrorist chemical agent incident. Aberdeen Proving Ground, MD; 1999 Nov. Domestic Preparedness Hotline: 1-800-368-6498.

U.S. Department of Defense, U.S. Army, U.S. Army Soldier and Biological Chemical Command. Chemical protective clothing for law enforcement patrol officers and emergency medical services when responding to terrorism with chemical weapons. Aberdeen Proving Ground, MD; 2000 Jan. Domestic Preparedness Hotline: 1-800-368-6498.

U.S. Department of Defense, U.S. Army, U.S. Army Soldier and Biological Chemical Command. Guidelines for mass casualty decontamination during a terrorist chemical agent incident. Aberdeen Proving Ground, MD; 2000 Jan. Domestic Preparedness Hotline: 1-800-368-6498.

U.S. Department of Health and Human Services, Office of Emergency Preparedness, American College of Emergency Physicians. Developing objectives, content, and competencies for the training of emergency medical technicians, emergency physicians, and emergency nurses to care for casualties resulting from nuclear, biological or chemical (NBC) incidents. Final report; 2001 Apr 23. p. ii.

U.S. Department of Justice, Office of Justice Programs, National Institute of Justice. Selection and application of police body armor. NIJ guide 100-98 (replaces NIJ guide 100-87); 1998 Oct. Available from: www.ojp.usdoj.gov/nij.

U.S. Department of Justice, Office of Justice Programs, National Institute of Justice. Guide for the selection of chemical agent and toxic industrial material detection equipment for emergency first responders. NIJ guide 100-00, vols. I and II. Law Enforcement and Corrections Standards and Testing Program; 2000 June. Available from: www.nlectc.org.

U.S. Department of Justice, Office of Justice Programs, National Institute of Justice. Guide for the selection of chemical and biological decontamination equipment for emergency first responders. NIJ guide 103-00, vols. I and II. Law Enforcement and Corrections Standards and Testing Program; 2001 Oct. Available from: www.nlectc.org.

U.S. Department of Justice, Office of Justice Programs, National Institute of Justice. Guide for the selection of personal protective equipment for the emergency first responders, vol. I (respiratory protection), vol. IIa (percutaneous protection—garments), vol. IIb, and vol. IIc (percutaneous protection—apparel). NIJ guide 102-00, vols. IIa, IIb, and IIc. Law Enforcement and Corrections Standards and Testing Program; 2001 Oct. Available from: www.nlectc.org.

U.S. Department of Transportation. IAFF training for radiation emergencies: first responder operations. Student text unit 8: Scene management, and student text unit 9: pre-incident planning; 1999 June.

U.S. Environmental Protection Agency, Office of Solid Waste and Emergency Response. First responders' environmental liability due to mass decontamination runoff. Chemical Safety Alert. EPA 550-F-00-009. 2000 July. Available from: www.epa.gov/ceppo/.

U.S. General Accounting Office. Combating terrorism: analysis of potential emergency response equipment and sustainment costs. Report to Congressional requesters. GAO/NSIAD-99-151. 1999 June. p. 2.

U.S. General Accounting Office. Chemical and biological defense: improved risk assessment and inventory management are needed. Report to the chairman, Subcommittee on Military Readiness, Committee on Armed Services, House of Representatives. GAO-01-667. 2001 Sep.

## ACTIVATION AND RESPONSE

Cordesman AH. Defending America: redefining the conceptual borders of homeland defense: the risks and effects of indirect, covert, terrorist, and extremist attacks with weapons of mass destruction—challenges for defense and response. Center for Strategic and International Studies, 1800 K Street NW, Washington, DC 20006; 17 Sept 2001. Ph.: (202) 775-3270. (See chemical, biological, radiological, and nuclear scenarios for risks and effects.)

Jones D. Guidelines for mailrooms. State of California Office of Emergency Services memorandum. 2001 Oct 12.

U.S. Department of Defense, Military Medical Operations Office, Armed Forces Radiobiology Research Institute. Medical management of radio logical casualties handbook. 1st ed. Bethesda, MD 20889-5603. 1999 Dec. Available from: www.afrri.usuhs.mil.

U.S. Department of Defense, U.S. Army Soldier and Biological Chemical Command, Domestic Preparedness Office. Improving local and state agency response to terrorist incidents involving biological weapons. Prepared in response to the Nunn-Lugar-Domenici domestic preparedness program; 2000 Aug 1. Ph.: (410) 436-3382.

U.S. Department of Health and Human Services, Division of Health Education and Promotion, Agency for Toxic Substances and Disease Registry. Report of the expert panel workshop on the psychological responses to hazardous substances. Prepared by Pamela Tucker, edited by Karen Resha. Atlanta, GA; 1995 Sep.

U.S. Department of Justice, Office of Justice Programs, Office for Victims of Crime. Responding to terrorism victims: Oklahoma City and beyond. NCJ 183949. 2000 Oct. Toll-free number: 1-800-627-6872. Available from: www.ncjrs.org.

U.S. Department of Transportation, Transport Canada, and the Secretariat of Transport and Communication Mexico. 2000 emergency response guidebook: a guidebook for first responders during the initial phase of a dangerous goods/hazardous materials incident; 2000 Jan. Ph.: (202) 366-4900.

U.S. General Accounting Office. Combating terrorism: observations on options to improve the federal response. Testimony before the Subcommittee on Economic

Development, Public Buildings, and Emergency Management; Committee on Transportation and Infrastructure; and the Subcommittee on National Security, Veterans Affairs, and International Relations; Committee on Government Reform; House of Representatives. Statement of Raymond J. Decker, director, Defense Capabilities and Management. GAO–01-660T. 2001 Apr 24.

## LEADERSHIP, AUTHORITY, AND COMMUNICATION

City of Santa Luisa, CA. Emergency operations checklist, generic checklist, standardized emergency management system, local government emergency operations center, positions checklists; 1997 Dec.

Cordesman AH. Defending America redefining the conceptual borders of homeland defense: the risks and effects of indirect, covert, terrorist, and extremist attacks with weapons of mass destruction—challenges for defense and response. Center for Strategic and International Studies, 1800 K Street NW, Washington, DC 20006. Ph.: (202) 775-3270. (See chemical, biological, radiological, and nuclear scenarios for risks and effects.)

de Borchgrave A, Cilluffo FJ, Cardash SL, Ledgerwood MM. Cyber threats and information security: meeting the 21st century challenge. Washington, DC: Center for Strategic and International Studies; 2000 Dec. Available from: www.csis.org.

Federal Emergency Management Agency. Guide for all-hazard emergency operations planning. State and local guide (SLG) 101; 1996 Sep. Note: also includes chapter 6, attachment G–Terrorism.

Federal Emergency Management Agency, Emergency Management Institute. Incident Command System: independent study course—basic; 1998 Jan. Available from: www.fema.gov/emi/ishome.htm.

Federal Emergency Management Agency, United States Fire Administration. Improving firefighter communications [special report]. Technical report series. 1999 June. Available from: usfa.fema.gov.

Imel KJ, Hart JW. Understanding wireless communications in public safety: a guidebook to technology, issues, planning and management. U.S. Department of Justice, Office of Justice Programs, National Institute of Justice, National Law Enforcement and Corrections Technology Center, rev. 2000 Aug. Available from: www.nlectc.org.

Jones D. Guidelines for mailrooms. State of California Office of Emergency Services memorandum; 2001 Oct 12.

Molander RC, Riddle AS, Wilson PA. Strategic information warfare: a new face of war. The RAND Corporation, prepared for the Office of the Secretary of Defense, National Defense Research Institute; 1996. Available from: www.rand.org or (310) 451-7002.

State of California Governor's Office of Emergency Services. 1998 law enforcement guide for emergency operations; 1998 Jan. Available from: www.oes.ca.gov. Ph.: (916) 262-1744.

U.S. Agency for International Development, Bureau for Humanitarian Response, Office of Foreign Disaster Assistance. Field operations guide for disaster assessment and response. 3rd ed. 1998 Aug. Available from: www. info.usaid.gov/ofda/.

U.S. Department of Defense, Military Medical Operations Office, Armed Forces Radiobiology Research Institute. Medical management of radiological casualties handbook. 1st ed. Bethesda, MD 20889-5603. 1999 Dec. Available from: www.afrri.usuhs.mil.

U.S. Department of Defense, U.S. Army Soldier and Biological Chemical Command, Domestic Preparedness Office. Improving local and state agency response to terrorist incidents involving biological weapons. Prepared in response to the Nunn-Lugar-Domenici domestic preparedness program; 2000 Aug 1. Ph.: (410) 436-3382.

U.S. Department of Health and Human Services, Division of Health Education and Promotion, Agency for Toxic Substances and Disease Registry. Report of the expert panel workshop on the psychological responses to hazardous substances. Prepared by Pamela Tucker, edited by Karen Resha. Atlanta, GA; 1995 Sep.

U.S. Department of Justice, Office of Justice Programs, National Institute of Justice. Guide for the selection of communication equipment for emergency first responders, vols. I and II. NIJ Guide 104-00, Law Enforcement and Corrections Standards and Testing Program. Rockville, MD 20849-1160. 2001 Oct. Available from: www.nlectc.org.

U.S. Department of Justice, Office of Justice Programs, Office for Victims of Crime. Responding to terrorism victims: Oklahoma City and beyond. NCJ 183949. 2000 Oct. 1-800-627-6872. Available from: www. ncjrs.org.

U.S. Department of Transportation. IAFF training for radiation emergencies: first responder operations. Student text unit 8: scene management; and student text unit 9: pre-incident planning. 1999 June.

U.S. Department of Transportation, Transport Canada, and the Secretariat of Transport and Communication Mexico. 2000 emergency response guidebook: a guidebook for first responders during the initial phase of a dangerous goods/hazardous materials incident; 2000 Jan. Ph.: (202) 366-4900.

U.S. General Accounting Office. Combating terrorism: observations on options to improve the federal response. Testimony before the Subcommittee on Economic Development, Public Buildings, and Emergency Management; Committee on Transportation and Infrastructure; and the Subcommittee on National Security, Veterans Affairs, and International Relations; Committee on Government Reform; House of Representatives. Statement of Raymond J. Decker, director, Defense Capabilities and Management. GAO–01-660T. 2001 Apr 24.

U.S. General Accounting Office. Critical infrastructure protection: comments on the national plan for information systems protection. Testimony before the

Subcommittee on Technology, Terrorism and Government Information; Committee on the Judiciary; U.S. Senate. Statement for the record by Jack L. Brock Jr, director, Governmentwide and Defense Information Systems, Accounting and Information Management Division. GAO/T-AIMD-00-72. 2000 Feb 1.

U.S. General Accounting Office, Accounting and Information Management Division. Information security risk assessment: practices of leading organizations. A supplement to GAO's May 1998 executive guide on information security management. GAO/AIMD-00-33. 1999 Nov.

U.S. Government, Office of the President of the United States. Interagency domestic terrorism concept of operations plan. 1995. Note: The CONPLAN was developed through the efforts of six primary departments and agencies with responsibilities as identified in Presidential Decision Directive/NSC-39 (PDD-39).

## ADDITIONAL SELECTED RESOURCES

## Books (from the Global Security Institute, Michigan State University, Critical Incident Protocol)

Disaster exercise manual. Emergency: guidelines on exercising emergency operations plans for local government. Emergency Management Division, Department of Michigan State Police. EMD PUB-702. Publication 09-99.

Emergency information procedures workbook. Emergency Management Division, Department of Michigan State Police. EMD PUB-401. Rev. 1991.

Emergency planning handbook. American Society of Industrial Security; 1994.

Keith GS. Pre-incident planning for industrial and commercial facilities fire protection handbook. 18th ed. Quincy, MA: National Fire Protection Association; 1997.

Michigan hazard analysis. Emergency Management Division, Department of Michigan State Police. EMD PUB-103. Publication 10-98.

Site emergency planning workbook. Emergency Management Division, Department of Michigan State Police. EMD PUB-602. Publication 5-95.

Wagoner WD. Comprehensive plan/hazard mitigation interface; integration of emergency management into the community planning. Planning Department Team, Livingston County Department of Planning. Winter, 1998–1999.

Warning. Evacuation and in-place protection handbook. Emergency Management Division, Department of Michigan State Police. EMD PUB-304. Publication 1-94.

Wright CJ. Managing the response to hazardous materials incidents. Fire protection handbook. 18th ed. Quincy, MA: National Fire Protection Association; 1997.

# Internet Resources (from the Global Security Institute, Michigan State University, Critical Incident Protocol)

dp.sbccom.armv.mil: This website, SBCCOM: Program Director for Domestic Preparedness, is dedicated to enhancing federal, state, and local emergency responders.

ns.noaa.gov: NOAA's website contains information on monitoring and analyzing hazards. Additional information on monitoring, responding to, and mitigating hazards is available.

www.atf.treas.gov: The Bureau of Alcohol, Tobacco, and Firearms website. Contains information on bomb threat and detection resources. A bomb and physical security planning link entitled "Bomb Threat Workbook" for the public sector is available, along with bomb threat checklists and information on detecting suspicious devices.

www.cbiac.apgea.army.mil: The Chemical and Biological Defense Command website. Provides information and analysis on CW/CBD.

www.cdc.gov: Information on infectious diseases from the Centers for Disease Control and Prevention.

www.disasterrelief.org: The Disaster Relief website is maintained by the American Red Cross, Cable News Network (CNN), and International Business Machines (IBM). It provides information on disasters and sources for recovery support.

www.doc.gov: Department of Commerce information on emergency/disaster mitigation.

www.doe.gov: Information on Department of Energy capabilities and support involving radiological materials and related emergencies.

www.dot.gov: U.S. Department of Transportation (DOT) information on hazardous materials.

www.dtic.mil/def: U.S. Department of Defense with links to domestic preparedness resources.

www.emforum.org/: The virtual forum for emergency management professionals' websites provides information on emergency management and links with professional organizations throughout the world. The Emergency Information Infrastructure Partnership is a voluntary association for exchanging information on disaster planning and recovery. The EMForum includes FEMA, the National Emergency Management Association (NEMA), the International Association of Emergency Managers (IAEM), the National Volunteer Fire Council (NVFC), the Congressional Fire Service Institute (CFSI), and the State and Local Emergency Management Data Users Group.

www.epa.gov: The U.S. Environmental Protection Agency website provides information on accident protection and risk management, and their role in counterterrorism. Links to other federal agencies and organizations involved in counterterrorism are provided.

www.fbi.gov: Information and services available from the Federal Bureau of Investigation, designated as the lead federal agency in events involving terrorism.

www.fbi.gov/ansir/an8ir.htm: FBI/Awareness of National Security Issues and Response (ANSIR). The website is the public voice for the FBI on espionage and physical infrastructure protection.

www.fbi.gov/programs/ndpo/default.htm: The National Domestic Preparedness Office (NDPO) website. Provides links to other federal WMD assets and expertise.

www.fema.gov: The Federal Emergency Management Agency website. Contains emergency response and planning information. Documents on various hazards can be downloaded along with fact and planning sheets.

www.iaem.com: The International Association of Emergency Managers (IAEM) website provides information on emergency management issues.

www.ibhs.org: The Institute for Business and Home Safety provides information on residence and business natural disaster safety. The website is an initiative of the insurance industry to reduce death, injury, and property damage.

www.info.gov/fed-directorv/phone.shtml: Directory assistance link for the Government Information Exchange site. The link has access to the Operation Respond Emergency Information System (OREIS) database designed to provide first responders with information on various hazards.

www.msp.state.mi.us/division/emd/emdwebl.htm: Michigan State Police Emergency Management Division. Contains publications on emergency management.

www.nemaweb.org: The National Emergency Management Association website concentrates on mitigation of hazards. Links to related sites are provided.

www.nrt.org: National Response Team Preparedness Committee website on the exchange of lessons learned during training exercises. Links to over 100 preparedness and response websites.

www.oep-ndms.dhhs.gov: The Department of Human Health Services website. Describes its role and function in emergency planning.

www.oip.usdi.gov/osldps: Office for State and Local Domestic Preparedness Support was established to administer grants to assist state and local public safety personnel in acquiring the specialized equipment and training to safely respond to and manage domestic terrorist activities, especially dealing with weapons of mass destruction.

www.osha.gov: Occupational Safety and Health Administration information on various human health and safety hazards.

www.redcross.org: The American Red Cross website. Contains information on community disaster planning, mitigation, management, and recovery from disasters.

www.statelocal.gov: The U.S. state/local gateway for state and local access to federal information.

www.usgs.gov: The U.S. Geological Survey (USGS) contains information on geologic hazards. The USGS also monitors and evaluates threats from a number of natural hazards.

www.usia.gov/topical/pol.terror: The U.S. Information Agency website on counterterrorism; with links to U.S. government sources.

www.weather.com/safeside: The website provides information on a joint project, Project Safeside, between the American Red Cross and Weather Channel to inform communities on meteorological hazards and the importance of preparing for natural disasters.

## Information: Biological Agents

Cordesman AH. Defending America redefining the conceptual borders of homeland defense: biotechnology and biological weapons. Center for Strategic and International Studies, 1800 K Street NW, Washington, DC 20006. Available from: www.csis.org, listed under Homeland Defense. Ph.: (202) 775-3270.

Cordesman AH. Defending America redefining the conceptual borders of homeland defense: the risks and effects of indirect, covert, terrorist, and extremist attacks with weapons of mass destruction—challenges for defense and response. Center for Strategic and International Studies, 1800 K Street NW, Washington, DC 20006. Ph.: (202) 775-3270.

U.S. Department of Defense, U.S. Army Soldier and Biological Chemical Command, Domestic Preparedness Office. Improving local and state agency response to terrorist incidents involving biological weapons. Prepared in response to the Nunn-Lugar-Domenici domestic preparedness program; 2000 Aug 1. Ph.: (410) 436-3382.

## Information: Chemical and Hazardous Agents

206.39.77.2/DMCR/dmrhome.html: Disaster Management Central resource

206.39.77.2/DMCR/dmrhome.html: NBC Medical Defense Library

206.39.77.2/dmcr/NBC/chemicas/Decontam.htm: Decontamination

aepo-xdv-www.epo.cdc.gov/wonder/prevguid: Medical management guidelines for acute chemical exposures; U.S. Department of Health and Human Services, Public Health Service, Agency for Toxic Substance and Disease Registry; Recommendations from their website entitled "Unidentified chemical prehospital management."

atsdr1.atsdr.cdc.gov:8080/hazdat.html: Agency for Toxic Substances and Disease Registry, Hazardous Substance Release/Health Effects Database

chemdef.apgea.army.mil/instbilb.htm: USAMRICD open literature publications and books, 1981–1996

Cordesman AH. Defending America redefining the conceptual borders of homeland defense: the risks and effects of indirect, covert, terrorist, and extremist attacks with weapons of mass destruction—challenges for defense and response. Center for Strategic and International Studies, 1800 K Street NW, Washington, DC 20006. Telephone: (202) 775-3270.

research.nwfsc.noaa.gov/msds.html: Northwest Fisheries Science Center. Material safety data sheet searches.

U.S. Department of Defense, U.S. Army Soldier and Biological Chemical Command, Domestic Preparedness Office, Chemical Team. Guidelines for responding to a chemical weapons incident. Prepared in response to the Nunn-Lugar-Domenici domestic preparedness program; 2001 Mar. Ph.: (410) 436-3382.

U.S. Department of Transportation, Transport Canada, and the Secretariat of Transport and Communication Mexico. 2000 emergency response guidebook: a guidebook for first responders during the initial phase of a dangerous goods/hazardous materials incident; 2000 Jan. Ph.: (202) 366-4900.

www.apgea.army.mil: CBDCOM website homepage

www.cbdcom.apgea.army.mil: ERDEC safety office material safety data sheets

www.cbiac.apgea.army.mil: CBIAC homepage

www.cdc.gov: Centers for Disease Control and Prevention

www.emergency.com: Emergency Response and Research Institute

www.emergency.com: HAZMAT information

www.emergency.com/hzmtpage.htm: Hazardous materials operations page

www.epa.gov/chemfact/: Chemicals in the environment: OPPT chemical fact sheets

www.firesci.com: Fire science information

www.infotrieve.com/healthworld/preview: Disaster preparedness, decontamination, and chemical warfare

www.nbc-med.org: Nuclear, biological, and chemical medical website with field manual 8-285

www.nbc-med.org/BioAgents.html: Biological agent information papers, USAMRIID

www.opcw.nl/chemhaz/decon.htm: Website from the Organization for the Prohibition of Chemical Weapons (OPCW) in The Hague, the Netherlands. OPWC is responsible for implementing the Chemical Weapons Convention (CWC); decontamination of chemical warfare agents: an introduction to methods and chemicals for decontamination.

www.os.dhhs.gov/: USAD Health and Human Services homepage

## Information: Radiological and Nuclear Crisis

U.S. Department of Defense, Military Medical Operations Office, Armed Forces Radiobiology Research Institute. Medical management of radiological casualties handbook. 1st ed. Bethesda, MD 20889-5603; 1999 Dec. Available from: www.afrri.usuhs.mil.

## SELECTED RESOURCES ON GENERAL DISASTERS AND COMMUNITY CRISES SINCE 1992

### History and Theory

Hewitt K. Regions of risk: a geographical introduction to disasters. Essex, UK: Longman, Ltd.; 1997.

Horlick-Jones T. Modern disasters as outrage and betrayal. International Journal of Mass Emergencies and Disasters 1995;13(3):305–15.

Kates RW. Human adjustment. In Hanson S, editor. Ten geographic ideas that changed the world. New Brunswick, NJ: Rutgers University Press; 1997. p. 87–107.

Kreps GA. Disaster as systematic event and social catalyst: a clarification of subject matter. International Journal of Mass Emergencies and Disasters 1995;13:255–84.

Mitchell K, editor. Crucible of hazard. Tokyo: UNU Press; 1998.

Quarantelli EL. What is a disaster? London: Routledge; 1998.

Stallings RA. Sociological theories and disaster studies. Preliminary paper no. 249. Newark, DE: University of Delaware, Disaster Research Center; 1997.

### Development and Mitigation

Aberly D, editor. Futures by design: the practice of ecological planning. Philadelphia, PA: New Society Publishers; 1994.

Bauman C, Greene M. Revision of the community safety element: The San Francisco experience. In: proceedings of the 5th International Conference on Seismic Zonation; 1995 Oct 17–19; Nice, France.

Berke PR. Natural hazard reduction and sustainable development: a global assessment. Center for Urban and Regional Studies Working Paper S95-02. Chapel Hill, NC: University of North Carolina; 1995.

Berke PR. Natural hazard reduction and sustainable development: a global assessment. Journal of Planning Literature 1995;9(4):370–82.

Clark K. Modelling catastrophic risk. In: U.S. National Committee for the Decade for Natural Disaster Reduction; Commission on Geosciences, Environment, and Resources; National Research Council, editors. Facing the challenge: The U.S. National Report to the IDNDR World Conference on Natural Disaster Reduction; 1994. Washington, DC: National Academy Press; 1994. p. 16–8.

Dalton LC, Burby RJ. Mandates, plans and planners: building local commitment to development management. Journal of the American Planning Association 1994;60:444–62.

Godschalk DR, Parham DW, Porter DR, Potapchuk WR, Schukraft SW. Pulling together: a planning and development consensus-building manual. Washington, DC: Urban Land Institute; 1994.

Groenwold J, Porter E, editors. World in crisis: the politics of survival at the end of the twentieth century. Prepared for Doctors Without Borders. London: Routledge; 1997.

May PM, Burby RJ, Dixon J, Ericksen N, Handmer J, Michaels S, et al. Environmental management and governance: intergovernmental approaches to hazards and sustainability. London and New York: Routledge Press; 1996.

Munasinghe M, Clarke C, editors. Disaster prevention for sustainable development: economic and policy issues. Washington, DC: The International Bank for Reconstruction and Development/The World Bank; 1995.

National Research Council. Preparing for the 21st century: the environment and the human future. Washington, DC: National Academy of Sciences; 1997.

Otero RC, Marti RZ. The impacts of natural disasters on developing economies: implications for the international development and disaster community. In: Munasinghe M, Clark C, editors. Disaster prevention for sustainable development: economic and policy issues. Washington, DC: World Bank; 1995.

Ronfeldt D, Thorup C. North America in the era of citizen networks: state, society and security. Santa Monica, CA: RAND Corporation; 1995.

U.S. Environmental Protection Agency. The National Response Team's integrated contingency plan guidance. National Register 1996;61(109):28642–64.

## Incidents

Blaikie P, Cannon T, Davis I, Wisner B. At risk: natural hazards, people's vulnerability, and disasters. New York: Routledge; 1994.

Cutter SL, Ji M. Trends in U.S. hazardous materials transportation spills. Professional Geographer 1997;49(3):318–31.

Dash N. A comparison of populations at risk for hurricanes and earthquakes. Miami: International Hurricane Center, Florida International University; 1996.

Hardin SB, Weinrich M, Weinrich S, Hardin TL, Garrison C. Psychological distress of adolescents exposed to Hurricane Hugo. Journal of Traumatic Stress 1994;7(3):427–40.

Hill C. Mayday! Weatherwise 1996;49(3):25–8.

International Federation of Red Cross and Red Crescent Societies. World disasters report: 1994. The Netherlands: Martinus Nijhoff Publishers; 1994.

Jones RT, Frary R, Cunningham P, Weddle JD. Psychological effects of Hurricane Andrew on an elementary school population. Quick response report no. 62. Boulder, CO: University of Colorado, Natural Hazards Research and Applications Information Center; 1993.

Munich Reinsurance. Topics: natural catastrophes. Munich, Germany: Munich Reinsurance Company; 1995.

National Climatic Data Center. Lightning statistics. 1996. Available from: www.ncdc.noaa.gov/.

National Institute for Building Sciences. HAZUS technical manual: earthquake loss estimation methodology. Prepared for the Federal Emergency Management Agency. NIBS #5203. Washington, DC: National Institute for Building Sciences; 1997.

National Oceanic and Atmospheric Administration, National Hurricane Center. The costliest U.S. hurricanes of this century (unadjusted). 1996. Available from: www.nhc.noaa.gov.

National Weather Service, Office of Meteorology. A summary of natural hazard fatalities for 1994 in the U.S. Washington, DC: U.S. Department of Commerce; 1995.

Noji EK, editor. The epidemiological consequences of disasters. New York: Oxford University Press; 1997.

Nuhfer EB. What is a geologic hazard? Geotimes 1994;4.

Property Claim Services. American Insurance Services Group, Inc. News 1996 Jan 14.

Rackers D. Heat surveillance summary—1995. Jefferson City, MO: Missouri Department of Health, Office of Epidemiology; 1996.

Rose A, Benavides J, Chang S, Szczesniak P, Lim D. The regional economic impact of an earthquake: direct and indirect effects of electricity lifeline disruption. Journal of Regional Science 1997;37(3): 437–48.

Rosenfield J. Cars vs. the weather. Weatherwise 1996 49(5):14–21.

Shah HC. Scientific profiles of the "big one." Natural Hazards Observer 1995;20(3):1–3.

Shannon M, Lonigan CJ, Finch AJ Jr, Taylor CM. Children exposed to a disaster: epidemiology of post-traumatic symptoms and symptom profiles. Journal of the American Academy of Child and Adolescent Psychiatry 1994;33(1):80–93.

Showalter PS, Myers MF. Natural disasters in the U.S. as release agents of oil, chemicals or radiological material between 1980–1989: analysis and recommendations. Risk Analysis: An International Journal 1994;14(2): 169–82.

United Nations Department of Humanitarian Affairs. Chernobyl: no visible end to the menace. DHA News 1995;(16):2–27.

U.S. Bureau of the Census. Statistical abstract of the U.S.: 1995. Washington, DC: U.S. Department of Commerce; 1995.

U.S. National Committee for the International Decade for Natural Disaster Reduction. Facing the challenge: U.S. national report to the International Decade of Natural Disaster Reduction. Washington, DC: National Academy Press; 1994.

## Human Consequences of Crisis

Adeola FO. Environmental hazards, health, and racial inequity in hazardous waste distribution. Environment and Behavior 1994;26(1):99–26.

Bedics B. The history and context of rural poverty. Human Services in the Rural Environment 1987;10(4) and 11(1):12–4.

Cook PJ, Mizer KL. The revised ERS county topology: an overview. Rural Development Research Report 89. Washington, DC: U.S. Department of Agriculture; 1994.

Cutter SL. The forgotten casualties: women, children, and environmental change. Global Environmental Change 1995;5(3):181–94.

Fothergill A. Gender, risk, and disaster. International Journal of Mass Emergencies and Disasters 1996;14(1):33–56.

Ginsberg L. An overview of rural social work. In: Ginsberg LH, editor. Social work in rural communities. Alexandria, VA: Council on Social Work Education; 1993. p. 2–17.

Rahnema M. Development and the people's immune system. In: Rahnema M, Bawtree V, editors. The post-development reader. London: Zed Press; 1997. p. 111–31.

U.S. Bureau of the Census. Statistical abstract of the U.S.: 1994. Washington, DC: U.S. Department of Commerce; 1994.

U.S. Bureau of the Census. Statistical abstract of the U.S.: 1995. Washington, DC: U.S. Department of Commerce; 1995.

U.S. Bureau of the Census. Census Bureau predicts 65+ population to double in eight states by 2020. Washington, DC: U.S. Department of Commerce; 1996.

U.S. Bureau of the Census. Population projections of the U.S. by age, sex, race, and Hispanic origin: 1995–2050. Washington, DC: U.S. Department of Commerce; 1996.

White GF, Bronzini MS, Colglazier EW, Dohrenwend B, Erikson K, Hansen R, et al. Socioeconomic studies of high-level nuclear waste disposal. Proceedings of the National Academy of Sciences 1994;91:10786–9.

## Infrastructure Consequences

Burby RJ, Dalton LC. Plans can matter! The role of land use plans and state planning mandates in limiting the development of hazardous areas. Public Administration Review 1994 May/June;54:229–38.

Comerio MC, Landis JD, Rofe Y. Post-disaster residential rebuilding. Working paper 608. Berkeley, CA: University of California, Institute of Urban and Regional Development; 1994.

Housner GW, Bergman LA, Caughey TK, Chassiakos AG, Claus RO, Masri SF, et al. Structural control: past, present and future. Journal of Engineering Mechanics 1997;123(9):897–971.

Insurance Institute for Property Loss Reduction. Opinions of building code officials on administrating and enforcing building codes. Boston, MA: Insurance Institute for Property Loss Reduction; 1995.

## Interactions of Systems

Erickson K. New species of trouble: explorations in disaster, trauma, and community. New York: W.W. Norton & Co; 1994.
Redclift M, Benton T, editors. Social theory and the global environment. New York: Routledge; 1994.
Risk Management Solutions, Inc. What if the 1923 earthquake strikes again? A five-prefecture Tokyo region scenario. Menlo Park, CA: Risk Management Solutions, Inc.; 1995.
Stallings RA. Promoting risk: constructing the earthquake threat. New York: Aldine de Gruyter; 1995.
Turner AK, Schuster RL, editors. Landslides: investigation and mitigation. Special Report 247 of the Transportation Research Board of the National Research Council. Washington, DC: National Academy Press; 1996.

## Metropolitan Statistical Areas and Megacities

International Decade for Natural Disaster Reduction Secretariat. Cities at risk: making cities safer . . . before disaster strikes. Geneva: International Decade for Natural Disaster Reduction Secretariat; 1996.
Parker D. Disaster vulnerability of megacities: an expanding problem that requires rethinking and innovative responses. GeoJournal 1995;37(3):295–301.
Steedman S. Megacities: the unacceptable risk of natural disaster. Built Environment 1995;21(2–3):89–83.
Uitto J. The geography of disaster vulnerability in megacities: a theoretical framework. Applied Geography 1998;18(1):7–16.

## Mitigation

Blanck PD. Disaster mitigation for persons with disabilities: fostering a new dialogue. Washington, DC: Northwestern University, Annenberg Washington Program in Communications Policy Studies; 1995.
Brown P, Ferguson FIT. "Making a big stink": women's work, women's relationships, and toxic waste activism. Gender and Society 1995; 9(2):145–71.
Duval TS, Mulilis JP, Lalwani N. Impact of the magnitude 4.5 aftershock of December 5, 1994, on San Fernando residents' levels of earthquake preparedness and selected psychosocial variables. Quick response report no. 75.

Boulder, CO: University of Colorado, Natural Hazards Research and Applications Information Center; 1995.

Hewitt K. The social space of terror: towards a civil interpretation of total war. In: Cutter S, editor. Environmental risks and hazards. Englewood Cliffs, NJ: Prentice Hall; 1994. p. 360–89.

Kone D, Mullet E. Societal risk perception and media coverage. Risk Analysis 1994;14(1):21–4.

Kunreuther H, Ericksen N, Handmer J. Reducing losses from natural disasters through insurance and mitigation: a cross-cultural comparison. Publication 93-10-01. Philadelphia: University of Pennsylvania, Risk Management and Decision Processes Center; 1993.

Lindell MK. Perceived characteristics of environmental hazards. International Journal of Mass Emergencies and Disasters 1994;12:303–26.

McDaniels T, Axelrod LJ, Slovic P. Characterizing perceptions of ecological risk. Risk Analysis 1995;15:575–88.

Mejer JH. Hazard perception and community change: cultural factors in Puna, Hawaii. International Journal of Mass Emergencies and Disasters 1994;12(2):199–213.

Mulilis J-P, Duval TS. The PrE model of coping and tornado preparedness: moderating effects of responsibility. Journal of Applied Social Psychology 1997;27:1750–66.

Pomerantz EM, Chaiken S, Tordesillas RS. Attitude strength and resistance processes. Journal of Personality and Social Psychology 1995;69:408–19.

Rohrmann B. Risk perception of different societal groups: Australian findings and cross-national comparisons. Australian Journal of Psychology 1994;46:150–63.

Scanlon J. Gender and disasters: a second look. Natural Hazards Observer 1997;21:1–2.

Sparks P, Shepherd R. Public perceptions of the potential hazards associated with food production and food consumption: an empirical study. Risk Analysis 1994;14:799–806.

Webler T, Rakel H, Renn O, Johnson B. Eliciting and classifying concerns: a methodological critique. Risk Analysis 1995;15:421–36.

## Individual and Collective Decision-Making Processes

Chaiken S, Maheswaran D. Heuristic processing can bias systematic processing: effects of source credibility, argument ambiguity, and task importance on attitude judgment. Journal of Personality and Social Psychology 1994;66:460–73.

Davis M. Ecology of fear: Los Angeles and the imagination of disaster. New York: Henry Holt (Metropolitan Books); 1998.

Payne JW, Bettman JR, Johnson EJ. The adaptive decision maker. New York: Cambridge University Press; 1993.

Pennebaker JW, Harber K. A social stage model of collective coping: the Loma Prieta earthquake and the Persian Gulf War. Journal of Social Issues 1993;49:125–45.

Rodrigue CM, Rovai E, Henderson A, Potter S, Hotchkiss J. El Niño and perceptions of the southern California floods and mudslides of 1998. Quick response report no. 107. Boulder: University of Colorado, Natural Hazards Research and Applications Information Center; 1998. Available from: www.Colorado.EDU/hazards/qr/qr107.html.

Thompson EP, Roman RJ, Moskowitz GB, Chaiken S, Bargh JA. Accuracy motivation attenuates covert priming: the systematic reprocessing of social information. Journal of Personality and Social Psychology 1994;66:474–89.

## Awareness Programs and Risk Communication

Federal Emergency Management Agency. A guide to preparing emergency public information materials. Washington, DC: Federal Emergency Management Agency; 1991.

Kasperson RE, Stallen PJM. Communicating risks to the public: international perspectives. Technology, risks, and society series. vol. 4. Boston: Kluwer Academic Publishers; 1991.

Margolis H. Dealing with risk: why the public and the experts disagree on environmental issues. Chicago and London: The University of Chicago Press; 1996.

Mazur A. A hazardous inquiry: the Rashomon effect at Love Canal. Cambridge, MA, and London: Harvard University Press; 1998.

Mileti DS, Darlington JD. Societal response to revised earthquake probabilities in the San Francisco Bay area. International Journal of Mass Emergencies and Disasters 1995;13:119–45.

Mileti DS, Darlington JD. The role of searching in shaping reactions to earthquake risk information. Social Problems 1997;44:89–103.

Mileti DS, Fitzpatrick C, Farhar BC. Risk communication and public response to the Parkfield earthquake prediction experiment. Fort Collins: Colorado State University, Hazards Assessment Laboratory; 1990.

Mileti DS, O'Brien PW. Warnings during disaster: normalizing communicated risk. Social Problems 1992;39:40–57.

Mileti DS, Sorensen JH. Communication of emergency public warnings: a social science perspective and state of the art assessment. ORNL-6609. Oak Ridge, TN: Oak Ridge National Laboratory; 1990.

Mulilis J-P, Lippa RA. Geopsychology: fear appeals and earthquake preparedness. Paper presented at the annual meeting of the American Psychological Association, Los Angeles, California; 1985.

O'Keefe DJ. Persuasion: theory and research. Newbury Park, CA: Sage; 1990.

Perry RW, Nelson LS. Ethnicity and hazard information dissemination. Environmental Management 1991;15:581–7.

Place SE, Rodrigue CM. Media construction of the "Northridge" earthquake in English and Spanish print media in Los Angeles. In: Proceedings of the International Geographical Union; 1995. Also available from: www.csulb. edu/~rodrigue/igu1994.html.

Rogers GO. Aspects of risk communication in two cultures. International Journal of Mass Emergencies and Disasters 1992;10(3):437–64.

Schulz P. Education, awareness, and information transfer issues. In: Federal Emergency Management Agency. Improving earthquake mitigation; a report to Congress on the National Earthquake Hazards Reduction Program. Washington, DC: Federal Emergency Management Agency; 1993. p. 159–75.

Showalter PS. Prognostication of doom: an earthquake prediction's effect on four small communities. International Journal of Mass Emergencies and Disasters 1993;11:279–92.

Sims JH, Baumann DD. Educational programs and human response to natural hazards. Environment and Behavior 1983;15:165–89.

Smith C. Media and apocalypse: news coverage of the Yellowstone forest fires, Exxon Valdez oil spill, and Loma Prieta earthquake. Westport, CT, and London: Greenwood Press; 1992.

## Planning

Bauman C, Greene M. Revision of the community safety element: the San Francisco experience. Paper presented at the Fifth International Conference on Seismic Zonation; 1995; Nice, France.

Bowonder B, Kasperson JX, Kasperson RE. Avoiding future Bhopals. Reprint no. 47. Worcester, MA: Clark University, Center for Technology, Environment and Development; 1985.

Burby RJ. Land use planning and development management for hazard mitigation: summary of research findings and use. New Orleans, LA: University of New Orleans, College of Urban and Public Affairs; 1994.

California Seismic Safety Commission. California at risk: reducing earthquake hazards, 1992–1996. Sacramento CA: California Seismic Safety Commission; 1991.

California Seismic Safety Commission. Research and implementation plan for earthquake risk reduction in California, 1995–2000. Report SSC 94-10. Sacramento, CA: California Seismic Safety Commission; 1994.

Federal Emergency Management Agency. National mitigation strategy. Washington, DC: U.S. Government Printing Office; 1995.

Godschalk DR, Beatley T, Berke P, Brower D, Kaiser E. Making mitigation work: recasting natural hazard planning and implementation. Washington, DC: Island Press; 1998.

Jamieson G, Drury C. Hurricane mitigation efforts at the U.S. Federal Emergency Management Agency. In: Diaz HF, Pulwarty RS, editors.

Hurricanes: climate and socioeconomic impacts. New York: Springer-Verlag; 1997. p. 251–60.

Kartez J, Faupel C. Factors promoting comprehensive local government hazards management. In: From the mountains to the sea—developing local capabilities: proceedings of the Nineteenth Annual Conference of the Association of State Floodplain Managers. Special publication 31. Boulder, CO: University of Colorado, Institute of Behavioral Science; 1995. p. 65–79.

Kunster JH. The geography of nowhere. New York: Touchstone; 1993.

Langdon P. A better place to live. New York: Harper Press; 1994.

May PM. Addressing natural hazards: challenges and lessons for public policy. Australian Journal of Emergency Management 1996;11(4):30–7.

National Research Council. A safer future—reducing the impacts of natural disasters. Washington, DC: National Academy Press; 1991.

Office of Technology Assessment, Congress of the United States. Reducing earthquake losses. Washington, DC: U.S. Government Printing Office; 1995.

Russell LA, Goltz JD, Bourque LB. Preparedness and hazard mitigation actions before and after two earthquakes. Environment and Behavior 1995;27: 744–70.

Setterberg F, Shavelson L. Toxic nation: the fight to save our communities from chemical contamination. New York: John Wiley & Sons, Inc; 1993.

Smith K. Environmental hazards: assessing risk and reducing disaster. New York: Routledge; 1992.

Smith RA, Deyle RE. Development of a risk-based mechanism for funding local government coastal storm hazard management services. Tallahassee, FL: Department of Urban and Regional Planning, Florida State University; 1994.

Tengs TO, et al. Five-hundred life-saving interventions and their cost-effectiveness. Risk Analysis 1995;15:3.

Tobin LT. Legacy of the Loma Prieta earthquake: challenges to other communities. In: Practical lessons from the Loma Prieta earthquake. Washington, DC: National Academy Press; 1994.

Topping KC. Lessons from the Oakland Hills. In: J. Schwab et al., editors. Pre-event planning for post-disaster recovery. Chicago, IL: American Planning Association; 1997.

# Engineering, Building Codes, Standards, Practice, and Regulations

Abrams DP, et al. Assessment of earthquake engineering research and testing capabilities in the U.S. Publication no. WP-01A. Oakland, CA: Earthquake Engineering Research Institute; 1995.

American Society of Civil Engineers. Minimum design loads for buildings and other structures. ASCE 7-1995. New York: ASCE; 1995.

Applied Technology Council. Dynamic vulnerability and impact of disruption of lifelines in the conterminous U.S. ATC-25. Redwood City, CA: Applied Technology Council; 1992.

Bowles DS. Reservoir safety: a risk management approach. Logan, UT: Utah State University, Utah Water Research Laboratory; 1996.

Brumbaugh R, Werick W, Teitz W, Lund J. Lessons learned from the California drought (1987–1992). IWR report 94-NDS-6. Fort Belvoir, VA: U.S. Army Corps of Engineers, Institute for Water Resources; 1994.

California Seismic Safety Commission. Research and implementation plan for earthquake risk reduction in California 1995–2000. Sacramento, CA: Seismic Safety Commission; 1994.

Committee on Experimental Research, Earthquake Engineering Research Institute. Assessment of earthquake engineering research and testing capabilities in the U.S. Oakland, CA: Earthquake Engineering Research Institute; 1995.

Cook RA, Soltani M, editors. Hurricanes of 1992. New York: American Society of Civil Engineers; 1994.

Elsayed EA. Reliability engineering. Reading, MA: Addison Wesley Longman, Inc.; 1996.

Federal Emergency Management Agency. Reducing losses of life and property through model codes. FEMA-209. Washington, DC: Federal Emergency Management Agency; 1991.

Federal Emergency Management Agency. Southern California firestorms. FEMA-1005-DR-CA. Washington, DC: Federal Emergency Management Agency; 1994.

Federal Emergency Management Agency. A nontechnical explanation of the 1994 NEHRP recommended provisions. FEMA-99. Washington, DC: Federal Emergency Management Agency; 1995.

Federal Emergency Management Agency. Multihazard identification and risk assessment. Washington, DC: Federal Emergency Management Agency; 1997.

Greeley-Polhemus Group, Inc. Guidelines for risk and uncertainty analysis in water resources planning. Vols. I and II, IWR reports 92-R-1 and 92-R-2. Fort Belvoir, VA: Institute for Water Resources, U.S. Army Corps of Engineers; 1992.

Harberg R, et al. Reliability of urban water systems. Denver, CO: American Water Works Association; 1997.

Heinrichs P, Fell R, editors. Acceptable risks for major infrastructure. Rotterdam: AA Balkema; 1995.

International Fire Code Institute. Urban-wildland interface code. Whittier, CA: International Fire Code Institute; 1996.

la Grega MD, Buckingham PL, Evans JC. Environmental Resources Management Group. Hazardous waste management. New York: McGraw-Hill; 1994.

Lind NC. Policy goals for health and safety. Risk Analysis 1995;15:1.

Magnell CO. Federal public works infrastructure R&D: a new perspective. Final report for the Federal Infrastructure Strategy Program. Ft. Belvoir, VA: Institute for Water Resources, U.S. Army Corps of Engineers; 1993.

Mays LW, Tung Y. Hydrosystems engineering and management. New York: McGraw-Hill; 1992.

McDonald JR. Damage mitigation and occupant protection. In: Church C, editor. The tornado: its structure, dynamics, prediction and hazards. Geophysical monograph 79. Washington, DC: American Geophysical Union; 1993. p. 523–8.

National Conference of States on Building Codes and Standards, Inc. Introduction to building codes. Herndon, VA: National Conference of States; 1994.

National Research Council. Uses of risk analyses to achieve balanced safety in building design and operations. Washington, DC: National Academy Press; 1991.

National Research Council. Wind and the built environment: U.S. needs in wind engineering and hazard mitigation. Panel on the Assessment of Wind Engineering Issues in the U.S. Washington, DC: National Academy Press; 1993.

National Research Council. Toward infrastructure improvement—an agenda for research. Washington, DC: National Academy Press; 1994.

National Research Council. Measuring and improving infrastructure performance. Washington, DC: National Academy Press; 1995.

National Research Council. Understanding risk: informing decisions in a democratic society. Washington, DC: National Academy Press; 1996.

National Safety Council. Accident facts. 1993 ed. Itasca, IL: National Safety Council; 1993.

National Safety Council. Accident facts. 1995 ed. Itasca, IL: National Safety Council; 1995.

National Science Foundation. Civil infrastructure systems research: strategic issues. Washington, DC: The National Science Foundation; 1993.

Pushing for a national standard. Engineering News Record 1993 Nov 8:8.

Robertson JAL. Policy goals for health and safety: another view. Risk Analysis 1995;15:3.

U.S. Environmental Protection Agency. A guidebook to comparing risks and setting environmental priorities. EPA 230-B-93-003. Washington, DC: Environmental Protection Agency; 1993.

West CT, Lenze DG. Modeling the regional impact of natural disaster and recovery: a general framework and application to Hurricane Andrew. International Regional Science Review 1994;17(2):121–50.

## Prediction, Forecasts, Warnings, and Warning Response

Bourque LB, Shoaf K, Russell LA. Community response to the January 17, 1994, Northridge earthquake. Paper presented at the 20th Natural Hazards Research and Applications Workshop, Boulder, CO; 1995.

Drabek TE. Anticipating organizational evacuations: disaster planning by managers of tourist-oriented private firms. International Journal of Mass Emergencies and Disasters 1994;9:219–46.

Federal Emergency Management Agency. Guide for the evaluation of alert and notification systems for nuclear power plants. Washington, DC: Federal Emergency Management Agency; 1985.

Gavin JP. Hurricane evacuation studies program overview. Philadelphia, PA: U.S. Army Corps of Engineers; 1996.

Gillespie DA, Murty SA. Setting boundaries for research on organizational capacity to evacuate. International Journal of Mass Emergencies and Disasters 1991;9:201–18.

Sorensen J. When shall we leave: factors affecting the timing of evacuation departures. International Journal of Mass Emergencies and Disasters 1991;9(2):153–65.

Vogt B, Sorensen J. Preparing EBS messages. ORNL/TM-12163. Oak Ridge, TN: Oak Ridge National Laboratory; 1992.

Vogt BM, Sorensen JH. Evacuation research: a reassessment. ORNL/TM-11908. Oak Ridge, TN: Oak Ridge National Laboratory; 1992.

## Insurance

Berz G. Natural disasters and insurance and reinsurance. Earthquakes and Volcanoes 1991;22(3):99–102.

Britton NR, Oliver J. Insurance and urban planning: partnering in risk resolution. In: Britton NR, Oliver J, editors. Insurance viability and loss mitigation: partners in risk resolution. Brisbane: Griffith University Press; 1995. p. 1–20.

Diaz HF, Pulwarty RS, editors. Hurricanes: climate and socioeconomic impacts. New York: Springer-Verlag; 1997.

Insurance Research Council. Public Attitude Monitor 1996 Jan;96.

Insurance Research Council and Insurance Institute of Property Loss Reduction. Coastal exposure and community protection: Hurricane Andrew's legacy. Wheaton, IL: Insurance Research Council; 1995.

Kunreuther H. Mitigating disaster losses through insurance. Journal of Risk and Uncertainty 1996;12:171–87.

Kunreuther H. Rethinking society's management of catastrophic risks. Working paper 96-06-04. Geneva Papers on Risk and Insurance 1997;83:151–76.

U.S. Congress. Federal disaster assistance report of the Senate Task Force on Funding Disaster Relief. Washington, DC: U.S. Government Printing Office; 1995.

White R, Etkin DA. Climate change, extreme events, and the Canadian insurance industry. Journal of Natural Hazards 1997;16(203):135–63.

## Disaster Management and Emergency Management

Bolin R, Stanford LM. Shelter and housing issues in Santa Cruz County. In: Bolin R, editor. The Loma Prieta earthquake: studies of short-term impacts. Boulder, CO: University of Colorado, Institute of Behavioral Science; 1990.

Bolin R, Stanford LM. Emergency sheltering and housing of earthquake victims: the case of Santa Cruz County. In: Bolton PA, editor. The Loma Prieta, California, earthquake of October 17, 1989—public response. U.S. Geological Survey Professional Paper 1553B. Washington DC: U.S. Government Printing Office; 1993. p. B43–50.

Britton NR, Lindsay J. Demonstrating the need to integrate city planning and emergency preparedness: two case studies. International Journal of Mass Emergencies and Disasters 1995;13(1):161–78.

Britton NR, Moran CC, Correy B. Stress coping and emergency disaster volunteers: a discussion of some relevant factors. In: Dynes RR, Tierney KJ, editors. Disasters, collective behavior, and social organization. Newark, DE: University of Delaware Press; 1994. p. 128–44.

Cooke D. Los Angeles earthquake puts city disaster services to the test. Disaster Recovery Journal 1995;7(1):10–4.

Drabek TE. Emergency management: strategies for maintaining organizational integrity. New York: Springer-Verlag; 1990.

Drabek TE, Hoetmer GJ, editors. Emergency management: principles and practice for local government. Washington, DC: International City Management Association; 1991.

Federal Emergency Management Agency and U.S. Department of the Army. Planning guidance for the Chemical Stockpile Emergency Preparedness Program. Oak Ridge, TN: Oak Ridge National Laboratory; 1996.

Goggin M, Bowman AO, Lester JP, O'Toole LJ. Implementation theory and practice: toward a third generation. Glenview, IL: Scott Foresman; 1990.

Kreps GA. The federal emergency management system in the U.S.: past and present. International Journal of Mass Emergencies and Disasters 1990;8:275–300.

Mileti DS, Sorensen JH, O'Brien PW. Toward an explanation of mass care shelter use in evacuations. International Journal of Mass Emergencies and Disasters 1992;10(1):25–42.

National Academy of Public Administration. Coping with catastrophe: building an emergency management system to meet people's needs in natural and manmade disasters. Washington, DC: National Academy of Public Administration; 1993.

Schneider SK. Flirting with disaster: public management in crisis situations. Armonk, NY: ME Sharpe; 1995.

Topping KC. Disaster field office information management action plan. Pasadena, CA: California Governor's Office of Emergency Services; 1995.

Vog B. Evacuation of institutionalized and specialized populations. ORNL/Sub-7685/1. Oak Ridge, TN: Oak Ridge National Laboratory; 1990.

Wiest RE, Mocellin JSP, Motsisi DT. The needs of women and children in disasters and emergencies. Winnipeg, Canada: University of Manitoba; 1992.

## Preparedness and Response

Bourque LB, Russell LA, Goltz JD. Human behavior during and immediately after the earthquake. In: Bolton PA, editor. The Loma Prieta, California, earthquake of October 17, 1989—public response. U.S. Geological Survey professional paper 1553-B. Washington DC: U.S. Government Printing Office; 1993. p. B3–22.

Britton NR, Lindsay J. Integrating city planning and emergency preparedness: some of the reasons why. International Journal of Mass Emergencies and Disasters 1995;13(1):93–106.

Committee on Earthquake Response and Recovery. Emergency response and recovery. Monograph 4. Memphis, TN: Central U.S. Earthquake Consortium; 1993.

Dahlhamer JD, D'Souza M. Determinants of business disaster preparedness in two U.S. metropolitan areas. International Journal of Mass Emergencies and Disasters 1997;15:265–81.

Drabek TE. Disaster evacuation and the tourist industry. Monograph no. 57. Boulder, CO: University of Colorado, Institute of Behavioral Science; 1994.

Drabek TE. Disaster responses within the tourist industry. International Journal of Mass Emergencies and Disasters 1995;13:7–23.

Duguay J. Safe in any language. Emergency Preparedness Digest 1996 Oct:12–4.

Faupel CE, Kelley SP, Petee T. The impact of disaster education on household preparedness for Hurricane Hugo. International Journal of Mass Emergencies and Disasters 1992;10(1):5–24.

Goltz JD, Russell LA, Bourque LB. Initial behavioral response to a rapid onset disaster: a case study. International Journal of Mass Emergencies and Disasters 1992;10(1):43–69.

Kartez JD, Lindell MK. Adaptive planning for community disaster response. In: Silves RT, Waugh WL Jr, editors. Cities and disaster: North American studies in emergency management. Springfield, IL: Charles C. Thomas Publishers; 1990. p. 5–31.

Kreps GA, Bosworth SL. Disaster, organizing, and role enactment: a structural approach. American Journal of Sociology 1993;99:428–63.

Lindell MK. Are local emergency planning committees effective in developing community disaster preparedness? International Journal of Mass Emergencies and Disasters 1994;12:159–82.

Lindell MK, Meier MJ. Effectiveness of community planning for toxic chemical emergencies. Journal of the American Planning Association 1994;60:222–34.

Lindell MK, Whitney DJ. Effects of organizational environment, internal structure and team climate on the effectiveness of local emergency planning committees. Risk Analysis 1995;15:439–47.

Lindell MK, Whitney DJ, Futch CJ, Clause CS. The local emergency planning committee: a better way to coordinate disaster planning. In: Silves RT, Waugh WL Jr, editors. Disaster management in the U.S. and Canada: the politics, policymaking, administration and analysis of emergency management. Springfield, IL: Charles C. Thomas Publishers; 1996. p. 274–95.

Lindell MK, Whitney DJ, Futch CJ, Clause CS. Multi-method assessment of organizational effectiveness in a local emergency planning committee. International Journal of Mass Emergencies and Disasters 1996;14:195–220.

Mileti DS, Fitzpatrick C, Farhar BC. Fostering public preparations for natural hazards: lessons from the Parkfield earthquake prediction. Environment 1992;33(3):16–20.

Mileti DS, O'Brien P. Warnings during disaster: normalizing communicated risk. Social Problems 1992;39:40–57.

O'Brien PW, Mileti DS. Citizen participation in emergency response following the Loma Prieta earthquake. Mass Emergencies and Disasters 1992;10(1):71–89.

O'Brien PW, Mileti DS. Citizen participation in emergency response. In: Bolton PA, editor. The Loma Prieta, California, earthquake of October 17, 1989—public response. U.S. Geological Survey Professional Paper 1553-B. Washington DC: U.S. Government Printing Office; 1993. p. B23–30.

Phillips BD. Cultural diversity in disasters: sheltering, housing, and long-term recovery. International Journal of Mass Emergencies and Disasters 1993;11(1):99–110.

Russell GW, Mentzel RK. Sympathy and altruism in response to disasters. Journal of Social Psychology 1990;130(3):309–16.

Simile C. Disaster settings and mobilization for contentious collective action: case studies of Hurricane Hugo and the Loma Prieta earthquake [dissertation]. Newark, DE: University of Delaware, Department of Sociology and Criminal Justice; 1995.

## Recovery and Long-Term Impacts

Baum A, Fleming I, Israel A, O'Keefe MK. Symptoms of chronic stress following a natural disaster and discovery of a human-made hazard. Environment and Behavior 1992;24:347–65.

Bay Area Regional Earthquake Preparedness Project. Putting the pieces to-gether: the Loma Prieta earthquake one year later. Oakland CA: Bay Area Regional Earthquake Preparedness Project; 1990.

Berke P, Beatley T. After the hurricane—linking recovery to sustainable devel-opment in the Caribbean. Baltimore, MD: Johns Hopkins University Press; 1997.

Berke PR, Kartez J, Wenger D. Recovery after disaster: achieving sustainable development, mitigation and equity. Disasters 1993;17(2):93–109.

Bolin R. Disaster impact and recovery: a comparison of black and white victims. International Journal of Mass Emergencies and Disasters 1986;4(1): 35–50.

Bolin RC. Household and community recovery after earthquakes. Monograph no. 56. Boulder, CO: University of Colorado, Institute of Behavioral Science; 1993.

Bolin R, Stanford L. Shelter, housing and recovery: a comparison of U.S. disas-ters. Disasters: The Journal of Disaster Studies and Management 1991;15(1):24–34.

Bolton PA, Liebow EB, Olson JL. Community context and uncertainty following a damaging earthquake: low-income Latinos in Los Angeles, California. The Environmental Professional 1993;15:240–7.

California Governor's Office of Emergency Services. Earthquake recovery: a survival manual for local governments. Sacramento, CA: California Office of Emergency Services; 1993.

Comerio MC. Disaster hits home: new policy for urban housing recovery. Berkeley and Los Angeles: University of California Press; 1998.

Greene M. Housing recovery and reconstruction: lessons from recent urban earthquakes. In: Proceedings of the 3rd U.S./Japan Workshop on Urban Earthquakes. Publication no. 93-B. Oakland, CA: Earthquake Engineering Research Institute; 1992. p. 11–5.

Mader GG, Tyler MB. Rebuilding after earthquakes, lessons from planners: re-port of an international symposium on rebuilding after earthquakes. Portola Valley, CA: William Spangle and Associates; 1991.

McDonnell S, Troiano RP, Barker N, Noji E, Hlady WG, Hopkins R. Evalu-ation of long-term community recovery from Hurricane Andrew: sources of assistance received by population sub-groups. Disasters: The Journal of Disaster Studies and Management 1995;19(4):338–47.

Miller K, Nigg JM. Event and consequence vulnerability: effects on the disaster recovery process. Paper presented at the annual meeting of the Eastern Sociological Society, Boston, Massachusetts; 1993.

Mitchell J, editor. The long road to recovery: community responses to indus-trial disasters. Tokyo, Japan: United Nations Press; 1996.

Peacock WG, Morrow BH, Gladwin H, editors. Hurricane Andrew and the reshaping of Miami: ethnicity, gender, and the socio-political ecology of disasters. Gainesville, FL: University Press of Florida; 1997.

Rodrigue CM, Rovai E, Place SE. Construction of the "Northridge" earthquake in Los Angeles' English and Spanish print media: damage, attention, and skewed recovery. Presentation to the Southern California Environment and History Conference, Northridge, California; 1997. Available from: www.csuchico.edu/geop/chr/scehc97.html.

Rubin CB. Recovery from disaster. In: Principles and practice of emergency management. Washington, DC: International City Management Association; 1991.

Rubin CB. Physical reconstruction: timescale for reconstruction. In: Wellington after the quake: the challenge of rebuilding cities. Christchurch, New Zealand: Centre for Advanced Engineering and the New Zealand Earthquake Commission; 1995.

Snarr DN, Brown EL. Post-disaster housing reconstruction: a longitudinal study of resident satisfaction. Disasters 1994;18(1):76–80.

Topping KC. Model recovery and reconstruction ordinance. In: J. Schwab, et al., editors Pre-event planning for post-disaster recovery. Planners advisory service report prepared for the Federal Emergency Management Agency. Chicago, IL: American Planning Association; 1998.

# Index

Second-order effect, 245
Secure Socket Layer, 229
Seeds of terrorism, 97, 98
Self stereotyping, 20, 22
Sexual terrorism, 97
Shell Oil Company, 295
Signal detection, 255, 257–58
Simple Network Management
    Protocol, 229, 239
Situational analysis, 277
Sleeper cells, 244
Smallpox, 201–2, 271, 278
Social capital, 308, 311–12,
    314–15
Social Capital Community
    Benchmark Survey, 314
Social identity, 7, 13, 15, 16, 20,
    24–25
Social Security, 106
Socialization, 7, 29–30, 39–41,
    43–44, 56
Somatoform disorder, 56, 60
Spontaneous self, 76
Sprint, 234–37, 239, 241
SPVC, 236
State Health Department, 180
Status quo, 104, 141, 169, 171–72,
    187
Strategic biodefense
    communication model,
    197–99
Sun, 167, 176
Superfund Amendments and
    Reauthorization Act, 129
Surveillance system, 202, 270,
    277, 283
SVC, 236
Synchronous Optical Networking
    (SONET (POS)), 229,
    235, 237, 239

Taliban, 109, 113
Telecommunication, 10, 228, 234,
    269, 275–77, 279–80, 283

Telecommunication tools, 10,
    277, 280
Telecommunications Industry
    Association, 228
Telecommunications Union, 228
Telemedicine, 279–80
Terrorism, 1–8, 10–26, 28–38,
    40–41, 43–44, 47–61,
    64–70, 72, 74–76, 81, 83,
    85–88, 96, 98–102, 105–8,
    111–18, 125–27, 131–33,
    135–36, 141–42, 145–47,
    150–51, 154–55, 158, 161,
    167–69, 175, 178, 185, 187,
    212–23, 243–47, 250, 252,
    258, 261, 270, 280, 295,
    303
Terrorist, 1–11, 13–25, 30–34, 36,
    38, 40, 42–44, 47–48,
    50–58, 60, 65–88, 96,
    98–101, 106–7, 109–13,
    116–18, 125–28, 132–34,
    136, 138, 140–42, 144, 147,
    150–51, 154–55, 157–58,
    161, 167–69, 175, 180,
    186–87, 200, 202, 211–23,
    243–45, 250–51, 253–64,
    269–70, 272, 283, 287–88,
    296, 302, 307–15, 320–21
Texaco, 299–300
Thematic frame, 31
Therapeutic, 54, 204
Therapy by walking around, 55
Thompson, Tommy, 179, 192
Three Mile Island, 128–29
Tibetan, 14
Time Division Multiplexing
    (TDM), 229–30, 233, 239
Time magazine, 109–10, 112
Tornado team, 288
Toxin, 269–70, 272
Traditional socialization
    institutions, 29
Transgression, 3, 77

# About the Editors and Contributors

KENNETH ALIBEK, MD, PhD, ScD (Tomsk Medical Institute, Russia), is a Distinguished Professor of Medical Microbiology and Immunology and the director for education, National Center for Biodefense, George Mason University. He is also the vice chairman and chief scientist at Advanced Biosystems, where he leads medical and scientific research programs dedicated to developing new forms of medical protection against biological weapons and other infectious diseases. Dr. Alibek served as first deputy chief of the civilian branch of the Soviet Union's offensive biological weapons program and has more than twenty years of experience in development, management, and supervision of high containment (BL-4) pathogen laboratories. He has extensive knowledge of biotechnology, including bioprocessing, biological weapons threat analysis, antibacterial and antiviral drug development, development of regimens for urgent prophylaxis and treatment of the diseases caused by biological weapons, and mass casualty handling. He is a former Soviet Army colonel. Dr. Alibek has published articles in a number of classified journals on developments in the field of biological weapons, biological weapons threat, and on medical aspects of biodefense. He holds many patents, both Russian and American. Dr. Alibek defected to the United States from the Soviet Union in 1992 and subsequently served as a consultant to numerous U.S. government agencies in the areas of industrial technology, medical microbiology, biological weapons defense, and biological weapons nonproliferation. He has worked with the National Institutes of Health, testified extensively before the U.S. Congress on nonproliferation of biological weapons and is the author of

*Biohazard.* Dr. Alibek holds an MD in epidemiology and infectious diseases, and holds additional degrees including a PhD in medical microbiology and an ScD in industrial biotechnology. Dr. Alibek has given more than 300 lectures, seminars, and presentations on biological weapons threat and defense, microbiology, and immunology for various military and civilian colleges and universities (including Princeton, Harvard, MIT, Brown, Dartmouth, Georgetown, Rockefeller, the University of Pennsylvania, the University of Virginia, National Defense University, Uniform Services University, and the Air Force, Naval, and Army Academies). He has delivered lectures and presentations to government agencies and academic units in Great Britain, Sweden, France, Japan, Singapore, the Netherlands, Germany, Switzerland, and Australia. Dr. Alibek specializes in medical and scientific research dedicated to developing new forms of protection against biological weapons and other infectious diseases, biodefense, mechanisms of pathogenesis by *Bacillus anthracis* (anthrax) and other pathogens, and new forms of protection against infectious diseases.

CHARLES BAILEY, PhD, is a Distinguished Professor of Biology and the executive director for research, National Center for Biodefense, George Mason University. Dr. Bailey is the former commander of the U.S. Army Medical Research Institute of Infectious Diseases. Dr. Bailey has twenty-five years of U.S. Army experience in research and development and management in infectious diseases and biological warfare defense. Over a continuous thirteen-year period, he served as a research scientist, deputy commander for research, deputy commander and commander at the U.S. Army Medical Research Institute of Infectious Diseases. Before joining George Mason University, Dr. Bailey helped lead a team of scientists at Advanced Biosystems, conducting medical and scientific research dedicated to developing new forms of protection against biological weapons and other infectious diseases. Dr. Bailey retired from the U.S. Army as a colonel. He holds BS, MS, and PhD degrees in biology and entomology from Oklahoma State University. He has written extensively on foreign biological warfare capabilities as an officer in the Defense Intelligence Agency. He conducts research on biodefense and new forms of protection against infectious diseases.

JENNIFER A. H. BECKER (MA, Ball State University, 1999) is a doctoral candidate in the Department of Communication at the University of Oklahoma. Her research interests are in interpersonal communication, particularly problematic communication in organizational and mental-health settings. She also investigates how interpersonal communication and personal relationships are related to the psychosocial health of those who have been impacted by terrorism.

SHANNON A. BOWEN earned her PhD in 2000 from the University of Maryland in communication. She is assistant professor of public relations in the School of Communication at the University of Houston. Dr. Bowen won the ICA Public Relations Division Outstanding Dissertation Award for her research on ethical decision-making in issues management. Her work has been published in major journals such as: *Journal of Public Relations Research, Journal of Mass Media Ethics, Journal of Public Affairs,* and *Public Relations Review.* She is assisting Glen Broom, PhD, with the ninth edition of the *Effective Public Relations* textbook, and she authored numerous entries for the *Encyclopedia of Public Relations.* Dr. Bowen is the principal investigator on a grant from the International Association of Business Communicators to study the ethics of communication professionals.

W. TIMOTHY COOMBS holds a PhD in public affairs and issues management from Purdue University. His crisis communication research focuses on the development and testing of the Situational Crisis Communication Theory (SCCT). His crisis communication work was awarded the 2002 Jackson, Jackson and Wagner Behavioral Research Prize from the Public Relations Society of America and the 2002 PRIDE Award for Best Article from the Public Relations Division of the National Communication Associations. His book, *Ongoing Crisis Communication,* won the PRIDE Award for Best Book in 2000. He has published over 20 articles and book chapters on crisis-related topics. Coombs gives presentations on crisis communication/management at a wide variety of academic and professional meetings in the U.S., Europe, and Australia. He consults on a variety of crisis-related topics, including media training, crisis plan preparation, and crisis response strategy selection. He sits on the editorial board of four journals and reviews for three others in the area of crisis communication.

PAUL DOUTE has worked in the communications industry since 1985 in a number of engineering roles with Motorola Information Systems Group, PictureTel, Nortel Networks, and Sprint. Paul's primary role has been as a Wide Area Network Specialist, and he has earned a number of industry certifications from places such as Control Data Institute, Nortel Networks, and PictureTel. He has a Bachelor of Arts degree from Siena Heights University. At Sprint, Paul has been the lead engineer on the MiCTA Service account for the past three years. As the lead engineer on the MiCTA account, he is responsible for working with Sprint engineers and MiCTA members all over the United States designing and implementing communication networking solutions. Paul is a great contributor to the success of the Sprint/MiCTA relationship. On a number of occasions, Paul has been asked to present technology reviews to the MiCTA membership during the MiCTA Spring and Fall Conferences. Most recently, he supported the joint effort of writing a chapter on "Convergence" for a soon-to-be-published series of books in conjunction with MiCTA and several other organizations. Paul has been recognized for his many achievements working with MiCTA. In the past two years, he received the Sprint Values Excellence Annual Award as a Distinguished Contributor during 2002 and 2003 for his contributions in representing Sprint and the MiCTA account.

GARY GREEN has been with MiCTA Service Corporation since May of 1997 and was named vice president of education services in June of 2000. He has held the offices of president, vice president, and ex officio of MiCTA and has been affiliated with the organization since September 1982. He received a BS in physical therapy with a minor in computer science from Wayne State University. Prior to joining the MiCTA, Gary was director of facilities and technical services at North Central Michigan College for 24 years, where he was responsible for all aspects of campus facilities as well as the management and development of the technical info-structure. Prior to his work at North Center Green, he worked at the Detroit Medical Center and St. Johns Hospital. From 1989 to 1992, Green, along with other colleagues from MiCTA, helped develop and deploy "Switched Dial-up Digitally Compressed Video" for distance learning, in partnership with Sprint, British Telecom, and Innovative Communications, Inc. The network now connects numerous states and has grown to nearly 200 locations in Michigan.

ROBERT L. HEATH is professor of communication at the University of Houston. He is the director of the Institute for the Study of Issues Management and has written extensively on rhetoric, communication theory, public relations, risk communication, and issues management.

EDWARD M. HOROWITZ (PhD, University of Wisconsin, Madison) is an assistant professor of communication at the Cleveland State

University. His research focuses on young adults and political communication in both the United States and central and eastern Europe. He received a grant in 2003 from The Center for Information and Research on Civic Learning and Engagement to study the mayoral primary election in Baltimore, Maryland, the first U.S. election allowing sixteen- and seventeen-year-olds to vote. He has presented his research at numerous professional conferences and at meetings of the European Youth Commission at the European Parliament in Strasbourg, France. His work has appeared in *Communication Research* and *Journalism and Mass Communication Quarterly*.

GARY L. KREPS (PhD, University of Southern California) is chief of the Health Communication and Informatics Research Branch at the National Cancer Institute (NCI), where he plans, develops, and coordinates major new national research and outreach initiatives concerning risk communication, health promotion, behavior change, technology development, and information dissemination to promote cancer prevention and control. His areas of expertise include health communication and promotion, information dissemination, organizational communication, information technology, multicultural relations, and applied research methods. He is an active scholar, whose published work includes more than twenty books and 160 scholarly articles and chapters concerning the applications of communication knowledge in society. He has received numerous honors, including the 2004 Lewis Donohew Outstanding Health Communication Scholar Award from the University of Kentucky, the Future of Health Technology Institute's 2002 Future of Health Technology Award, the Ferguson Report's 2002 Distinguished Achievement Award for Outstanding Contributions in Consumer Health Informatics and Online Health, the 2000 Outstanding Health Communication Scholar Award from both the International Communication Association and the National Communication Association, and the 1998 Gerald M. Phillips Distinguished Applied Communication Scholarship Award from the National Communication Association.

DAVID B. McKINNEY is manager of external affairs for the Shell chemical plant and refinery in Deer Park, Texas. He has been with Shell since 1980 and has held a variety of communications positions at Shell facilities throughout the United States. A former newspaper reporter, McKinney holds a BA in journalism and an MA in mass communications. He is an adjunct professor of mass communications and public relations at the University of Houston. He is accredited by both the Public Relations Society of America and the International Association of Business Communicators.

RONALD C. MERRELL, MD, FACS, is director of the Medical Informatics and Technology Applications Consortium at Virginia Commonwealth University, where he is also a professor of surgery. He has been an educator and telemedicine innovator with extensive international experience.

LINDA NEUHAUSER, DrPH, is clinical professor in the Division of Public Health Biology and Epidemiology at the University of California, Berkeley. She researches and teaches the effectiveness of health interventions, especially health communication and new media technologies. Her specialty is the collaborative design and evaluation of mass communication. She is a principal investigator in the UC Berkeley Center for Community Wellness, and she heads the risk communication and media relations component of the CDC-funded UC Berkeley Center for Infectious Disease Preparedness. She is a member of several task forces on the Internet and health, funded by the U.S. Department of Health and Human Services and the National Cancer Institute. She formerly served as a health officer in the U.S. State Department in west and central Africa and trained health researchers at World Health Organization regional training centers in Africa. Dr. Neuhauser's current research interests include participatory design of educational interventions, health communication (including risk communication for emergency preparedness and response), interventions research (practice and policy), food security and hunger (measurement and policy), and longitudinal study of impacts of parenting education.

H. DAN O'HAIR received his PhD in 1982 from The University of Oklahoma in communication. He is a professor in the Department of Communication at The University of Oklahoma. He has published more than seventy research articles in communication, business, management, and psychology journals and volumes, and has authored and edited ten books in the areas of communication, business, and health. He has been the principal investigator for several grants from business, nonprofit, and government institutions totaling more than $2 million. He has served on the editorial boards of eighteen research journals and is the immediate past editor of the *Journal of Applied Communication Research*, published by the National Communication Association. Articles published in *JACR* have been referenced or reviewed by such publications as the *Wall Street Journal* and the *Harvard Communication Letter*. He was recently elected second vice president of the National Communication Association and will assume the office of president in 2006.

BOLANLE A. OLANIRAN (PhD, University of Oklahoma, 1991) is a professor in the Department of Communication Studies at Texas Tech University. His areas of research include organization, communication technology, and intercultural communication. His work has appeared in several journals and as book chapters.

MICHAEL J. PALENCHAR recently joined the faculty at the University of Tennessee's School of Advertising and Public Relations (ABD-PhD, University of Florida; MA, University of Houston; BA, University of Texas). Research interests include risk communication and issues management related to industrial chemical production, community relations and community awareness of emergency response protocols and manufacturing risks, crisis communication, health communication, and general public relations. Teaching areas include risk communication, issues management, public relations campaigns, principles of public relations, and public relations cases, strategies, and tactics. He has more than a decade of professional experience working in corporate, nonprofit, and agency areas. He has also been a risk communication and issues management research consultant for clients ranging from Fortune 500 companies to local government agencies. He has coauthored two journal articles that have been published in the *Journal of Public Relations Research* and two book chapters in print on risk communication, terrorism, and professional ethics. Along with his coauthor, he was the recipient of the 2000 National Communication Association's Pride Award for the top national published article in public relations. He has authored or coauthored fifteen regional, national, or international communication conference papers, winning nine top paper awards. He currently sits on the editorial board of *Communication Studies.*

AZHAR RAFIQ, MD, EMBA is chief scientific officer of the Medical Informatics and Technology Applications Consortium at Virginia Commonwealth University. He is also assistant professor in the Department of Surgery and coinvestigator for the bioterrorism training initiative at VCU, which is funded by the Department of Health and Human Services.

JOHN RHOADS completed his bachelor's degree in communication from the University of Texas at Austin and attended law school at

South Texas College of Law in Houston, Texas. Additionally, Rhoads holds a master's degree from the University of Houston at University Park in public relations, specializing in the areas of employee relations and corporate culture. He earned a Six Sigma Certification from Southern Polytechnic State University (at the University of Georgia) in Atlanta, Georgia in 2002, working on corporate culture and human resource issues. Since 1998, Rhoads has worked with the law firm of Haynes & Boone, LLP as a consultant to firm clients in the areas of employee satisfaction, risk management, and corporate culture. To further his passion for cultural and individual development, Rhoads is a lecturer to local and national industry groups using the Six Sigma and S.H.A.P.E. curricula. Currently, Rhoads serves as an industry representative to the training and education committee of the International Association of Security and Investigative Regulators and is an active member of the International Association of Business Communicators and the Risk Insurance Management Society. Rhoads lives in Houston, Texas with his wife, Sandra, and two sons, Addison and Leyton.

KATHERINE E. ROWAN, PHD is an associate professor of communication at George Mason University, Fairfax, VA. Her research concerns the public relations challenges of earning trust and explaining complexities in the contexts of risk and crisis communication. She also studies the teaching of mass-media writing, particularly writing to communicate intellectually and emotionally challenging subjects. At George Mason University, she heads the public relations curriculum and codirects instruction in writing across mass media. Dr. Rowan received her bachelor's degree from George Mason University's English Department in 1975. After graduation, she worked for the Smithsonian Institution's Office of Public Affairs. Her master's degree was earned in communication and journalism from the University of Illinois and her doctorate in the teaching of rhetoric and composition from Purdue's English Department. She joined Purdue's Communication Department in 1985, earning tenure in 1991 and full professor status in 1996. Dr. Rowan became interested in risk communication through studies of science communication in the mass media. She has authored or edited more than forty scholarly and governmental publications concerning effective methods for earning trust and explaining complex science. During the last fifteen years, she has given presentations on risk and science communication for organizations such as the National Library of Medicine, Agricultural Communicators in Education, the Indiana Arborists, the Garden Writers of America, the U.S. Department of Agriculture, the National Academy of Sciences, and the U.S. Environmental Protection Agency.

MICHAEL RYAN, a professor of communication at the University of Houston, has taught research methods, theory, and writing at Houston, Temple University, and West Virginia University. His teaching and research interests are in media ethics, communication pedagogy, public relations, media and terrorism, and new communication technologies. He has coauthored two books and published more than 100 scholarly and professional articles. Ryan's work has appeared in *Journalism and Mass Communication Quarterly*, *Journalism and Mass Communication Monographs*, *Public Relations Review* and the *Journal of Communication*, among many others.

JULIANN C. SCHOLL (PhD, University of Oklahoma, 2000) is assistant professor of communication studies at Texas Tech University. Much of her research emphasizes problematic interpersonal interactions as they are influenced by organizational structures such as workplace settings and health contexts. This emphasis has focused on deception, conflict, and humor.

MATTHEW W. SEEGER (PhD, Indiana University, 1982) is professor and director of speech communication in the Department of Communication at Wayne State University. His work on communication and crisis management has appeared in *Communication Yearbook*, the *Handbook of Public Relations*, *Communication Studies*, the *Southern Communication Journal*, *Journal of Applied Communication Research*, *Communication Research Reports*, *Journal of Health Communication Research*, the *Journal of Business Ethics*, and in several edited books. His most recent book, *Communication Organization and Crisis*, was recently published by Quorum Press. His commentaries on organizations, crisis, and leadership have appeared in the *Detroit Free Press* and *Detroit News*. Dr. Seeger has also served as a communication consultant for AT&T, DaimlerChrysler, General Motors, and K-Mart Corporation among others. He has worked with the CDC on issues of crisis communication, warnings regarding infectious disease and bioterrorism, and community leadership during crisis. He has also worked with the Michigan Department of Public Health, Office of Public Health Preparedness.

TIMOTHY L. SELLNOW (PhD, Wayne State University, 1987) is a professor of communication at North Dakota State University. Sellnow's research focuses primarily on crisis and risk communication. He has published his research in such journals as *Journal of Applied Communication Research*, *Communication Education*, *Critical Studies in Media Communication*, *Communication Studies*, *Communication Quarterly*, *Argumentation and Advocacy*, *Journal of Business Communication*, *Communication Reports*, and *Public Relations Review*. He has written chapters for *Communication Yearbook* and *Handbook of Public Relations*. Dr. Sellnow's funded research blends organizational communication strategies with crisis and risk issues. He has worked on several projects with the U.S. Department of Agriculture in the areas of staffing and risk communication. He and colleagues at North Dakota State University have received more than $2 million in federal funding for these projects. Dr. Sellnow has also recently consulted with the CDC regarding its crisis-communication planning. Most recently he contributed to the development of a reference tool to be used by all state public information officers as they plan and train for bioterrorism episodes.

LISA SPARKS (PhD, University of Oklahoma, 1998) is an associate professor of communication at George Mason University. Her research primarily focuses on communication with, by, and about older adults and how such communication relates to healthy and successful aging outcomes. Her research draws on theories of lifespan development, social identity, communication accommodation, and intergroup behavior. She has published five books including *Cancer Communication and Aging* (forthcoming), and *Communication and Cancer Care* (forthcoming), both coedited with H. Dan O'Hair and Gary L. Kreps. She has published more than thirty journal articles and book chapters related to the intersection of aging, communication, and health/risk issues. Her publications have appeared in *Health Communication*, *Journal of Applied Communication Research*, *Journal of Health Communication*, *Journal of Gerontology: Medical Sciences*, *Journal of Cross-Cultural Gerontology*, *Case Studies in Health Communication*, and *Handbook of Communication and Aging*. She has served as a cancer communication research fellow and an external scientific reviewer for the Health Communication and Informatics Research Branch, Behavioral Research Program, Division of Cancer Control and Population Sciences, National Cancer Institute, National Institutes of Health. Dr. Sparks serves on the editorial board for *Communication Studies* and as a guest editor for a number of peer-reviewed journals in communication and gerontology. She served as guest editor of health communication for *Special Issue on Cancer Communication and Aging* (2003), which featured papers presented at a symposium held at George Mason University.

LES SWITZER, a professor emeritus at the University of Houston, was a journalist for nine years on three continents and an academic for thirty-three years. Switzer, having completed the requirements for a master's degree in divinity, entered the chaplaincy program at a hospital in the Texas Medical Center in 2004. Switzer's teaching and research interests are in journalism and media studies, development studies, critical theory, media and terrorism, cultural studies, religious studies, and southern African studies. He is the author of seven books and monographs, and more than twenty-five book chapters, articles, and essays in scholarly journals.

SHARLENE THOMPSON (MA, George Mason University, 2001) is a doctoral student in the Department of Communication at the University of Oklahoma, studying health communication. Her interests include cancer communication, sexual health communication, and doctor-patient communication.

ROBERT R. ULMER (PhD, Wayne State University, 1998) is associate professor of speech communication at the University of Arkansas at Little Rock. His research and teaching interests focus on crisis communication, communication and ethics, and issues related to stakeholder involvement in environmental, risk, and crisis communication. His work has appeared in *Management Communication Quarterly*, *Journal of Business Ethics*, *Journal of Applied Communication Research*, *Communication Yearbook*, and *Public Relations Review*, among others. He is also a coauthor of *Communication and Organizational Crisis*, a recent book on crisis communication. He serves as a consultant on issues of crisis preparedness and effective crisis and risk communication.

JOHAN WANSTROM is a graduate student in communication at the University of Oklahoma. His research interests include communication in democracy and civic education.

DAVID E. WILLIAMS (PhD, Ohio University, 1990) is an associate professor of communication studies at Texas Tech University. Dr. Williams has been conducting research in crisis communication for several years.